Caring for the
Perioperative Patient

Paul and Joy would like to dedicate this book to:
Our teachers, our students, our colleagues, our friends
Claire Campbell
Kate, Mairi and Neil Wicker
Barry and Nicola O'Neill
Beth Lynch

Caring for the Perioperative Patient

Paul Wicker

Programme Leader
Diploma of Higher Education in Operating
Department Practice
Edge Hill College of Higher Education,
Liverpool

AND

Joy O'Neill

Training and Development Co-ordinator
Theatre Department, Royal Oldham Hospital
Pennine Acute NHS Hospital Trust

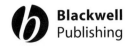

Blackwell
Publishing

Blackwell Publishing Ltd
Editorial offices:
Blackwell Publishing Ltd, 9600 Garsington Road, Oxford OX4 2DQ, UK
    Tel: +44 (0)1865 776868
Blackwell Publishing Inc., 350 Main Street, Malden, MA 02148-5020, USA
    Tel: +1 781 388 8250
Blackwell Publishing Asia Pty Ltd, 550 Swanston Street, Carlton, Victoria
3053, Australia
    Tel: +61 (0)3 8359 1011

First published 2006 by Blackwell Publishing Ltd
2   2007

ISBN: 978-1-4051-2802-5

Library of Congress Cataloging-in-Publication Data
Wicker, Paul.
        Caring for the perioperative patient / Paul Wicker and Joy O'Neill.
            p. ; cm.
        Includes bibliographical references and index.
        ISBN-13: 978-1-4051-2802-5 (alk. paper)
        ISBN-10: 1-4051-2802-X (alk. paper)
        1. Operating room nursing.   2. Preoperative care.   3. Postoperative
    care.   I. O'Neill, Joy.   II. Title.
        [DNLM: 1. Perioperative Care–nursing. 2. Perioperative Nursing
    –methods.   WY 161 C2778 2006]
        RD32.3.W53 2006
        617'.9192—dc22

2005017356

A catalogue record for this title is available from the British Library

Set in 9 on 11 pt Palatino by SNP Best-set Typesetter Ltd, Hong Kong
Printed and bound in India by Replika Press Pvt. Ltd

For further information on Blackwell Publishing, visit our website:
www.blackwellnursing.com

Contents

Foreword

In recent years the NHS has seen unprecedented change, resulting in significant healthcare improvement for patients and increased career opportunities within the NHS and its partners. These developments in innovative and advancing levels of practice are also reflected across Europe and many parts of the world.

The dynamic pace of this change has presented significant challenges for clinicians as they endeavour to acquire high-level clinical skills and deliver care while adapting to many new ways of working.

The United Kingdom National Health Service has had to respond dramatically to the changing demographics of its workforce and to high-level policy to drive down waiting times for patients and to increase the capacity for surgery. The perioperative workforce has been at the forefront of such changes and has had to undergo significant transformation in the way it works, crossing traditional healthcare boundaries. The aspirations of health professionals, structured NHS career frameworks, pay modernisation, working practice legislation, advancing levels of practice and the skills escalator concept of skills progression all contribute to the complexity of delivering care to patients.

The provision of education to health professionals giving perioperative care has also undergone significant change, with much more cross-profession delivery of core skills, increased e-learning opportunities and the development of nationally led Advanced Practitioner programmes. This education and exposure to hands-on learning is against a backdrop of increasing workload and advances in technology that now support clinical intervention.

Clinical input for trainees is a vital component in the education of our perioperative workforce, but both students and teachers within the many specialisms that encompass perioperative practice need access to a knowledge base that is modern, comprehensive and fit for purpose. The publication of such a clinically based and up-to-date resource is well overdue, and this book promises to fill that gap.

This text is well structured for easy reference and lends itself to detailed underpinning of knowledge while at the same time being suitable for use as a quick reference guide. I am confident that it will fulfil a need for both learners and teachers within perioperative care.

Mary Moore
Associate Director, National Orthopaedic Project
Department of Health
London

Preface

Perioperative care has been through a number of changes and has now developed into a truly patient-centred, holistic, evidence-based speciality that offers practitioners challenges and opportunities that are rarely seen outside the perioperative environment. Perioperative practitioners are defined in this book as nurses or operating department practitioners (ODPs) who perform scrub, circulating and recovery roles while caring for perioperative patients.

The pressures brought about by initiatives such as the NHS Plan, Clinical Governance and Agenda for Change mean that the care of the patient undergoing surgery is now carried out by many different professionals. Old technique-centred practice has given way to a patient-centred, evidence-based approach. A diverse and challenging perioperative environment has therefore developed, with subsequent challenges for the practitioners who work there.

The development of this book was informed by the document produced by the National Board for Nursing for Scotland (now NHS Education Scotland) entitled *Perioperative Care: A Route to Enhanced Competence*. This document is available online at: http://www.nes.scot.nhs.uk/docs/publications/qacpd/portfolios/periop.html

The purpose of this book is to identify and discuss the essential skills and knowledge required by perioperative practitioners in order to care for their patients. It is aimed primarily at the period following registration but before the development of advanced surgical skills, such as those displayed by advanced practitioners. As such it is also a useful source of information for nursing and ODP students working in perioperative care.

This book has been written to take on board the changes in the perioperative role discussed above. It is skills-orientated and uses examples of techniques or procedures to illustrate how those skills can be applied. It refers to 'perioperative practitioners' rather than ODPs and nurses, and it is evidence-based and innovative.

The book is arranged in two sections: core issues and more specific perioperative practices. Chapter 1 describes the practitioner's role in the delivery of therapeutic interventions required because of the anatomical and physiological influences of anaesthesia and surgery. The chapter reviews the concept of homeostasis in the context of holistic perioperative care and identifies the impact of anaesthesia and surgery on the systems of the body. Topics include principles of perioperative homeostasis, fluid balance, cardiovascular homeostasis, the respiratory system, wound healing and trauma.

Chapter 2 discusses the overall management of perioperative equipment, with specific reference to the most common items of equipment currently in use. There is a discussion on the safe use and maintenance of specific items of equipment. Topics include discussion about electrosurgery, the anaesthetic machine, the use of surgical instruments and other common pieces of equipment found in the operating department.

Chapter 3 discusses the implications of the use of various drugs on perioperative care. There is discussion on the metabolism of drugs and the uses, administration and side effects of common perioperative drugs. Drugs included in this chapter include opiates, muscle relaxants, analgesics, local anaesthetic agents, general anaesthetic agents and anti-emetics.

Chapter 4 considers ways to enhance communication in the perioperative environment. There is an exploration of important aspects of communication in relation to perioperative patients. There is also reference to the role of the practitioner within the perioperative team. Topics include clinical governance, change management, information technology and principles of record keeping.

Chapter 5 looks at risk management in the perioperative environment. It explores the main principles of risk management and identifies some of the common perioperative risks to patients. Topics include discussion about specific perioperative risks such as infection control, pressure area care, DVT prophylaxis, inadvertent hypothermia, latex allergy and smoke inhalation.

Chapter 6 presents the competencies associated with the role of the perioperative practitioner. It is based on the work carried out by an NHS Education Scotland (NES) working party in 2001–2002. This chapter provides a comprehensive list of perioperative competencies and their associated indicators. The indicators are measurable markers of the achievement of the competencies and are provided as examples of the indicators that practitioners develop in specific clinical areas. The next chapters explore indicators further and discuss some of the important skills and knowledge displayed by practitioners in anaesthesia, surgery and recovery.

Chapter 7 considers the role of the practitioner in the preoperative preparation of perioperative patients. It explores the techniques and methods of preoperative assessment and the role of the perioperative practitioner in preoperative visiting and care planning. Topics include selection of patients for surgery, assessment of patient's condition, common concurrent diseases, illnesses and conditions, and preoperative planning to prevent postoperative complications.

Chapter 8 explores the skills and knowledge required by anaesthetic practitioners. It discusses many of the clinical techniques used in anaesthesia and looks at the role of the practitioner in the anaesthetic team. Content includes the care of the patient undergoing general and local anaesthesia, patient monitoring and airway management.

Chapter 9 discusses the roles of the scrub and circulating practitioners. It explores some of the clinical techniques that practitioners use during surgery and the part that the practitioner plays in the surgical team. Content includes discussion on surgical scrubbing, haemostasis, wound closure, positioning the patient, dressings and wound care.

Finally, Chapter 10 considers unique aspects of the role of the recovery practitioner and the main clinical techniques used in recovery. Content includes discussion on the principles of care of the patient after clinical intervention, patient assessment, discharge criteria, airway maintenance in postoperative patients, pain management and managing complications such as shock, postoperative nausea and vomiting.

We hope that you enjoy using this book to enhance your practice and help you to provide the best patient care possible.

Paul Wicker and Joy O'Neill

Readers' note: every effort has been made to check the accuracy of drug and product information and nursing content. However, readers should check the manufacturer's product information and local protocols before undertaking any intervention.

Acknowledgements

We would like to say thank you to several people for helping us to produce this book. First, thank you to Caroline MacDonald, Joanne Wildman and Linda Faulkener for their help reviewing the book proposal. We also thank all the people who have read, reviewed, edited and commented on our work as it has developed including Rachel Astle, Janet Bidwell, Samantha Mills, Caroline Macdonald, Amanda Clarke, Andrew Clancy, Robert Hughes, Jonathon Kenworthy, Shahid Mirza, Mujahid Zaheer, Janet Barrie, Brian Allsop for the photographs, Beth Lynch for help with the illustrations, and all our colleagues at work. Finally thank you to Beth Knight for her confidence in us and for the role she has played in helping us to achieve our goal.

Section 1

Core Issues

1 Perioperative Homeostasis

LEARNING OUTCOMES

❑ Understand *homeostasis*.

❑ Discuss *fluid and electrolyte balance* in the perioperative patient.

❑ Describe the *structure, function and regulation of the cardiovascular and respiratory system*.

❑ Describe *blood pressure regulation*.

❑ Discuss the implications of the *metabolic response* and the *stages of wound healing*.

INTRODUCTION

Teamwork is the focus of good perioperative practice. Nowhere is teamwork more obvious than within the human body itself, where the close and efficient functioning of all the individual parts is essential for survival.

The purpose of this introductory chapter is to set the context of perioperative care and to identify links between the patient's anatomy and physiology, and perioperative care. Everything that happens to the perioperative patient during surgery and anaesthesia has an effect on his or her anatomy and physiology. This makes it important to understand the internal maintenance and control of the body's systems, and the external control through medical interventions.

The human body is a complex system of parts which can protect itself against major changes to its own internal environment. It does this by preserving a fine balance between all its major organs and systems, by maintaining fluids and electrolytes, blood pressure and oxygenation between particular limits to ensure efficient functioning. Every part of the system is related: the lungs absorb oxygen which is transported by the blood to muscles such as the heart, allowing it to beat and maintain blood pressure. The blood pressure in turn pushes the oxygenated blood around the body to the tissue cells. The blood then progresses back to the lungs where it supplies the lung tissue itself, as well as going on to provide a further source of oxygenated blood to all the cells of the body.

The term homeostasis is often used to refer to the maintenance of a constant environment. In perioperative care, however, it is better to see homeostasis as a dynamic process that results in a peak state for the body under existing circumstances (Clancy *et al.* 2002). Hence, for example, blood pressure may or may not be maintained at preoperative levels during the perioperative experience, and during surgery a low blood pressure may be helpful to reduce bleeding, ensuring a bloodless field. However, the main principles of control still hold true – maintaining an ideal environment for body processes to take place under current circumstances. The aim of medical interventions, as external homeostatic controllers, is to support the body's natural ability to maintain this dynamic homeostatic environment.

The topics associated with homeostasis are huge and this chapter will highlight selected areas of interest and relate them to clinical issues raised later in the book. This chapter therefore, describes some of the ways in which the human body maintains equilibrium, how anaesthesia and surgery affect this balance, and how medical interventions support the return to normal homeostasis. Finally, this chapter will book at the body's response to stress and the process of wound healing.

PRINCIPLES OF HOMEOSTASIS

To maintain homeostasis naturally, the body needs to:

- detect and analyse changes;
- take measures to address the changes;
- evaluate the effect of measures taken.

Control mechanisms carry out these processes, acting as receptors (detecting the changes), analysers (interpreting the changes) and effectors (acting on the changes to minimise, maximise or regulate them). These mechanisms detect changes in normal values and try to bring them back within the normal homeostatic range. An example of this system is the acid–base balance, where the buffer systems (described later in this chapter) act in unison to maintain the pH of body fluids within a normal range of around 7.35–7.45. Under normal circumstances, the body's buffer systems are able to maintain this balance, however, during illness, disease or because of trauma such as surgery or anaesthesia, the body may need support from external controls (medical interventions) to regain equilibrium.

Most of the body's own control mechanisms work through negative feedback – a change occurs to the body's environment and then mechanisms to cancel the changes are activated. Blood glucose regulation, for example, involves either the release of insulin to lower blood glucose or the release of glucagon to raise it. In either case, blood sugar levels are brought back to within the normal range.

Occasionally the control mechanisms work through positive feedback and a control mechanism to promote changes is activated – for example blood clotting, where the blood undergoes changes that allow it to clot and therefore reduce blood loss. Once the need has passed, the blood then returns to normal.

Internally, the organs act as both independent and interactive homeostatic controllers. This topic goes beyond the scope of this book. However, in the perioperative patient, several systems are specifically important because they are critical to the patient's immediate survival and are also the target of many perioperative interventions. Fluid and electrolyte balance are important perioperative considerations because of the potential for blood loss and possible hypovolaemia. Medical interventions that support the effects of blood and fluid loss, and help maintain electrolyte balance, merit consideration. The regulation of the respiratory and cardiovascular systems is also crucial in both the long and the short term. The aim of many anaesthetic functions is to control these systems to provide the optimum physiological environment during surgery.

WATER AND ELECTROLYTE HOMEOSTASIS

Table 1.1 describes the fluid compartments of the body. Total body water is distributed among all the fluid compartments of

Table 1.1 Terminology associated with fluid compartments.

Fluid compartment	Description
Extracellular (extracellular fluid = ECF)	Outside cells
Intracellular (intracellular fluid = ICF)	Inside cells
Interstitial	Between cells
Intravascular	Inside blood vessels (this is also extracellular)
Extravascular	Outside blood vessels (this may be intracellular, interstitial or transcellular)
Transcellular	Within hollow spaces, such as cerebrospinal fluid, the joints, the gastrointestinal tract, the urinary tract and the ducts of glands. Also called the 'third space'

the body. Of the 40 litres present in a 68 kg (150 lb) male, 65% is intracellular and 35% is extracellular. Extracellular fluid is composed of 25% tissue fluid, 8% blood plasma and lymph and 2% transcellular fluid such as cerebrospinal fluid (CSF) and synovial fluid.

Osmosis is the main process that distributes fluid throughout these compartments (Watson & Fawcett 2003). Osmosis is a special form of diffusion which involves the passage of water across a selectively permeable cell membrane that is freely permeable to water but not freely permeable to solutes. In osmosis, water will flow across a membrane toward the solution that has the higher concentration of solutes, because that is where the concentration of water is lowest (Figure 1.1).

An important effect of the movement of ions and water across cell membranes is the development of an electrical charge across the membrane. The resting potential is the charge across the membrane of an undisturbed cell. When the cell is stimulated, the electrical charge may be increased causing an 'action potential'. In nerves, for example, this represents the movement of information away from the cell body and down the nerve. In

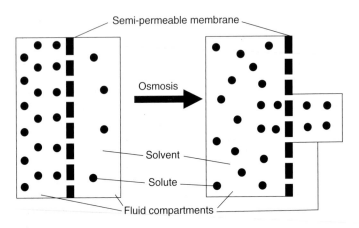

Semi-permeable membrane

Osmosis

Solvent

Solute

Fluid compartments

Fig. 1.1 Osmosis.

muscles, the action potential causes the contraction of muscle fibres.

Other methods which the cell uses to transport water and electrolytes include:

- filtration, which is a passive process where hydrostatic pressure (blood pressure) forces fluid and solutes across a membrane barrier;
- carrier-mediated transport, which involves specialised cell proteins binding to ions or organic substances facilitating their entry to or exit from the cell;
- vesicular transport, which involves the movement of materials within small membranous sacs, or vesicles.

Fluid balance

A person is in a state of fluid balance when water gain equals water loss; for example a water intake of 2.5 litres a day, taken in by food and drink, is balanced by water loss via routes such as faeces, expired air, sweat and urine.

Fluid intake is mainly controlled by the thirst centre in the hypothalamus which causes the sensation of thirst. Water output is regulated by varying urine volume. This system is mainly controlled by the antidiuretic hormone ADH, but also to a lesser extent by aldosterone and atrial natriuretic factor (ANF). Blood osmolarity is maintained because both sodium and water are retained or excreted.

Changes in the osmotic pressure exerted by plasma influence the release of ADH. High osmotic pressure (i.e. dehydration) leads to release of ADH; low osmotic pressure (i.e. hydration) reduces excretion of ADH. This system is so efficient that under normal conditions water balance is maintained to within 2% of the normal homeostatic range (Clancy *et al*. 2002).

Atrial natriuretic factor is a peptide released by walls of the cardiac atrium in response to high sodium chloride (NaCl) concentration, high extracellular fluid volume, or high blood volume. ANF inhibits NaCl reabsorption in the distal convoluted tubule and cortical collecting duct of the kidneys. It also dilates the afferent glomerular arteriole and constricts the efferent glomerular arteriole. This increases the glomerular filtration rate, which increases NaCl excretion, raises urinary filtration rate and therefore increases the rate of urine production.

Volume depletion (hypovolaemia) is a loss of total body water volume when osmolarity remains normal. Vomiting, diarrhoea, burns, haemorrhage or renal failure can cause this. Addison's disease results in dehydration leading to loss of total body water volume with an associated rise in osmolarity. This condition can also be caused by lack of drinking water, diabetes, profuse sweating or diuretics. Infants are more vulnerable to this condition.

Electrolyte balance

The balance of major electrolytes such as sodium (Na^+), potassium (K^+), calcium (Ca^{2+}), hydrogen (H^+) and bicarbonate (HCO_3^-) is essential to ensure homeostasis and the proper functioning of the body's processes (Saladin 2001).

Maintaining electrolyte and water balance are three major hormones: ADH, which promotes water retention independently of Na^+ and K^+ concentration; aldosterone which promotes retention of water and Na^+, and secretion of K^+; and ANF which increases NaCl secretion.

Electrolyte metabolism

Sodium and potassium

Sodium and potassium levels are critical to homeostasis because of their many roles. These two electrolytes contribute to maintaining membrane potentials, a major role of the sodium–potassium pump. Sodium is also responsible for 90–95% of osmolarity of ECF and potassium is the primary cation in ICF.

The normal sodium intake of around 3–7 g/day exceeds the 0.5 g/day needed for survival. Normal blood level ranges are:

Na^+, 130–145 mmol/litre
K^+, 3.5 to 5.5 mmol/litre

The homeostasis of water, sodium and potassium levels occurs by various linked systems:

- aldosterone/ANF;
- ADH;
- oestrogen/progesterone;
- salt craving.

Intercalated cells in the collecting duct of the kidneys also control potassium levels (Saladin 2001).

Calcium

Extracellular fluid contains a low concentration of calcium, however calcium exerts great influence on the body systems. Low calcium concentration increases the excitability of cells and in muscle cells this may lead to tetany. High concentrations of calcium ions make the cells less excitable and may lead to symptoms such as muscle weakness and bowel stasis. Other roles of calcium include skeletal mineralisation, muscle contraction, exocytosis (release of substances such as hormones from the vesicles of certain tissue cells) and blood clotting. Blood levels of 2.25–2.9 mmol/litre are normal.

Calcitonin is a hormone that takes part in calcium and phosphorus metabolism and affects bone deposition and resorption. Low intracellular Ca^{2+} levels influences calcitonin. The thyroid gland produces most calcitonin.

Phosphate

Phosphate is concentrated in ICF and variations in levels are well tolerated. Roles include being an ingredient of nucleic acids, phospholipids and some enzymes and co-enzymes such as adenosine triphophate. Phosphate also activates enzymes in metabolic pathways, and buffers pH. Maintenance and control of phosphate homeostasis is by tubular reabsorption in the kidneys.

Chloride

Sodium and chloride homeostasis are linked to each other. Chloride preserves osmolarity of ECF and plays a part in stomach acid production. The so-called 'chloride shift' (influx of chloride ions into cells) helps to maintain pH and electrical neutrality within cells. Chloride has a strong attraction to Na^+, K^+ and Ca^{2+} and is retained or secreted with Na^+ by the kidneys.

Acid–base balance

The acid-base balance is a critical part of homeostasis – the normal pH range of ECF (including blood) is 7.35–7.45. Several processes within the body affect acid–base balance maintenance. For example, normal metabolism produces substances such as lactic acids, phosphoric acids, fatty acids, ketones and carbonic acids which all affect pH. Even absorption of acidic foods may alter blood pH (Saladin 2001). Maintenance of acid-base balance is through buffer systems in the blood, respiration and renal systems.

Blood based buffers

The blood itself contains three buffering systems that help to stabilise pH – the bicarbonate buffer, the phosphate buffer and the protein buffer. The bicarbonate buffering system works through the association and disassociation of carbon dioxide, water, hydrogen, carbonic acid and bicarbonate, according to the following formula:

$$CO_2 + H_2O \leftrightarrow H_2CO_3 \leftrightarrow HCO_3 + H^+$$

One molecule of carbon dioxide (CO_2) combines with one molecule of water (H_2O) to become one molecule of carbonic acid

(H_2CO_3). The release of hydrogen ions from the carbonic acid increases the acidity of blood.

The carbonic acid molecule is not especially stable, and will break down in one of two ways. The carbonic acid molecule may break down back to carbon dioxide and water; the equation moves to the left, resulting in alkalosis. Alternatively it could break down into one molecule of bicarbonate and one hydrogen ion and the equation moves to the right, resulting in acidosis. The chemical reactions have the effect of equalising the levels of bicarbonate/hydrogen and carbon dioxide/water – so regulating the balance between alkalinity and acidity.

The phosphate buffer system works as follows:

$$H_2PO_4 \leftrightarrow HPO_4^{2-} + H^+$$

Again, an increase hydrogen ions increases acidity.

The protein buffer system works because the acidic side groups of protein molecules release hydrogen ions (increasing acidity) and amino side groups bind hydrogen ions (increasing alkalinity).

Respiratory buffer

The second main buffering system is a bicarbonate buffer within the respiratory system. This system is nearly three times more powerful as a buffer system than blood. The process is the same as the bicarbonate system in blood.

Renal buffer

The third and most powerful buffer system to adjust pH is renal control. The renal tubules secrete H^+ into urine and this secretion involves chemical processes using ammonium chloride and phosphate. The pH of urine affects the pH of blood by the diffusion of hydrogen ions through the membranes of the renal tubules into the kidney's capillaries (Saladin 2001).

Acidosis and alkalosis

Increasing acid or a significant loss of bicarbonate results in acidosis. H^+ ions diffuse into cells where they are buffered by the protein buffer system, and simultaneously K^+ ions are driven into the ECF. The result is membrane hyperpolarisation, which affects for example, muscle and nerve cells function. Alkalosis is essentially the opposite of this: H^+ ions diffuse out of the cells, K^+ ions diffuse in and the membrane becomes hypopolarised.

Acidosis has several possible causes, for example carbon dioxide retention (leading to increased carbonic acid); ketone or organic acid production (such as ketoacidosis or lactic acidosis); the use of acidic drugs; or renal failure resulting in the inadequate excretion of H^+ ions. The patient may suffer symptoms of headache, blurred vision, fatigue and weakness.

Metabolic alkalosis may be the result of various conditions including for example inadequate generation of metabolic acids, overuse of antacids or severe vomiting. Symptoms may include weakness, muscle cramps and dizziness.

Perioperative implications of fluid and electrolyte balance

Various factors present during anaesthesia and surgery can lead to water imbalances which must either be controlled by the body systems or supported through medical interventions (Sheppard 2000).

Preoperative fasting, while necessary to reduce the risk of aspiration of stomach contents during induction or recovery from anaesthesia, may also result in dehydration in susceptible patients, such as the elderly, the young or the sick.

Surgery may have a significant effect on water balance because of rapid changes in water level and distribution. High blood loss, for example, and resulting hypovolaemia can be quickly fatal. Hypovolaemia can also develop because of acute renal failure following disruption of perfusion of the kidneys, respiratory losses during ventilation or insensible losses through sweating because of postoperative pyrexia or disturbances in temperature. Other reasons include blood loss from wound drains, loss of peritoneal fluid and loss by vomiting, diarrhoea and evaporation by exposed moist tissues.

Surgery also has an effect on other systems of the body, especially the endocrine system, which can lead to changes in the homeostasis of water and electrolytes. For example, ADH is released because of hypotension, blood loss or dehydration, leading to water retention. Adrenaline (epinephrine) is released because of surgical stress and can lead to sodium and water retention by the kidneys (Clancy *et al.* 2002).

Management of the water balance is necessary because of these perioperative challenges. Fluid balance charts are the most common means of recording and estimating the fluid needs of patients. Consumed or infused fluids are matched against fluid losses such as urine output, exudates from wounds, blood loss and so on. Weighing swabs during surgery gives a rough idea of the volume of blood loss. The continuing assessment of patients to guard against dehydration or overhydration is therefore essential during all phases of their care (Hatfield & Tronson 1998).

Conditions such as renal depression, blood loss, vomiting or diarrhoea are likely to affect the perioperative electrolyte balance. Vomiting in particular leads to the loss of Na^+, Cl^- and K^+ ions, and gastric acids, leading to metabolic alkalosis. Anaesthetic drugs, such as morphine can stimulate vomiting, and so anti-emetics (such as metochlopramide and ondansetron) are often administered concurrently.

Diarrhoea is common following abdominal surgery for various reasons, such as the use of enemas, use of anti-emetic drugs, and following trauma or excision of the large or small bowel. When there is diarrhoea the bowel secretes several litres of fluid a day, which is high in bicarbonate, and may therefore lead to metabolic acidosis and overall electrolyte loss (Bellman & Manley 2000).

Intravenous replacement

The perioperative infusion of fluid and blood products supports homeostasis. Using fluid replacement therapies it is possible to influence the water and electrolyte content of the fluid compartments to achieve the desired result. It is important to realise that surgery and anaesthesia may have altered the body's needs either permanently, because of anatomical and physiological changes, or temporarily during the recovery phase and period of return to normality. The continuing assessment of the patient's needs is part of the science of anaesthesia and is beyond the scope of this book. However, following diagnosis and establishment of the patient's requirements, fluid and electrolyte replacement therapy will involve the practitioner in the use of colloids, crystalloids and blood products.

Colloids are plasma expanders – they selectively increase fluid in plasma while having a small effect on the intracellular compartments. Colloids include the protein-based gelatin (Gelofusine) and the carbohydrate-based dextran. They work by increasing or restoring the colloid pressure of plasma, resulting in increased fluid movement into the intravascular space. Infusion provides a short-term increase in plasma volume and their effects reduce as they are excreted.

Crystalloid infusates provide electrolytes and water and support both intracellular and extracellular compartments. Crystalloids can be hypertonic, hypotonic or isotonic. Hypertonic solutions draw water out of cells causing them to shrink. Mannitol is an example of such an infusate that shrinks brain cells and reduces pressure inside the cranium. Hypotonic solutions draw water into cells causing them to swell. There is a potential danger of lysis, where the cell membranes burst, and therefore it is rare to use hypotonic solutions. Cells suspended in an isotonic solution would neither increase nor decrease in size because the osmotic pressure of the fluid inside the cells is equal to that outside the cells. Isotonic solutions are widely used because they support both the intracellular and extracellular compartments.

Isotonic solutions, such as saline 0.9%, dextrose 5% and Hartmann's solution have an osmotic pressure similar to that of plasma and therefore move between the compartments in a similar way to normal body fluids. In hypovolaemia, isotonic crystalloids, the most common of which is sodium chloride 0.9% (normal saline) replace fluid in the intravascular compartment and will slowly diffuse into the intracellular space.

Dextrose 5% is a solution of glucose in water. At a concentration of 5% it has an equal osmolarity to body fluids and so on infusion it remains largely in the intravascular compartment since it cannot diffuse rapidly into the cells. However, the body's normal metabolic processes use up the glucose, leaving behind water, which is hypotonic. Intracellular volume increases as this water is drawn into the cells. Dextrose 5% is therefore effective at increasing both extracellular and intracellular fluid. The 25 g of glucose in 0.5% solution also provides a little energy – roughly equivalent to two chocolate biscuits per 500 ml!

Hartmann's solution provides a more complex mix of electrolytes, which closely resembles that of extracellular fluid, except for the presence of lactate rather than the bicarbonate normally found in blood. Other less common infusates include potassium chloride infusion, combinations such as dextrose/saline infusions and hyper/hypotonic variations of these solutions, such as 2.5% sodium chloride (Hatfield & Tronson 1998).

THE CARDIOVASCULAR SYSTEM

For the body to stay alive, each of its cells must receive a continuous supply of nutrition and oxygen. Simultaneously, the body removes carbon dioxide and other materials produced by the cells. The body's circulatory system – the heart and blood vessels – continuously support this process of nutrition delivery and waste removal. The circulatory system pumps blood from the heart to the lungs to receive oxygen. Blood then returns to the heart to be pumped throughout the body and then returns to the heart to begin again. The lymphatic system, which is an important constituent of the circulatory system, collects interstitial fluid and returns it to the blood. The cardiovascular system and the respiratory system are linked and could be seen as interlocking and interdependent systems. They are jointly responsible for carrying oxygen from the air to the bloodstream and tissues, and expelling the waste product of carbon dioxide.

Arteries and veins

Both arteries and veins consist of three major layers called 'tunica' (Figure 1.2). Endothelium lines the inner layer of the vessel, the tunica intima. The tunica media is the middle layer, which is much thicker in arteries and contains an extra thick layer of smooth muscle that can constrict to reduce the diameter of the vessel. Blood vessels have an outer layer called the tunica adventitia. Arteries use smooth muscle contractions to alter their internal diameter, which increases or decreases the resistance to the flow of blood provided by pressure from the

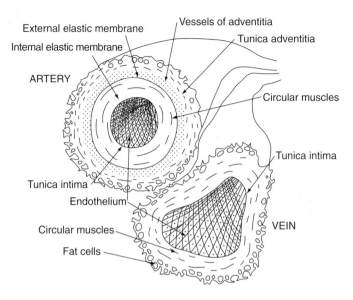

Fig. 1.2 Anatomy of an artery and a vein.

heart. Smooth muscle in veins can only contract weakly and so there are one-way valves that aid the flow of blood. Squeezing veins, by contracting muscles (such as calf muscles in the leg), produces blood flow through the one-way valves. Venous pressure is low in comparison with arterial pressure because the blood has lost the pressure exerted by the heart after moving through the smaller blood vessels and capillaries.

Arteries carry blood loaded with oxygen and nutrients away from the heart to all parts of the body. The only exception to this rule is the pulmonary artery which in fact carries deoxygenated blood from the heart to the lungs. Eventually arteries divide into smaller arterioles and then into even smaller capillaries, the smallest of all blood vessels. The network of tiny capillaries is where the exchange of oxygen and carbon dioxide between blood and body cells takes place.

The return of blood via the heart to the lungs for reoxygenation is of equal importance. Capillaries join to form venules and then veins, which flow into larger main veins, until finally they deliver deoxygenated blood back to the heart.

The heart

The heart consists mainly of cardiac muscle which works like a pump and contracts automatically (without conscious thought) to send blood to the lungs and the rest of the body. The heart consists of four chambers: each half of the heart consists of an upper chamber (called the atrium) and a larger lower chamber (called the ventricle). The major blood vessels entering and leaving the heart are shown in Figure 1.3.

The aorta is the largest artery in the body. It extends upward from the left ventricle of the heart, arches over the heart to the left, and descends just in front of the spinal column. The first portion of the aorta is the ascending aorta, which curves into the arch of the aorta. Three major arteries originate from the aortic arch: the brachiocephalic artery (which then branches into the right common carotid artery and the right subclavian artery), the left common carotid artery, and the left subclavian artery.

The cardiac cycle

Each heartbeat consists of a 'cardiac cycle'. As the heart relaxes, both atrium chambers fill with blood: deoxygenated blood comes into the right side from the superior and inferior vena cava, and oxygenated blood returns to the left side from the lungs via the pulmonary veins. The heart valves open and the atria contract (systole) and force the blood into the ventricles. The ventricles then contract to pump the deoxygenated blood through the pulmonary valve into the lungs and the oxygenated blood through the aortic valve into the body's main circulatory system. The atria relax once more (diastole) and fill with blood to restart the cycle. As the valves slap shut to prevent the blood's backflow, they make a noise described as the 'lub-dub' sound of a heartbeat (Tortora & Grabowski 1996).

Conduction of impulses within specialised muscle tissue in the heart itself largely control this process. The sinuatrial node, found in the right atrium starts an impulse which spreads throughout the atrium causing atrial contraction. It then arrives

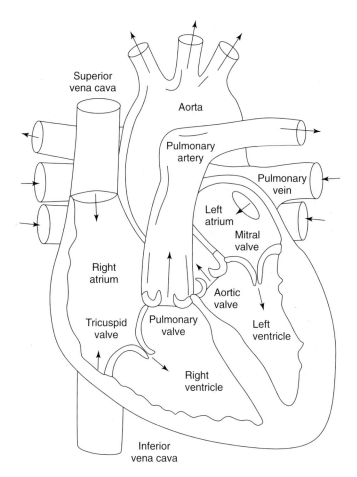

Fig. 1.3 The heart.

at the atrioventricular (AV) node which 'forwards' it to the bundles of His and the Purkinje fibres spreading the signal throughout the ventricles, which cause these parts to contract. The intrinsic properties of these nodes normally control the rate of heartbeat, however the autonomic nervous system (producing emotions such as anxiety or fear), and hormones such as thyroxine and adrenaline also influence the rate of the heartbeat. The electrical activity of the heart produces the signals that can be picked up by electrocardiographs.

This outline of the cardiovascular system serves only to show the complexity of the system. Reference to texts on anatomy and physiology are essential for a full understanding of this system (for example *Principles of Anatomy and Physiology* by Tortora and Grabowski).

The cardiovascular system delivers oxygen and nutrients to the cells of the body, and removes waste products. This system is inextricably linked to the survival of the patient and is thus vitally important in perioperative care (Clancy *et al.* 2002). Two important areas for the perioperative patient will now be considered – interpreting cardiac rhythms and the homeostasis of blood pressure.

The electrocardiogram

The electrocardiogram (ECG) measures the electrical changes of the heart as it goes through the cardiac cycle. It is therefore useful for diagnosis of abnormal cardiac rhythms and other cardiac pathology. Therefore ECG machines provide early warning of cardiac problems during anaesthesia and surgery.

Normal sinus rhythm (NSR)

The sinus node produces an electrical impulse that launches a normal heart rhythm. This signal radiates through the right and left atrial muscles producing electrical changes represented by the P-wave on the electrocardiogram. The electrical impulse stimulates the atria causing them to contract. This contraction of cardiac muscle is known as systole. The electrical impulse then continues to travel into and through specialised cardiac tissue known as the atrioventricular node, which conducts electricity at a slower pace, and forwards the impulse into the ventricles causing ventricular systole. The slower conduction rate will create a pause (PR interval) before stimulation of the ventricles. The pause between atrial and ventricular systole allows blood to empty into the ventricles from the atria before ventricular contraction, which propels blood out towards the aorta

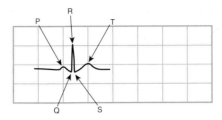

Fig. 1.4 ECG of a single cardiac cycle.

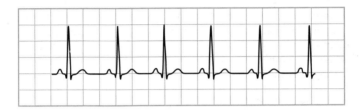

Fig. 1.5 Nornal sinus rhythm.

and the pulmonary artery. The QRS complex of waves on the ECG represents ventricular contraction. The T-wave follows, representing the electrical changes in the ventricles as they are relaxing. The QRS complex hides the electrical changes produced by atrial relaxation. The cardiac cycle then repeats itself after a short pause (Jevon & Ewens 2002).

Therefore, a cardiac cycle is represented on an ECG by P-waves which are followed after a brief pause by a QRS complex, then a T-wave (Figure 1.4).

Normal sinus rhythm (Figure 1.5) suggests that the rhythm produced by the sinus node is travelling through the tissues of the heart in a normal fashion and rate. The normal range of heart rate varies by individual and is influenced by factors such as age, health, body mass index, fitness and emotional state. An adult's heart rate is around 60–80 beats per minute at rest. A newborn infant may have a heart rate up to 150 beats per minute, while a child of 5 years old may have a heart rate of 100 beats per minute.

Tachycardia

Sinus tachycardia is a fast heart rate which occurs with a normal heart rhythm (Figure 1.6). This means that although the impulses producing the heartbeats are normal, they are occurring at a faster pace. This occurs because of conditions such as shock and drug actions as well as exercise, excitement, anxiety or as a reaction to stress.

Supraventricular tachycardia (SVT)

This is an abnormal heart rhythm because the sinus node does not produce the impulse stimulating the heart, which instead comes from tissues around the atrioventricular (AV) node. Rapid generation of these abnormal electrical impulses leads to a heartbeat that may reach up to 280 beats per minute (Figure 1.7).

Ventricular tachycardia is similar; however, it results from abnormal tissues in the ventricles producing a rapid and irregular heart rhythm. Poor cardiac output usually accompanies

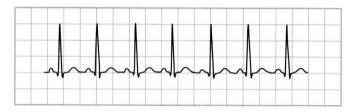

Fig. 1.6 Tachycardia.

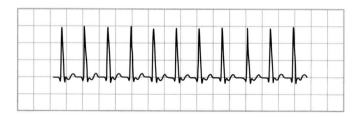

Fig. 1.7 Supraventricular tachycardia.

this rapid heart rhythm and can therefore be significant during surgery.

Atrial flutter

This abnormal rapid heart rhythm arises because the impulse which arises from the abnormal tissue in the atria bypasses the atrioventricular node. Without the dampening effect of the AV node, the impulse is repeated rapidly resulting in the faster abnormal rhythm (Figure 1.8).

Sinus bradycardia

Sinus bradycardia presents as a slow heart rate with a normal sinus rhythm (Figure 1.9). It is usually benign although in some circumstances it may need treatment, for example when caused by stimulation of the vagus nerve during surgery. It is also a result of using medications such as beta-blockers (see Chapter 3).

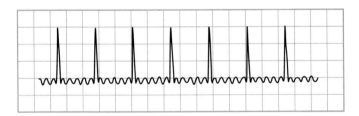

Fig. 1.8 Atrial flutter.

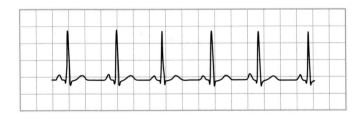

Fig. 1.9 Sinus bradycardia.

Atrioventricular block (AVB)

This abnormal rhythm occurs because of a block in conduction between the sinus node and the atrioventricular node. There are various types of AV block depending upon the mechanism of block. For example, second-degree heart block occurs when some signals from the atria don't reach the ventricles, resulting in 'dropped beats' (Figure 1.10). Third-degree or complete AV block results in a total lack of atrial impulses passing through the atrioventricular node and the ventricles therefore create their own rhythm. This rhythm is usually extremely slow and so the heartbeat must be raised to within the normal range with a pacemaker.

Premature atrial contraction (PAC)

The sinoatrial node fires early, causing the atria to contract early in the cycle, resulting in an irregular rhythm (Figure 1.11).

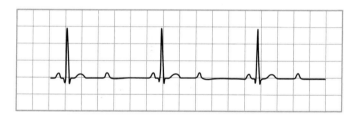

Fig. 1.10 Atrioventricular block.

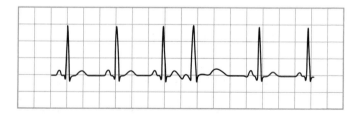

Fig. 1.11 Premature atrial contractions.

Premature ventricular contraction (PVC)

The AV node fires early, causing the ventricles to contract early in the cycle, resulting in an irregular rhythm (Figure 1.12).

Atrial fibrillation

This is a result of many sites within the atria firing electrical impulses in an irregular fashion causing irregular heart rhythm (Figure 1.13). This abnormal heart rhythm is unusual in children.

Asystole

Asystole represents the lack of electrical activity of the heart and therefore the ending of heartbeats. Note the absence of a completely straight line which signals continuing residual electrical activity (Figure 1.14).

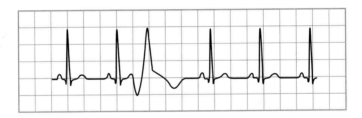

Fig. 1.12 Premature ventricular contractions.

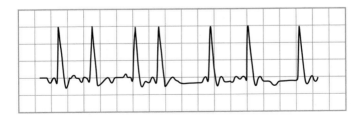

Fig. 1.13 Atrial fibrillation.

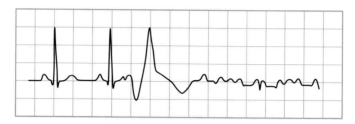

Fig. 1.14 Asystole.

Blood pressure homeostasis

There are two basic mechanisms for regulating blood pressure: short-term mechanisms, which regulate blood vessel diameter, heart rate and contractility; and long-term mechanisms, which regulate blood volume (Clancey *et al.* 2002).

Nervous control of blood pressure

The sympathetic and parasympathetic nervous systems mainly provide the nervous control of the blood pressure. The vagus nerve provides the parasympathetic nerve supply to the heart. Stimulation of the vagus nerve (for example during surgery on the vagus such as a vagotomy) leads to a paradoxical decrease in sympathetic nervous system activity. Blood pressure falls because of vasodilation, a lower heart rate (bradycardia) and lower cardiac output.

Sympathetic nerve fibres stimulate vasomotor fibres within the smooth muscle of arteries resulting in vasoconstriction; this causes blood pressure to rise. Lack of sympathetic stimulation results in relaxation of the arteries, an increased arterial diameter, and therefore reduces blood pressure.

In the heart, sympathetic activity stimulates the sympathetic cardiac nerves, which results in increased heart rate and contractility, higher cardiac output and increased blood pressure. Simultaneously the vagus (parasympathetic) nerve displays decreased activity.

Hormonal control of blood pressure

Increased sympathetic impulses to the adrenal glands lead to the release of adrenaline (epinephrine) and noradrenaline (norepinephrine) into the bloodstream. These hormones act on chemoreceptors to increase heart rate, contractility and vaso-constriction. The effect is slower-acting and more prolonged than nervous system control.

Short-term regulation of rising blood pressure

Baroreceptors, specialised areas of tissue which are sensitive to pressure, provide short-term control of rising blood pressure. Rising blood pressure leads to stretching of arterial walls and stimulation of baroreceptors in the carotid sinus, aortic arch, and other large arteries of the neck and thorax. The barorecep-tors send an increased frequency of impulses to the brain which leads to increased parasympathetic activity and decreased sym-pathetic activity. This results in a decreased heart rate and an increase in arterial diameter which aim to reverse the increas-ing blood pressure (Jevon & Ewens 2002).

Short-term regulation of falling blood pressure

Falling blood pressure inhibits the baroreceptors leading to a decrease in impulses sent to the brain. This causes a paradoxi-cal increase in sympathetic activity leading to three effects:

- increased heart rate and increased contractility;
- increased vasoconstriction;
- release of adrenaline (epinephrine) and noradrenaline (nor-epinephrine) from the adrenal glands which increases heart rate, contractility, and vasoconstriction.

The combined effect helps to increase blood pressure.

Long-term regulation of blood pressure

Long-term control of blood pressure is primarily accomplished by altering blood volume. The loss of blood through haemor-rhage, accident or donating a pint of blood will lower blood pressure and trigger processes to restore blood volume and therefore blood pressure back to normal. Long-term regulatory processes conserve body fluids by renal mechanisms and stimulate intake of water to normalise blood volume and blood pressures. (See section on water/electrolyte balance pages 6–8.)

Haemorrhage (loss of blood)

When there is loss of blood, blood pressure and blood volume decrease. Juxtaglomerular cells (a small endocrine organ associated with individual nephrons within the kidneys) monitor changes in the blood pressure. If blood pressure falls too low, these specialised cells release the enzyme renin into the bloodstream and launch the renin/angiotensin mechanism. This process consists of a series of steps aimed at increasing blood volume and blood pressure.

The first step of this process is angiotensin I formation. As renin travels through the bloodstream, it binds to an inactive plasma protein, angiotensinogen, activating it to become angiotensin I.

The second step is the conversion of angiotensin I to angiotensin II as it passes through the lung capillaries. Angiotensin II is a vasoconstrictor and therefore raises blood pressure in the body's arterioles, however, its main effect is on the adrenal gland. Here, in the third step, it stimulates the cells of the adrenal cortex to release the hormone aldosterone.

Aldosterone stimulates increased sodium reabsorption from the tubule cells. The increased sodium levels in the tubules make sodium move into the bloodstream, closely followed by water.

Increase in osmolarity

Dehydration resulting from sweating, diarrhoea or excessive urine flow will cause an increase in osmolarity of the blood and result in a decrease in blood volume and blood pressure. As osmolarity increases there is both a short- and long-term effect. In the long term, the hypothalamus sends a signal to the posterior pituitary to release ADH, which increases water reabsorption in the distal convoluted tubules and collecting tubules of the kidney. Water moves back into the capillaries, decreasing the osmolarity of the blood, increasing the blood volume, and therefore increasing the blood pressure.

A short-term effect of increased osmolarity is the activation of the thirst centre in the hypothalamus. The thirst centre stimulates the individual to drink more water and thus rehydrates the blood and the extracellular fluid, restoring blood volume and therefore blood pressure.

Pharmacology and blood pressure homeostasis

There are many chemicals that influence blood flow and blood vessel diameter and therefore have a direct action on blood pressure. Table 1.2 gives some examples of drugs that act on the cardiovascular system.

See Chapter 3 on pharmacology for further discussion of drugs acting on the cardiovascular system.

Shock

Shock is a condition that arises as a failure of the circulatory system to deliver oxygen and nutrients to the tissues of the body, and to remove waste products. Before going into shock in detail it is important to understand the relationship between cardiac output, peripheral resistance and blood pressure. Control of blood circulation is through the interaction of blood volume (provided via cardiac output), blood vessel diameter (vasoconstriction – especially peripherally), and the pressure gradient that 'pushes' blood through the tissues (blood pressure).

Cardiac output is the volume of blood ejected from the heart every beat (this is the stroke volume), per minute:

Cardiac output = stroke volume × heart rate
　　　　　　　 = 140 ml × 60 beats per minute
　　　　　　　 = 8400 ml per minute

This is the cardiac output for an average heart beating 60 times per minute with a stroke volume per ventricle of 70 ml (so 140 ml total).

Various factors affect stroke volume. For example, low venous return reduces the volume of blood refilling the heart between beats (end-diastolic volume) and therefore reduces stroke volume. Cardiac contractility affects the percentage of blood ejected from the heart on every beat – a stronger contraction will empty the heart more efficiently than a weak contraction. A huge variety of factors such as autonomic nervous stimulation, hormones and drugs affect the heart rate.

Table 1.2 Examples of drugs acting on the cardiovascular system.

Drug	Action	Uses
Adrenaline (epinephrine)	α agonist – coronary and peripheral vasoconstriction β agonist – increased heart rate and myocardial contractility	Used in cardiac arrest to stimulate the heart muscles
Isoprenaline, dopamine	β agonist – increased rate and force of heart beat, vasodilation	Cardiogenic shock in infarction or cardiac surgery
Ephedrine	Increases heart rate and myocardial activity. Increases peripheral vasoconstriction	Reversal of hypotension, for example from spinal or epidural anaesthesia
Phentolamine	α antagonist – vasodilation and myocardial stimulant. Overall effect of reducing blood pressure	Used as a vasodilator in cardiobypass surgery and in cardiogenic shock
Atenolol	Slows the heart beat and reduces myocardial oxygen demand	Prophylaxis of angina, treatment of dysrhythmias and hypertension
Propranolol (also oxprenolol and atenolol)	β antagonist – reduces heart rate and output, reduces myocardial oxygen demand	Control of ectopic heartbeats and tachycardia. Reduces incidence of angina
Digoxin	Cardiac glycoside – increases the force of myocardial contraction and reduces conductivity within the atrioventricular (AV) node	Most useful in the treatment of supraventricular tachycardias, especially for controlling ventricular response in persistent atrial fibrillation
Atropine	An antimuscarinic drug which blocks acetylcholine	Prevention and reversal of excessive bradycardia

Peripheral resistance refers to the tissue's resistance to blood flow. The diameter of blood vessels directly influences the resistance to blood flow – narrow vessels conduct blood at a slower rate than wide vessels. Control of blood vessel diameter occurs at a local tissue level through the release of lactic acid and other metabolites of normal cellular function. These metabolites cause local vasodilatation and therefore reduce peripheral vasoconstriction. Control of peripheral resistance occurs centrally through neural and hormonal activity, in particular the sympathetic nervous system.

Blood pressure is also subject to many controls. The higher the pressure gradient the faster blood will flow. The difference between the heart contractions (systole) and the relaxation phase (diastole) produces a pressure gradient. In humans, systolic pressure is normally around 120 mmHg and diastolic pressure is around 80 mmHg. The difference between these two measurements is the pulse pressure and it is this pressure that represents the pressure gradient. Pulse pressure is influenced by a combination of the contractility of the heart, the circulating volume and the peripheral resistance.

Shock, therefore, can be defined as acute circulatory failure leading to inadequate tissue perfusion, resulting in generalised cellular hypoxia and end organ injury. It is caused by a disruption to the cardiovascular system, and inadequate compensation to maintain tissue perfusion (Jevon & Ewens 2002).

Shock can be classified according to its three known causes:

- a fault of the heart, which is cardiogenic shock;
- a fault of the vascular system, which is distributive shock;
- a fault of fluid regulation, which is hypovolaemic shock.

Keeping in mind the previous discussion on blood pressure regulation, it can be seen that hypotension and shock are therefore caused by a problem with heart rate, stroke volume or peripheral resistance.

A clinical approach to shock (Table 1.3) identifies the main clinical problems associated with shock that can be treated by medical interventions such as drugs or surgery:

- low blood pressure, because of inadequate cardiac output or low peripheral resistance;

- low cardiac output, caused by a problem with heart rate or stroke volume;
- heart rate abnormalities – too fast (tachycardia) or too slow (bradycardia);
- stroke volume abnormalities, caused by failure to receive blood, failure to eject blood, or inadequate volume;
- low peripheral vascular resistance, because of inappropriate vasodilation.

Table 1.3   A clinical approach to shock.

Overall effect		Physiological problem	Clinical focus
Failure of cardiac output	Heart rate	Inappropriate heart rate	• Heart block/pacemaker • Hypotension • Bradycardia
	Stroke volume	Inadequate filling time	• Tachycardia • Arrhythmias
		Failure to receive blood	• Haemorrhage • Hypovolaemia • Dehydration • Inadequate fluid intake • Excessive fluid loss • Interstitial fluid loss (e.g. bowel surgery, pancreatitis) • Inflow obstruction • Mitral stenosis • Tamponade
		Failure to eject blood	• Muscle dysfunction • Myocardial ischaemia or fibrosis • Valvular/septal damage • Ventricular damage • Aortic regurgitation • Septal defects • Outflow obstruction • Pulmonary obstruction • Aortic/pulmonary stenosis
Failure of peripheral resistance		Inappropriate vasodilation	• Anaphylaxis • Shock • Sepsis

Hypovolaemic shock

During shock, the body protects itself from hypovolaemia by a series of reflex mechanisms involving the cardiovascular and neurohormonal systems as described previously. The result is a decrease in cardiac output and increased peripheral resistance. The selective shunting of blood occurs to essential organs such as brain, heart and kidneys, which are further protected by autoregulatory reflexes. This state is 'compensated shock' and may occur with up to 20% of blood loss (approximately 1 litre) (University of Pennsylvania 2004).

The clinical signs of compensated shock may be subtle: blood pressure may be normal; there is tachycardia, cold and clammy peripheries, decreased capillary refill; and a widened gap between core and peripheral temperature (Astiz *et al.* 1993).

As circulating volume decreases (1–2 litres blood loss) blood pressure begins to fall, resulting in increased peripheral vasoconstriction and tachycardia. Blood pressure may become unrecordable and there are signs of end organ failure (oliguria and confusion) following the loss of more than 40% (2 litres) of circulating volume. The drop in urinary output is a reliable way of identifying progressive loss of circulating volume.

Treatment of hypovolaemic shock

Treatment of shock addresses the cause by replacing lost fluids and supporting the body's essential systems against the effects of hypovolaemia. Techniques and protocols are constantly being reviewed as new research evidence becomes available.

Replacement of lost fluids by colloids and crystalloids is normally a priority for treating shock. Progressively worsening shock necessitates monitoring of arterial and central venous pressure (CVP) to assess the effects of fluid replacement. The end point of fluid replacement will be: blood pressure within normal limits; urinary output of greater than 1 ml/kg; CVP of over 12 mmHg; and lactate readings of less than 2 mmol/litre (University of Pennsylvania 2004). If the patient remains hypotensive after the volume replacement, then the problem lies with the cardiovascular system which must be supported through medical interventions. Noradrenaline and low dosage vasopressin may increase stroke volume, which can be measured with a pulmonary artery catheter or oesophageal Doppler. Dobutamine may be useful at this point to increase the efficiency of the heart pump.

The stroke volume, CVP and pulmonary capillary wedge pressure (PCWP) and venous oxygen saturation may guide fluid resuscitation. Since over-transfusion of patients rarely occurs during shock, non-invasive monitors such as the oesophageal Doppler may provide more rapid and less dangerous measurement of stroke volume. Close monitoring is essential since the patient's fluid status may change as the body recovers from shock or as the effects of medical interventions progress (Soni & Welch 1996).

RESPIRATORY SYSTEM

The respiratory system transports gasses between the bloodstream and the outside air. Blood delivers oxygen to the tissues of the body, while carbon dioxide from tissue activity is returned to the lungs. The carbon dioxide waste leaves the body during exhalation.

Breathing is the process of moving air into and out of the lungs. An adult normally breathes from 14 to 20 times per minute, rising to 80 breaths per minute on effort and dropping to 8 or 10 breaths per minute at rest. A child's rate of breathing at rest is faster than an adult's at rest, and a newborn baby has a rate of about 40 breaths per minute. In adults the tidal volume (amount of air taken in a normal breath) is about 0.5 litres. The vital capacity (the maximum amount) is about 4.8 litres in an adult male.

The process of breathing comprises two phases, inspiration and expiration. The lungs themselves have no muscle tissue so the ribcage and the diaphragm control their movements.

The diaphragm is a large, dome-shaped muscle that lies just under the lungs, which flattens when stimulated. This expands the volume of the thoracic cavity. The rib muscles also contract on stimulation, pulling the ribcage up and out, also expanding the thoracic cavity. The increased volume of the thoracic cavity creates a partial vacuum which sucks air into the lungs. The diaphragm and rib muscles relax when the nervous stimulation ends, the thoracic cavity shrinks and exhalation occurs.

Conscious control and overriding of the respiratory centre alter the rhythm, for example when singing or whistling, or when holding the breath.

Structure

The respiratory system extends from the nose to the lungs and is divided into the upper and lower respiratory tracts. The upper respiratory tract consists of the nose and the pharynx, or throat. The lower respiratory tract includes the larynx, or voice box; the trachea, or windpipe, which splits into two main branches called bronchi; tiny branches of the bronchi called bronchioles; and finally the lungs. The nose, pharynx, larynx, trachea, bronchi and bronchioles conduct air to and from the lungs. The lungs interact with the cardiovascular system to deliver oxygen and remove carbon dioxide.

Nose and nasal cavity

Capillaries in the nose and nasal cavity warm and humidify the air. Hairs and mucus inside the nasal cavity help to trap dust and other particles to protect the lungs. Stimulation of chemoreceptors inside the nose activates the olfactory nerve which eventually leads to the sensation of smell.

Pharynx

The pharynx is a short, funnel-shaped tube about 13 cm long that links the nose and the larynx. The pharynx transports air to the larynx and is lined with a protective mucous membrane and ciliated cells to remove impurities. The pharynx also houses the tonsils, which are lymphatic tissues that contain white blood cells. The tonsils help to protect against upper respiratory tract infections. High in the rear wall of the pharynx are the adenoids. Located at the back of the pharynx on either side of the tongue are the palatine tonsils. The lingual tonsils are found at the base of the tongue. The tonsils can become swollen with infection (tonsillitis) causing various symptoms associated with airway blockage and sepsis.

Viral infections such as the common cold, influenza, German measles (rubella), herpes and infectious mononucleosis cause pharyngitis, giving symptoms of a sore throat. Infection can also be caused by diphtherial, chlamydial, streptococcal and staphylococcal bacteria.

Larynx

Air moves from the pharynx to the larynx and on to the trachea. The larynx is about 5 cm long and consists of several layers of cartilage. The Adam's apple is a prominent bulge visible on the neck formed by a projection in the cartilage.

The larynx also produces sound, prevents food and fluid from entering the trachea and helps filter air. The presence of food or fluid in the larynx produces a cough reflex. If the cough reflex does not work, a person can choke.

The larynx houses two pairs of vocal cords made of elastic connective tissue covered by folds of mucous membrane. One pair, the false vocal cords, narrows the glottis (the pharyngeal opening of the larynx) during swallowing. Below this and extending as far as the thyroid cartilage are the true vocal cords. Sound is created when this pair of cords vibrates as air passes through them.

Laryngitis, which often accompanies colds, is the larynx's most common affliction and can lead to voice loss. Other diseases include croup, diphtheria and cancer. Cancer is often treated by radiotherapy and surgery – partial or total laryngectomy.

Trachea

The trachea extends from the larynx to the right and left primary bronchi in the lungs (Tortora & Grabowski 1996). The trachea is lined by ciliated mucous membrane; the mucus traps tiny particles and the cilia move the mucus up and out of the respiratory tract. Rings of cartilage reinforce the trachea and prevent it from collapsing. If the airway blocks above the larynx, a tracheostomy may be performed to bypass the blockage and ease breathing. Alternatively, the patient may need intubation using an endotracheal tube.

Bronchial tree and lungs

The trachea divides into the right and left primary bronchi which transport air to and from the right and left lungs respectively. Inside the lungs, each bronchus divides into smaller bronchi, bronchioles, terminal bronchioles, and finally the respiratory bronchioles.

The lungs, two pink and spongy sacs, occupy the chest cavity from the collarbone down to the diaphragm, which separates the contents of the abdominal cavity from the chest cavity. At birth the lungs are pink but as a person ages they become grey and mottled from tiny particles breathed in with the air.

The visceral pleura lines the outside of lungs and the parietal pleura lines the inside walls of the chest. The narrow space between the visceral and parietal pleurae is called the pleural cavity. A thin layer of pleural fluid in this cavity causes the visceral pleura to stick to the parietal pleura so the lungs stick to the chest wall. This causes them to expand and contract with the chest during breathing, drawing air in on inspiration and forcing it out on expiration.

Air entering the lungs contains about 21% oxygen and 0.04% carbon dioxide. Air leaving the lungs contains about 14% oxygen and about 4.4% carbon dioxide.

Alveoli

The bronchioles divide many more times in the lungs to end in tiny air sacs called alveoli. Each lung is composed mostly of about 150 million alveoli. Alveoli resembling tiny, collapsed balloons are arranged in grapelike clusters surrounded by tiny capillaries. The air in the wall of the alveoli is only about 0.1 to 0.2 μm from the capillary blood. The alveoli are where gaseous exchange occurs between the air in the alveoli and the blood in the capillaries in their walls (Figure 1.15). In the capillary beds of the lungs, carbon dioxide diffuses down its concentration gradient into the air inside the alveoli and is exhaled from the body during the next breath. Oxygen in the alveoli diffuses down its own concentration gradient into the blood. The oxygenated blood leaves the lungs, returns to the heart by the pulmonary arteries and then continues out of the heart into the body to restart the process (Figure 1.16).

The role of surfactant

Some of the cells forming the alveoli secrete a chemical called surfactant, which decreases surface tension of the fluid

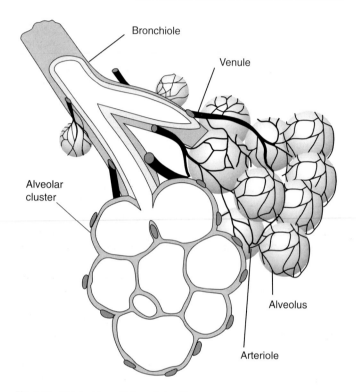

Fig. 1.15 Terminal bronchiole and alveoli.

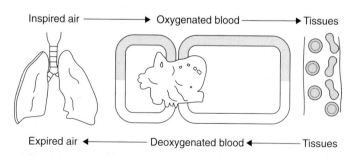

Fig. 1.16 Exchange of oxygen and carbon dioxide between the blood and lungs.

in the alveoli. This reduces the attraction between water molecules and prevents the walls of the alveolus from collapsing.

Infant respiratory distress syndrome (IRDS) is caused by a deficiency in surfactant. This syndrome is often seen in premature babies who may be unable to produce adequate amounts of surfactant. The alveoli collapse on exhalation making reinflation difficult. Giving surfactant and hormones can stimulate the surfactant-producing cells.

Regulation of breathing

Aerobic respiration is the process within cells in which nutrients and oxygen build the energy molecule adenosine triphosphate (ATP) through a process known as the Krebs' cycle. The overall effect of aerobic respiration is that body cells use oxygen to metabolise glucose, forming carbon dioxide as a waste product.

The oxygen and carbon dioxide concentrations in various parts of the body are measured as partial pressures – the pressure exerted by any one gas absorbed within a fluid. For example, pO_2 is the partial pressure of oxygen in the blood – the pressure exerted by oxygen which contributes to the entire pressure of all the absorbed gases.

The rate and pattern of breathing is controlled by a cluster of nerve cells in the brain stem called the respiratory centre – a circuit of neurons in the base of the brain (the medulla oblongata and pons). Motor neurons from the respiratory control centre innervate the diaphragm and chest muscles. When stimulated, they contract and change the volume of the thoracic cavity. The respiratory control centre also receives input from many other neurons.

Nerves from the higher brain centres controlling emotion stimulate or depress the respiratory control centre and cause changes in the rate and depth of breathing when the person is excited or relaxed. Sensory neurons such as proprioceptors from the joints and chemoreceptors from the arteries also interact with the respiratory control centre. On exercising, action potentials from proprioceptors in joints stimulate the respiratory control centre and increase the rate of breathing.

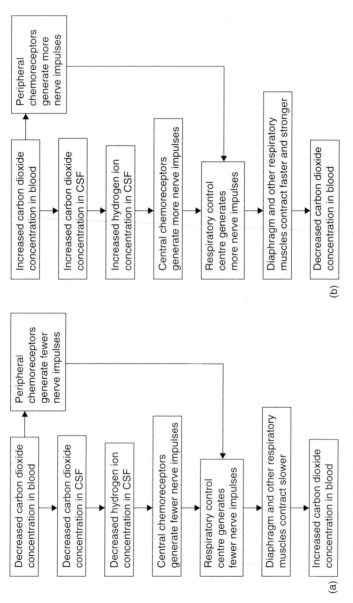

Fig. 1.17 Regulation of breathing and respiration by carbon dioxide concentration in the blood: (a) decreased; (b) increased. (Eberly College of Science, 2004)

However, the levels of carbon dioxide in the blood and cerebrospinal fluid (CSF) are the major factors regulating both the rate and depth of breathing (Figure 1.17). If carbon dioxide levels in the blood increase, the carbon dioxide will diffuse into the CSF. Central chemoreceptors in the medulla oblongata of the brain stimulate the respiratory control centre, increasing the rate and depth of breathing and so reducing pCO_2.

Hypercapnia is caused by high carbon dioxide concentration in blood. The carbonic acid equation moves to the right and the hydrogen ion concentration increases (see page 9). The increase in hydrogen ion concentration increases the acidity of blood and CSF, and can cause respiratory acidosis. The respiratory control centre will respond by increasing the speed and depth of breathing, causing carbon dioxide to diffuse from blood to the lungs more rapidly.

Hypocapnia is caused by low partial pressure of carbon dioxide in blood. In this case, the carbonic acid equation moves to the left, and hydrogen ion concentration will decrease as a new equilibrium is reached (see page 9). The decrease in blood hydrogen ion concentration causes respiratory alkalosis. The respiratory control centre reacts by decreasing the respiratory rate causing carbon dioxide from cellular respiration to build up in the bloodstream. The carbonic acid equation moves to the right again, reversing the respiratory alkalosis. The respiratory control centre constantly adjusts the depth and rate of breathing to maintain the proper balance. Although some degree of conscious control can be exerted over the amount of air inhaled, the most important factors controlling breathing are the carbon dioxide and hydrogen ion concentrations of the blood and cerebral spinal fluid (Eberly College of Science 2004).

Diseases and disorders

There are many diseases and disorders of the respiratory system which can affect any part of the respiratory tract.

Infection by a huge variety of cold viruses is one of the most common ailments affecting the membranes of the nasal passages and pharynx. The immune system fights back by increasing blood flow to the area, bringing numerous white blood cells to the scene. This inflammatory reaction causes the membranes to swell and increase the secretion of mucus, resulting in the stuffy and runny nose associated with colds. The infection can spread to the lower respiratory tract, to the middle ear, or to the sinuses where it causes sinusitis.

The respiratory system is prone to allergic reactions, such as hay fever and asthma, which are caused when the immune system is stimulated by pollen, dust or other irritants. A runny nose, watery eyes and sneezing characterises hay fever. In asthma, temporary constriction and inflammation of the bronchi and bronchioles causes difficulty in breathing. An asthma attack is typically mild in otherwise healthy patients, but can be severe enough to be life-threatening when anaesthesia and surgery, or other concurrent conditions compromise the patient.

Laryngitis is an inflammation of the larynx resulting from causes such as viral infections, trauma caused by endotracheal tubes, irritants such as cigarette smoke or by overuse of the voice. Laryngitis may result in hoarseness or whispering until the swelling subsides. Bronchitis, caused by viral or bacterial infection or by irritating chemicals, is an inflammation of the membranes that line the bronchi or bronchioles. Infections with bacteria or viruses can lead to pneumonia, a potentially serious condition of the lungs where fluid and inflammation prevent the flow of oxygen and carbon dioxide between the capillaries and the air in the alveoli.

Tuberculosis bacteria attack the lungs and sometimes other body tissues as well. Untreated infections in the lungs destroy lung tissue. In the past, antibiotics have controlled tuberculosis, but recently, new antibiotic-resistant strains of the tuberculosis bacterium have evolved. These new strains now pose a significant public health problem. Immunocompromised patients are particularly prone to tuberculosis.

In emphysema the alveolar bundles coalesce resulting in an overall smaller surface area for the exchange of gases. Weakened bronchioles collapse on exhalation, trapping air in the alveoli. This eventually hinders the exchange of oxygen and carbon dioxide with the circulatory system, leading to hypoxia and difficulty in breathing. Emphysema is a non-contiguous disease that can result from various causes including a genetic tendency to the condition, smog, cigarette smoke or infection.

Exposure to cancer-causing agents, such as tobacco smoke, asbestos or radiation, can lead to lung cancer in individuals with a genetic inclination to the disease. Cancerous tumours can start in the bronchi, bronchioles or in the alveolar lung tissue. Treatments are more effective on early detection of lung cancer, before it has spread to other parts of the body, and provide a good prognosis for full recovery. The prognosis is poor if the cancer has had the opportunity to spread.

Respiratory distress syndrome (RDS) is the name for a cluster of symptoms that suggest severe failure of the lungs. In infants, RDS is termed infant respiratory distress syndrome (IRDS). IRDS is commonly found in premature infants when the alveoli fail to expand fully during inhalation. Expansion of the alveoli requires surfactant, but in many premature infants the alveoli cannot produce this substance. Treatment of IRDS is by artificial ventilation and giving surfactant until the alveoli begin producing surfactant on their own. Severe damage to the lungs caused by, for example, trauma, poisonous gases or as a response to inflammation in the lungs, causes acute (adult) respiratory distress syndrome (ARDS). ARDS is a life-threatening condition with a survival rate of about 50%.

TRAUMA AND WOUND HEALING
Anaesthesia and surgery cause stress to the body, so it comes as no surprise that the perioperative patient presents many of the responses found with naturally occurring stressors. This section describes the body's metabolic response to anaesthesia and surgery and then, the process of wound healing.

Stressors such as surgery and anaesthesia, as well as others such as injury, burns, vascular occlusion, dehydration, starvation, sepsis, acute medical illness, or psychological stress, may launch the metabolic response to trauma. The body responds locally by an inflammatory response designed to protect tissues from further damage and to encourage repair. The purpose of the somatic response is to conserve fluid and provide energy for tissue repair.

Two phases characterise the somatic response. Initially the body produces an *acute catabolic reaction* where the patient is in shock, characterised by:

- depression of enzymatic activity;
- decreased oxygen consumption;
- low cardiac output;
- low core temperature;
- lactic acidosis.

An *anabolic phase* follows where fat and protein stores are regained and weight increases, characterised by:

- increased cardiac output;
- increased oxygen consumption;
- increased glucose production;
- lactic acid may be normal.

The state of normal homeostasis returns as the triggers resolve and the body returns to its normal metabolic balance (Orthoteers 2004a).

The form of the metabolic response depends chiefly on the degree of trauma suffered. Other contributing factors include the influence of drugs, sepsis, underlying systemic disease, the underlying nutritional state and the efficacy of the medical interventions. Although the metabolic response is protective, it can become harmful if excessive or prolonged. The aim of medical interventions is to revive body systems, control pain and temperature, and provide acceptable fluid and nutrition.

Factors starting the metabolic response

The factors that start the metabolic response include hypovolaemia, factors exuded by the wound, hormonal responses, sepsis and the inflammatory response.

Hypovolaemia is common in major surgery but the body's own response and the early use of fluid replacement therapy may significantly reduce the metabolic response. Pain and anxiety can also initiate a hormonal response but this can be adjusted by analgesia so that a metabolic response is not stimulated.

Tissue injury activates two specific responses, inflammatory (humoral) and cellular. Products of these responses play a role in organ dysfunction. For example, the inflammatory mediators of injury have been implicated in membrane dysfunction, leading to various conditions affecting every organ of the body.

The inflammatory response is a complex collection of reactions involving macrophages, polymorphonuclear leucocytes and phagocytic cells such as neutrophils and eosinophils. Normal phagocytosis (engulfing of foreign bodies by phagocytes) is one of the primary activations of the metabolic response. This results in responses such as neutrophil aggregation, and secretion of histamine and serotonin, which may increase vascular permeability and vasodilation. A combination of these reactions results in the inflammatory response.

The action and release of adrenaline, noradrenaline, cortisol and glucagon are increased, while other hormones are decreased during trauma. The hypothalamus has a major role in coordinating the stress response through endocrine actions by the pituitary and the sympathetic and parasympathetic nervous systems. The pituitary gland responds to trauma by increasing adrenocorticotrophic hormone (ACTH), prolactin and growth hormone levels.

Pain receptors, osmoreceptors, baroreceptors and chemoreceptors stimulate the hypothalamus to induce sympathetic nerve activity. Stimulus of the pain receptors results in the secretion of endogenous opiates, which adapt the response to pain.

Hypotension, hypovolaemia and hyponatraemia stimulate the anterior pituitary to secrete ACTH. ACTH stimulates the secretion of antidiuretic hormone (ADH) from the anterior hypothalamus, aldosterone from the adrenal cortex, and renin from the juxtaglomerular apparatus of the kidney. This has the overall effect of increasing water reabsorbtion and thereby increasing blood volume.

Reactions to changes in glucose concentration include the release of insulin from the cells of the pancreas, while high amino acid levels stimulate the release of glucagon from the pancreatic cells.

Result of the metabolic response

The stress of major surgery can lead to the initiation of the metabolic response. Many of the interventions carried out on the perioperative patient are aimed at moderating the metabolic response, which if untreated may rapidly prove fatal.

As can be seen from the above, the metabolic response results in systemic inflammatory responses which increase the activity of the cardiovascular system, reflected as tachycardia, widened pulse pressure and a greater cardiac output. As metabolic rate increases, there is an increase in oxygen consumption, increased protein catabolism and hyperglycaemia.

The resting energy expenditure can rise to more than 20% above normal, if the patient is well enough to respond. In an inadequate response, oxygen consumption may fall and endotoxins and anoxia may injure cells and limit their ability to utilise oxygen. Cellular injury, impaired hepatic gluconeogenesis and lack of oxygen may result in rapid deterioration of processes requiring energy. As a result of the inefficient energy-making process lactate is produced, causing a severe metabolic acidosis.

The oliguria, which often follows major surgery, is a consequence of the release of ADH and aldosterone. As well as promoting the reabsorption of water, aldosterone also releases large quantities of intracellular potassium into the extracellular fluid, possibly causing a significant rise in serum potassium especially if renal function is impaired. Retention of sodium and bicarbonate may contribute to metabolic alkalosis with impairment of the delivery of oxygen to the tissues.

Critically ill postoperative patients may develop a glucose intolerance which resembles that found in pregnancy and in diabetic patients. This is as a result of both increased mobilisation and decreased uptake of glucose by the tissues. The turnover of glucose is increased and the serum glucose is higher than normal.

The glucose level following surgery should therefore be carefully monitored since hyperglycaemia may exacerbate ventilatory insufficiency and may provoke an osmotic diuresis. The optimum blood glucose level is between 4 and 10 mmol/litre. Control of blood glucose is best achieved by titration with intravenous insulin, based on a sliding scale. However, because of the degree of insulin resistance associated with trauma, the quantities required may be considerably higher than normal.

The principal source of energy following trauma is adipose tissue and as much as 200–500 g of fat may be broken down daily after major surgery. High levels of ketones are produced as free fatty acids are broken down to provide energy. Because of the possible problems with glucose metabolism, nutritional support of traumatised patients requires a mixture of fat and carbohydrate.

The intake of protein by a healthy adult is between 80 and 120 g of protein, or around 1–2 g protein/kg/day. Lack of protein intake leads to the breakdown of skeletal muscle in order to produce essential amino acids. After major surgery, or with sepsis, as much as 20 g/day of urea nitrogen from protein breakdown may be excreted in the urine. A severely ill patient may lose over 600 g of muscle mass per day, leading to marked muscle wasting. Depletion of amino acids also results in atrophy of the intestinal mucosa and failure of the mucosal antibacterial barrier. This may lead to systemic infection and multisystem failure after severe trauma. This is normally fatal in patients who lose more than 40% of body protein because of failing immunocompetence. The protein intake can be improved dramatically by parenteral or enteral feeding, as long as adequate liver function is present.

Survival after trauma such as surgery depends on a balance between the extent of cellular damage, the efficacy of the metabolic response and the effectiveness of supporting treatment. Hypovolaemia is a major initiating trigger for the metabolic sequence, therefore, adequate fluid resuscitation to shut off the hypovolaemic stimulus is important during and following surgery. Fear and pain, tissue injury, hypoxia and toxins from infection add to the initiating factor of hypovolaemia and so it is important that these are also moderated by perioperative interventions in order to reduce the metabolic response.

Patient support during perioperative care should be aimed at reducing the factors triggering the metabolic response. During surgery, important aspects of patient care include adequate fluid volume, maintenance of oxygen delivery to the tissues, careful handling of tissues and removal of pus or devitalised tissue, combined with control of infection, respiratory and nutritional support to aid defence mechanisms.

Wound healing

Wound healing is the process of tissue repair. It involves the interaction of epithelial, endothelial and inflammatory cells, platelets and fibroblasts which are activated and act together in order to repair the damaged tissue. The overall process can be divided into the three overlapping phases of inflammation, proliferation and maturation (Figure 1.18) (Orthoteers 2004b).

Inflammatory phase (day 0–5)

Tissue healing follows essentially the same process regardless of the tissue involved or the type of injury sustained, although healing times and the duration of each phase depend on a variety of factors such as health of the individual, nutritional status, mode of injury, tissue type, blood supply, moisturisation and so on.

The healing response is initiated from the moment that the surgical incision is made. Blood filling the wound interacts with collagen and leads to platelet degranulation and activation of

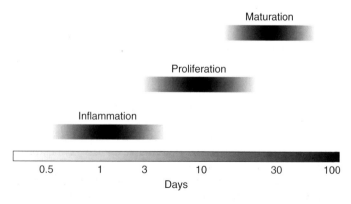

Fig. 1.18 Phases of wound repair: inflammation, proliferation and maturation.

Hageman factor (factor XII). This factor in turn sets into motion the clotting cascade, which serves to bind the wound and also alerts the systemic system to a local injury.

Kinins and prostaglandins produced by the process cause local vasodilatation and oedema and are responsible for the pain and swelling which occurs after injury. Leucocytes enter the wound site shortly after injury and their numbers increase steadily, peaking at 24–48 hours. Their main function appears to be phagocytosis of the bacteria that have been introduced into the wound during injury.

The next cells to enter the wound are macrophages, which are derived from circulating monocytes. They first appear within 48–96 hours post-injury and persist in the wound until healing is complete. T lymphocytes appear around the fifth day post-injury, peaking about 7 days after injury. The presence and activation of both macrophages and lymphocytes in the wound is critical to the progress of the normal healing process because they phagocytose and digest pathological organisms and tissue debris. Macrophages, platelets and lymphocytes also release growth hormone and other biologically active substances known collectively as cytokines. Cytokines are small proteins released by cells that communicate with, and affect the behaviour of, other cells. In the context of wound repair, they initiate and support granulation tissue formation.

Proliferative phase (day 3–14)

The proliferative phase of healing commences once the wound has been successfully cleared of devitalised and unwanted material. This phase is characterised by the formation of granulation tissue in the wound. Granulation tissue consists of a combination of cellular elements, including fibroblasts and inflammatory cells, along with new capillaries embedded in a loose extracellular matrix of collagen, fibronectin and hyaluronic acid. In a process of fibroblast proliferation and synthetic activity known as fibroplasia, fibroblasts are induced to proliferate and are attracted into the wound by cytokines. Fibroblasts are responsible for tissue reconstruction through the production of structural proteins, in particular the glycoprotein collagen, which forms the main constituent of the wound matrix and which imparts tensile strength to the scar. The collagen forms into an organised matrix along the wound's stress lines.

Wound revascularisation also occurs at this time. In response to a variety of local mediators, capillary buds sprout from venules, form capillary loops, connect to the bloodstream and then join together to form a capillary plexus.

Re-epithelialisation of the wound surface begins within a couple of hours of the injury. Epithelial cells from the periphery of the wound begin to migrate under the scab and over the underlying viable connective tissue, filling the wound. Once the defect is bridged the migrating epithelial cells proliferate through mitosis and the surface layer eventually becomes keratinised. Re-epithelialisation is normally complete in less than 48 hours in approximated surgical wounds, but will take longer in larger wounds where there is tissue loss. Epithelialisation can also take place in the absence of fibroplasia and granulation tissue formation in wounds (such as skin graft donor sites) where only the epithelium is damaged. Again, the mediators for re-epithelialisation include a variety cytokines and other local cellular products.

Maturation phase (day 7 to 1 year)

Almost as soon as the extracellular matrix is laid down it becomes cross-linked and aggregated into fibrillar bundles, which gradually provide the healing tissue with increasing stiffness and tensile strength through collagen fibrogenesis. The wound develops 20% of its final strength after 3 weeks, with the maximum breaking strength of the scar reaching 70% of that of the intact skin.

This gradual gain in tensile strength is due not only to continuing collagen deposition, but also to collagen remodelling. Collagen synthesis and catabolism leads to the formation of larger collagen bundles and increased crosslinking. As this occurs, a thin pale scar is formed from collagen which is relatively avascular and acellular.

Wounds healed by primary intention are those which require minimal granulisation tissue and minimal loss of wound volume. Large and complex wounds, associated with significant tissue loss, heal by secondary intention. Granulation tissue gradually fills the defect and epithelialisation proceeds slowly from the wound edges. The wound area starts to contract rapidly through the inward movement of the uninjured skin edges caused by an interaction between fibroblast locomotion and collagen reorganisation. The result of the healing process is a scar that helps to restore tissue continuity, strength and function.

REFERENCES

Astiz, M.E., Rackow, E.C. & Weil, M.H. (1993) Pathophysiology and treatment of circulatory shock. *Critical Care Clinics* **9** (2), 183–203.

Bellman, L. & Manley, K. (2000) *Surgical Nursing Advancing Practice.* Churchill Livingstone, Edinburgh.

Clancy, J., McVicar, A.J. & Baird, N. (2002) *Perioperative Practice: Fundamentals of Homeostasis.* Routledge, London.

Eberly College of Science (2004) *The Respiratory System.* www.bio.psu.edu/Courses/Fall2002/Biol142/respiratory/respiratory.html Accessed: 8 June 2004.

Hatfield, A. & Tronson, M. (1998) *The Complete Recovery Book.* Oxford University Press, New York.

Jevon, P. & Ewens, B. (eds) (2002) *Monitoring the Critically Ill Patient.* Blackwell Science, Oxford.

Orthoteers (2004a) Metabolic Response to Trauma. www.orthoteers.co.uk/Nrujp~ij33lm/Orthtraumametab.htm Accessed: 1 June 2004.

Orthoteers (2004b) Wound healing. www.orthoteers.co.uk/Nrujp~ij33lm/Orthwound.htm Accessed: 1 June 2004.

Saladin, K.S. (2001) *Anatomy and Physiology: The Unity of Form And Function.* William C Brown, New York.

Sheppard, M. (2000) Monitoring fluid balance in critically ill patients. *Nursing Times* **96** (21), 39–40.

Soni, N. & Welch, J. (1996) *Invasive Haemodynamic Monitoring.* Ohmeda, Hatfield.

Tortora, G.J. & Grabowski, S.R. (1996) *Principles of Anatomy and Physiology,* 8th edn. Addison Wesley Longman, New York.

University of Pennsylvania (2004) *Critical Care Medicine Tutorials: Cardiovascular System.* www.ccmtutorials.com/cvs/index.htm Accessed: 27 May 2004.

Watson, R. & Fawcett, T.N. (2003) *Pathophysiology, Homeostasis and Nursing.* Routledge, London.

2 | Managing Perioperative Equipment

LEARNING OUTCOMES
❏ Understand the principles underlying the *safe use of equipment* in the operating room.
❏ Understand the principles of the *efficient checking of perioperative equipment* before and after use.
❏ Understand the *use and preparation of anaesthetic and surgical equipment*.
❏ Describe the *measures to be taken if equipment is faulty*.
❏ Discuss the *need for infection control* and the implications of not undertaking such measures.

INTRODUCTION
Surgical equipment is expensive and represents a major investment for the NHS. Surgical procedures have become more complicated and intricate and, as a result, equipment has become more technical, more precise in design and more delicate in structure. Misuse, inadequate cleaning and rough handling can cause damage, reduce life expectancy and produce safety risks due to malfunction.

Perioperative practitioners need to keep up-to-date with the continually changing technology and legislation to ensure their professional competence and accountability in their perioperative practice. It is essential that they have the knowledge and an understanding of the use of operating room equipment. It is the responsibility of the perioperative team to ensure the availability of all relevant equipment, to check it before use and to ensure that it is in full working order for the surgical procedures.

Competent use of equipment is an important part of risk management. Practitioners should continuously monitor the operating room for potential hazards to patients during surgical procedures.

DUTIES OF THE EMPLOYER

The legislation identified in the Health & Safety at Work Etc. Act 1974, places a duty on the employer to maintain a working environment for employees that is as safe as reasonably practicable. This duty extends to incorporate the working environment, equipment and safe working practices, as well as education, training and supervision (NATN 2004).

In addition, hospitals also develop their own policies and procedures for equipment use, safety and training, which are reviewed and revised as necessary. Perioperative practitioners need to know the location of the local policies in their department so they have easy access to them for reference.

The operating department manager has a responsibility to set up a planned maintenance programme agreed between the operating room department and the electrical and biomedical department (EBME). Training and regular updates on equipment use are essential and the operating room manager must keep documentation of attendance as proof in case of an inquiry following an incident. The EBME marks all operating room equipment and they undertake annual equipment audits in liaison with the operating room manager.

DUTIES OF THE EMPLOYEE

Local policies govern the use and safety of the operating room equipment for the perioperative practitioners. They should be familiar with all operating room equipment, its use and potential hazards, to ensure a safe environment for patients and members of the perioperative team. Practitioners check all equipment before an operating list, identify any faults and follow the proper local procedures to ensure effective maintenance and/or repair of the faulty item.

Standards are set at an operational level for safe use of equipment and must relate to the manufacturer's guidelines (NATN 2004). Instructions for assembly, use, cleaning, moving and storing the equipment may be written in procedures or may be referenced to a manufacturer's manual (Gruendemann & Fernsebner 1995).

Practitioners should not operate any item of equipment without instruction or knowledge of its use, as this could be dangerous for the practitioner, other perioperative personnel and especially to the patient.

Before an operating list

Before an operating list it is vital that the perioperative team checks all the equipment and formalises this check by signing a checklist as illustrated in Box 2.1.

NATN (2004) identify that the standards for the provision and use of electrical equipment within the perioperative setting should comply within the recommendations of the Medical Devices Agency Code of Practice (1997). Equipment should therefore:

- be checked by the approved designated personnel on delivery and before use;
- be used in accordance with manufacturer's recommendations;
- only be used by the employee who has been instructed in the use and setting up of that equipment;
- have a planned preventive maintenance programme including a regular maintenance contract.

Ensure that all on loan or trial electrical equipment has a current certificate of indemnity and checks are carried out before its use.

Box 2.1   Procedure before an operating list

- Select the correct equipment and accessories according to the needs of the operating list and the patients' individual needs.
- Identify promptly any faults or malfunctioning equipment, take it out of use and report the fault to the relevant personnel or the EBME department. Do not return it to the operating room theatre until it is repaired and ready for use.
- Calibrate equipment in line with the manufacturer's instructions.
- Monitor equipment while in use according to the manufacturer's instructions.

ANAESTHETIC EQUIPMENT

The anaesthetic machine

Anaesthetists must have a sound understanding and knowledge of all anaesthetic equipment in common use (Aitkenhead & Smith 1996). All anaesthetic practitioners need to have an understanding of the principles of use of the anaesthetic machine, its components, how to troubleshoot any problems and report faults in line with local policies.

The anaesthetic machine is checked before use by the anaesthetic practitioner to maintain patient safety. They should follow the local protocol using the guidelines described by the Association of Anaesthetists of Great Britain and Ireland, (AAGBI 2004), and the manufacturer. The misuse and failure of the machine can have serious consequences for the patient. A typical anaesthetic machine is illustrated in Figure 2.1.

The components of an anaesthetic machine are:

- gas supply: via pipeline or cylinder supply;
- pressure regulators;
- oxygen pressure failure devices;
- flow control valves and flowmeters;
- scavenger systems;
- vaporisers;
- ventilators;
- oxygen analysers;
- suction.

Gas supply

The gas supply of an anaesthetic machine consists of a pipeline or cylinder source. The anaesthetic practitioner checks both types of gas supply before each operating session.

The common units of pressure used in the operating room environment are:

- bar pressure (bar);
- kilopascals (kPa);
- pounds per square inch (psi);
- pounds per square inch gauge (psig) (this is the pressure above atmospheric pressure).

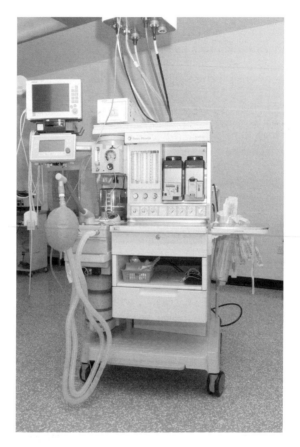

Fig. 2.1 Anaesthetic machine.

Their relationship is illustrated below:

- 1 bar = 14.5 pounds per square inch (psi);
- 1 bar = 100 kilopascals (kPa) (SI unit).

As a rule of thumb 1000 psi approximately equals 70 bar and 100 bar equals 1450 psi (Meyer 1998).

Pipeline

Hospital stores supply medical gases from a central store via pipelines or by large cylinders or tanks. The gases are delivered to specific ports located in the wall or from the ceiling, via a boom in the operating and anaesthetic rooms (Figure 2.2). Non-interchangeable spring-loaded valves are inserted into the wall ports and connect to the anaesthetic machine via flexible non-crushable tubing. The pipes are colour coded and are bonded to the valve. The pressure in the anaesthetic gas pipeline is 4 bar

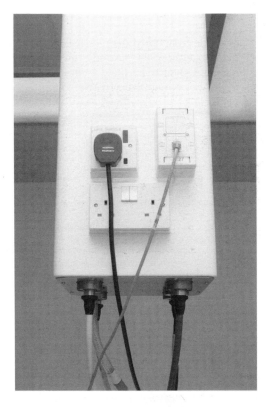

Fig. 2.2 Gas pipelines attached to an anaesthetic boom.

(400 kPa) and is the same as the working pressure of the anaesthetic machine.

While the nitrous oxide and medical air lines directly connect with the flowmeters, the oxygen line passes via pressure-failure devices, the oxygen flush valve and the ventilator power outlet. If oxygen pressure falls below 25 psig (roughly 50% of normal) a fail-safe valve automatically closes the nitrous oxide flow and other gas lines to prevent accidental delivery of a hypoxic mixture to the patient. In this event the oxygen gas alarm sounds (Morgan & Mikhail 1996). Safety checks are illustrated in Box 2.2 and pipeline details are summarised in Table 2.1.

Cylinders

Cylinders are made from molybdenum steel, are colour coded (same as pipelines) and consist of a body and a shoulder which contains threads into which are fitted a pin-index valve block, a bull-nosed valve or a hand-wheel valve. The pin index is to ensure correct installation and interchangeability of gas cylin-

---

Box 2.2   Safety checks for pipeline gas supply

- Check all pipeline connections.
- Perform the Westminster tug test to ensure connections are secure. Take care because the high-pressure of the gas from the boom can cause the pipeline to disconnect at speed.
- Check the pressure of gas (400 kPa) on the front of the anaesthetic machine.
- Check the individual gas bobbins rotate on the anaesthetic machine with gas flow and they do not stick throughout the range.
- Check the nitrous oxide flow falls before the oxygen flow (on disconnection of the oxygen pipe) to prevent a hypoxic mixture occurring.
- Check the oxygen alarm sounds to identify no flow of oxygen gas.

Table 2.1   Pipeline colours and gas pressures.

Gas	Pipe colour	Gas pressure
Oxygen	White	400 kPa
Nitrous oxide	Blue	400 kPa
Medical air	Black	400 kPa
Suction vacuum	Yellow	53 kPa

Box 2.3   Safety checks for cylinder gas supply

- Ensure correct installation of the cylinders. Open and close the cylinders slowly to prevent a surge of gas pressure and damage to the machine.
- Check for any leaks from the cylinders, check the Bodok seal and change if necessary.
- If the gas cylinder registers as empty or almost empty, change it before the beginning of the operating list.
- Turn off cylinders when not in use.
- Check that individual bobbins are rotating with gas flow, will rotate throughout the range and do not stick.
- Check that the nitrous oxide flow falls before the oxygen flow to prevent hypoxic mixture being delivered to the patient.
- Check the oxygen alarm sounds to identify no flow of oxygen gas.
- To prevent slippage or accidents such as burns, do not use hand cream before handling cylinders.

Table 2.2   Cylinder colours and gas pressures.

Gas	Body	Shoulder	Pressure
Oxygen	Black	White	137 bar
Nitrous oxide	Blue	Blue	44 bar
Medical air	Grey	White & black	137 bar

ders. The washer at the pin index is called a Bodok seal and its function is to prevent leakage. The anaesthetic practitioner or operating room support worker should change the seal if it shows signs of wear or damage.

Full cylinders are supplied with dust covers and they should be stored separately from empty cylinders in the relevant store cupboard. The anaesthetic practitioner or operating room support worker should take care when they change any gas cylinder. They should ensure that they close the cylinder valve before disconnection from the machine. Safety checks are outlined in Box 2.3 and cylinder details are summarised in Table 2.2. Figure 2.3 shows anaesthetic gas cylinders.

Pressure regulators
Pressure regulators have two important functions:

- they reduce high pressures of compressed gases to manageable levels acting thus as pressure-reducing valves;

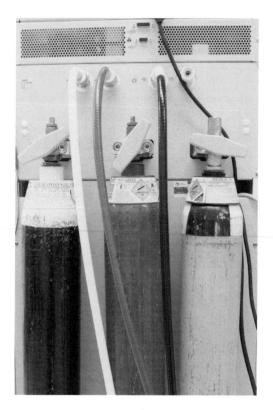

Fig. 2.3 Anaesthetic gas cylinders. Left to right: oxygen (black), nitrous oxide (blue), medical air (grey).

- they minimise fluctuations in the pressure within an anaesthetic machine, which would otherwise necessitate frequent manipulations of flowmeter controls (Aitkenhead & Smith 1996).

Piped gases are delivered to the anaesthetic machine at pressures of between 45 and 50 psig through the pin-index system. The high pressure in the gas cylinder makes the flow difficult and dangerous and the pressure regulator ensures a safe delivery of gas to the patient at a pressure of less than 50 psig.

Oxygen pressure failure devices

The nitrous oxide and medical air gas flows connect directly with the flowmeters but the oxygen gas flow passes via the pressure-failure devices, the oxygen flush device and the ventilator power outlet.

If oxygen gas (piped or cylinder) fails, a fail-safe valve automatically closes off the nitrous oxide flow and prevents the patient receiving an hypoxic mixture of gas. An alarm should sound to alert the anaesthetist or anaesthetic practitioner of this event. Anaesthetic practitioners should check the alarm works before the operating list begins. The anaesthetist can give emergency oxygen by pressing or pushing the oxygen flush valve. The oxygen flush provides a high flow of oxygen to the patient direct from the common gas outlet.

Flow control valves and flowmeters

Gas flows from the anaesthetic machine to the patient through a breathing system. When the anaesthetist switches on the gas flow controls (e.g.: oxygen, nitrous oxide, medical air) by turning them anti-clockwise, the gas flows through the valve and the bobbin turns, indicating that the gas is on. The ball or bobbin rises or falls depending on the level of gas delivered to the patient.

Scavenger systems

The scavenging system removes waste gases from the operating room environment by a system of valves and tubing and a pump. This is essential for the well-being of the members of the operating room team. Anaesthetic practitioners should check that they have connected all attachments into the boom in the operating room and into the fitting in the wall of the anaesthetic room. The valve attaches to the expiratory valve of the breathing system or the ventilator (in the anaesthetic room or operating room). Safety checks to be carried out are summarised in Box 2.4.

Box 2.4   safety checks for the scavenging system

- Check the security and fitting of attachments.
- Check the tubing is not too long or the resistance will be high and it can become a safety issue for the perioperative team.

The anaesthetic machine supports the control of the patient's inspired gas mixture and gas exchange.

Vaporisers

A vaporiser is a device for adding clinically useful concentrations of anaesthetic vapour to a stream of carrier gas. The saturated vapour pressure of volatile anaesthetic agents at room temperature is many times greater than that required to produce anaesthesia, and so a vaporiser mixes gas passing through a vaporising chamber with gas containing no vapour to produce a final mixture with the appropriate concentration (Davis *et al.* 1995).

There are two types of vaporiser. In one type (drawover) the anaesthetic agent is vaporised by the negative pressure generated by the patient's respiratory effort and in the other type (plenum) the positive pressure of the gas supply is used to vaporise the anaesthetic agent.

In a drawover vaporiser the gas is pulled through the vaporiser when the patient inspires, creating a subatmospheric pressure. In a plenum vaporiser the gas is forced through the vaporiser by the pressure of the gas supply (Aitkenhead & Smith 1996).

There are different types of vaporising agent and each type has its own vaporiser and filling outlet to prevent incorrect filling with the wrong agent. The vaporising agents (coloured bottles) are stored away from the light to prevent breakdown of the consistency of the agent. There may be one, two, three or more vaporisers on the anaesthetic machine but the anaesthetist will only use one vaporiser at a time. Each vaporiser fits onto the back bar of the anaesthetic machine and will not lock onto this bar if not fitted properly. The back bar incorporates a safety interlock mechanism to prevent simultaneous use of agents (Morton 1997). A checklist for vaporisers is given in Box 2.5.

Properties and side effects of vaporising agents are discussed in Chapter 3. A vaporiser is illustrated in Figure 2.4.

Ventilators

The goals of ventilation are to deliver oxygen to the alveoli and to remove carbon dioxide. Ventilators collect gas and the

---

> **Box 2.5   Checklist for vaporisers**
>
> • Check the security and fitting of individual vaporisers. Remove and refit if the vaporiser is not seated properly.
> • Ensure there is sufficient anaesthetic agent within each vaporiser (up to the indicated line for full).
> • Check only one vaporiser will turn on at a time.
> • Check that gas flowmeter moves when the vaporiser is switched on.
> • Check for leaks within the breathing circuit.

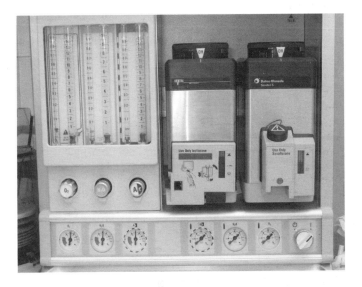

Fig. 2.4   Anaesthetic gas vaporiser.

vaporising agent into a bag or bellows and deliver these to the patient's lungs. They create a pressure gradient between the proximal airway and the alveoli and there are four phases during the ventilation cycle:

• inspiration;
• the transition from inspiration and expiration;
• expiration;
• the transition from expiration to inspiration.

Anaesthetists may use different ventilators in conjunction with the insertion of an endotracheal (ET) tube and the rapid sequence induction procedure. These are described in Chapter 8. Ventilators can be of two types – mechanical and power driven. Anaesthetic practitioners should familiarise themselves with the different types of ventilator and their checking procedures.

A mechanical ventilator applies the gas or agent mixture at an intermittent positive pressure to the airway to overcome the elastic resistance of the lungs and chest wall and the frictional airways resistance (Illingworth & Simpson 1994). The gases are pneumatically driven into a bag or a bellows and are compressed. The bellows takes the place of the breathing bag used in spontaneous breathing.

The power source of power driven ventilators can be either compressed gas, electricity or both.

The possible hazards with ventilators are:

- no available alarm;
- disconnection of electricity or tubing can occur;
- failure of oxygen gas supply and delivery of ventilation.

Before anaesthesia, and at any appropriate time during anaesthesia, the anaesthetic practitioner must check all aspects of the ventilator to prevent occurrence of these hazards. These checks are outlined in Box 2.6.

Box 2.6   Checklist for ventilators

- Check the efficient working of the ventilator before the operating list.
- Check the correct configuration as per the local anaesthetic checklist.
- Check the attachment of the breathing bag to the ventilator tubing and check that the ventilator works efficiently on the set configuration.
- Check all connections, leak test and ventilator alarm.
- During ventilation of the patient:
  — Observe the colour of the patient, chest movements and bellow movements or sound of the ventilator.
  — Observe the waveform of end-tidal carbon dioxide on the monitor.

Total intravenous anaesthesia (TIVA)

TIVA can be used both with patients who are breathing spontaneously and those who are being ventilated. The anaesthetist uses syringe pumps and an anaesthetic drug (propofol) in conjunction with an opiate (remifentanil) to ensure anaesthesia. No volatile agents or nitrous oxide are used with this technique. TIVA equipment is illustrated in Figure 2.5.

Syringe pumps use a driver that pushes the preferred drug out of the syringe (50 ml) by advancing its plunger while the barrel is kept stationary.

The important features of the syringe pump are:

- a bolus facility which gives the ability to increase quickly the plasma concentration;
- flow rate – the pump should be able to function accurately on small flows of gas (oxygen or oxygen and medical air);
- battery – there should be an indication of the status of the battery;
- tight syringe fitting – the syringe plunger must fit securely in the clamp.

(Yuill & Simpson 2002).

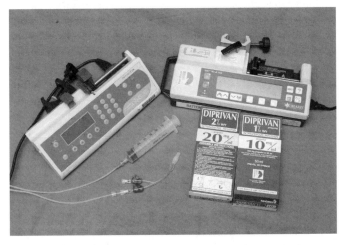

Fig. 2.5 TIVA equipment.

Box 2.7 TIVA checklist

- Locate the appropriate syringe pumps, drug infusion set (propofol) and accessories (connecting tubing and a Y-connector) to deliver the induction agent and opiate through the venous cannula.
- Attach the syringe pumps to a drip stand and plug them in.
- Give the anaesthetist the opiate and record it in the controlled drugs book.
- Have other propofol infusion sets available for a long surgical procedure.
- Ensure that vaporisers are filled in case the anaesthetist changes from TIVA to an inhalational anaesthesia technique.
- After use syringe pumps should be plugged in to ensure that they are charged up and ready to use again.

The role of the anaesthetic practitioner in TIVA is illustrated in Box 2.7.

Oxygen analyser

The anaesthetist uses an oxygen analyser to ensure that the patient receives a correct concentration of oxygen. There is 21% of oxygen in the air and the anaesthetic practitioner checks and calibrates the oxygen analyser before each operating list to ensure it has the correct setting. For instructions on how to calibrate the analyser for 21% and 100% see Box 2.8b, page 66.

Suction

A pipeline vacuum suction is available with the anaesthetic machine. It is controlled by an on and off switch and it usually has a medium and a high setting. Operating support workers or anaesthetic practitioners insert new disposable linings into the suction machine for each patient. Relevant suction catheters are used for the patients.

Checking the anaesthetic machine

The checking procedure for the anaesthetic machine covers all aspects of the anaesthetic delivery system including the gas supply pipelines, machine, breathing systems (filters, connectors and airway devices), ventilators, suction monitoring and ancillary equipment (AAGBI 2004). This is outlined in Box 2.8a and b.

Box 2.8a   Anaesthetist's check list for the anaesthetic machine (AAGBI guidelines)

- The anaesthetic machine is connected to the electricity supply and switched on.
- All monitoring devices, oxygen analyser, pulse oximeter and capnograph are functioning and have appropriate alarm limits.
- Gas sampling lines are attached and free from obstructions.
- An appropriate frequency of recording of blood pressure is selected.
- Correct insertion of pipeline gases and perform Westminster tug test for all gases.
- The anaesthetic machine is connected to a supply of oxygen and there is an oxygen cylinder with an adequate supply fitted to the back of the machine.
- All pipeline gas pressure gauges indicate 400–500 kPa.
- Operation of flowmeters.
- Each flow operates smoothly and bobbins move freely throughout the range.
- The anti-hypoxic device is working correctly.
- The emergency oxygen bypass control.
- Vaporisers are fitted correctly, filled and leak tested.
- Breathing circuit, leak test and patency of flow of gas.
- Face mask, filter and catheter mount are available.
- Ventilator tubing is securely attached, leak tested and works efficiently on set configuration and alarms are set.
- Alternative ventilation means is available (breathing circuit and oxygen cylinder).
- Scavenging tubing is attached to appropriate exhaust port of the breathing system, ventilator or workstation and is in set limits.
- Ancillary equipment is available (intubation equipment as described Chapter 8, page 249).
- Recording of the anaesthetic machine check by anaesthetic team.

(AAGBI 2004).

Box 2.8b   Anaesthetic practitioner's check list for the anaesthetic machine (Pennine Acute NHS Hospitals Trust guidelines)

- Observes the machine for damage and that the mains cable is plugged in.
- Checks that all accessories are present.
- Presses the drain button if appropriate.
- Disconnects all pipeline supplies and turns off any fitted gas cylinders.
- Ensures all flow controls are off (fully clockwise).
- Opens slowly the oxygen cylinder valve. Checks amount of oxygen in the cylinder.

Cont.

Box 2.8b *Continued.*

- Closes the oxygen cylinder valve and observes the gauge. The gauge must not fall by more than 690 kPa (100 psi) in one minute.
- Repeat for air and nitrous oxide cylinders.
- Drain all cylinders.
- Check there is a 'No oxygen pressure' audible alarm
- Change cylinders if necessary.
- Full cylinders:

  Oxygen – 2175 psi, nitrous oxide – 725 psi, medical air – 1450 psi.

- Plug in all pipeline gases.
- Ensure each gauge registers approximately 400 kPa.
- Perform the Westminster tug test.
- Ensure the scavenging system is connected and efficient.
- Remove the oxygen sensor from the circuit.
- Calibrate the cell to 21%. This will take up to 3 minutes.
- Once calibrated refit the oxygen cell to the circuit.
- Once a month calibrate the cell to 100%.
- After fitting the cell flow 5 litres of oxygen through the system.
- Calibrate to 100%

Negative leak test

- Switch off the machine.
- Turn all controls to 1.5 turns anti-clockwise.
- Switch on auxiliary common gas outlet (ACGO).
- Test the leak device to the ACGO by squeezing the bulb and blocking the end off (the bulb should stay collapsed).
- Fit the test device to the ACGO and squeeze the hand bulb several times until the bulb collapses.
- If the bulb reinflates within 30 seconds there is a leak on the anaesthetic machine.
- Initially the gas flow bobbins will rise.
- The bulb should not inflate within 30 seconds.
- Turn one vaporiser on initially to 0%.
- Re-squeeze the bulb several times until the bulb collapses. Ensure the bulb does not reinflate.
- Repeat this with any other vaporiser.
- Ensure that only one vaporiser can be turned on at one time.
- Remove the hand bulb from the ACGO and turn the flow controls off.
- Return the ACGO to the off position.

Breathing system leak tests

- Occlude the patient breathing circuit at the end remembering to remove any filters or gas sampling lines.
- Switch the bag/vent switch on the absorber to vent mode.

Box 2.8b *Continued.*

- Use the oxygen flush to fill the bellows.
- Turn on the machine and switch the vent to bag mode.
- The bellows should not fall by more than 100 ml in 30 seconds.
- While in bag mode turn the adjustable pressure limiting (APL) valve to 30 cmH$_2$O.
- Ensure a 2-litre bag is connected to the side arm.
- While pressing the flush button observe the pressure guage dial to ensure that it reads approximately 30 cmH$_2$O. ($\pm$5% i.e 28.5–31.5 cmH$_2$O).
- Release the flush button.
- Following an initial drop in pressure ensure the dial stabilises at a pressure of approximately 30 cmH$_2$O ($\pm$5% i.e 28.5–31.5 cmH$_2$O).
- Check the 2-litre bag for any leaks.
- Open the APL valve to ensure that it is not sticking.

Hypoxic guard test

- Use the oxygen analyser for this test.
- Turn all controls fully clockwise and observe the flows:

  oxygen – 25–75 ml, nitrous oxide – zero, medical air – zero.

- Adjust the nitrous oxide flow from 900 ml, 1.5 litres, 3 litres, 6 litres and 9 litres and the oxygen flow from 300 ml, 500 ml, 1 litre, 2 litres and 3 litres.

  The oxygen analyser percentage should stay within 21–30% to ensure there is no hypoxic flow.

Oxygen failure test

- Turn all the gas flows to mid range. Disconnect the oxygen pipeline and ensure the following:
  — An oxygen failure alarm appears on the ventilator.
  — Nitrous oxide and oxygen flows stop. The small oxygen bobbin must reach the bottom of the flow tube after the nitrous oxide bobbin. The medical air will still flow.
- Reconnect the oxygen and all flows should reinstate themselves.
- Turn off the medical air and nitrous oxide controls (fully clockwise).

Vaporiser back pressure test

- Turn the oxygen flow to 6 litres.
- Slowly turn the first vaporiser to 1%.
- The oxygen flow should not drop by more than 1 litre.
- Repeat for each vaporiser fitted.

Ventilator operation

- Connect a re-breathe bag to the patient circuit.
- Set the ventilator to the required settings.

Cont.

Box 2.8b *Continued.*

- Switch to mechanical ventilation.
- Press the oxygen flush button to completely fill the bellows.
- The ventilator should reach within 10% of the set readings within seven cycles.
- Check the absorber valves are working.
- Turn off the ventilator flow controls.

Suction

- Ensure the suction is connected and working efficiently.

Auxiliary oxygen meter

- Check the bobbin flows throughout the range.

ANAESTHETIC MONITORING EQUIPMENT

During anaesthesia the anaesthetic team observes the patient and monitors his or her physiological status throughout the perioperative stage and throughout transfer to the intensive care ward or to another hospital. They document the recordings on the patient's anaesthetic record and the care plan. See Chapter 8 (page 278) for an example of the anaesthetic record of the care plan. Anaesthetic practitioners should attach all monitoring devices before the commencement of anaesthesia and record the first physiological readings on the patient's care plan.

During the establishment and maintenance of anaesthesia the patient's physiological state, depth of anaesthesia and functioning of the equipment need continual assessment. To achieve this, monitoring devices are used to supplement clinical observation.

The anaesthetist observes:

- mucosal colour;
- pupil size;
- response to surgical stimuli;
- movement of the chest wall.

The anaesthetist can also undertake palpation of the pulse, auscultation of breath sounds and, if appropriate, measurement of urine and blood loss.

The anaesthetist observes physiological monitoring (AAGBI 2004):

- pulse oximetry;
- non-invasive blood pressure;
- electrocardiography;
- capnography;
- vapour analyser;
- temperature

Monitoring devices

For all monitoring devices the anaesthetic team set appropriate parameters before use and these include:

- cycling times;
- frequency of recordings;
- alarm settings.

Pulse oximetry

The pulse oximeter measures the oxygen saturation of the patient's blood. The pulse oximeter probe is attached to the patient's finger, toe or ear. The probe contains a light source and, when it is attached to a monitor, the patient's oxygen saturation percentage is displayed as a light absorption trace and a reading on the monitoring machine. It is non-invasive and easy to apply.

The functioning of pulsoximetry is based on the absorption of light and the ratio of oxyhaemoglobin to deoxyhaemoglobin. As both forms of haemoglobin are present within a sample of blood the saturation may be calculated by measuring the absorption at two different wavelengths (Aitkenhead & Smith 1996).

The anaesthetic practitioner should check the probe, during a long anaesthetic or with patients who have impaired circulation, to identify any pressure on the probe site and should change the probe site if necessary. Details of any pressure should be documented on the patient's care plan and the appropriate operating personnel informed.

Non-invasive blood pressure measurement

The anaesthetic practitioner attaches the appropriate size of blood pressure cuff to the patient. The cuff is usually fitted to the dominant arm of the patient, unless the identified surgery is on that arm. In this circumstance the anaesthetist should be asked for their preference and the cuff may be positioned on the leg instead.

The tubing is attached to the monitor and the blood pressure reading will be displayed on the monitor. The cuff inflates and deflates, the machine detects arterial wall motion and calculates systolic, mean and diastolic pressures. Most machines have a trend setting where the anaesthetic team can read blood pressure readings from the first reading until disconnection from the monitor machine.

Electrocardiograph (ECG)
The anaesthetic practitioner attaches the ECG electrodes to the patient before the induction of anaesthesia. The leads are attached to the monitor and the ECG reading is displayed on the monitoring machine. See Chapter 1 (pages 18–24) for discussion of these physiological readings.

Capnography
A capnograph measures end-tidal carbon dioxide and this helps the anaesthetist to confirm correct placement of the ET tube and ventilation. The anaesthetic practitioner should check correct attachment of the gas sampling lines and that they are free from obstruction or kinks before the start of the operating list and between surgical procedures if necessary. The carbon dioxide gas sampling line connects to the distal end of the breathing circuit or ventilator tubing and the other end attaches to the monitoring machine. Carbon dioxide absorbs infra-red light. The amount of carbon dioxide present is given by the absorption reading on the monitor as a waveform. The shape of this waveform determines the level of expired carbon dioxide.

Capnography provides indications of:

- correct placement of the laryngeal mask airway (LMA) or ET tube if the patient is breathing and has a circulation.

Fall in end-tidal carbon dioxide indicates:

- disconnection of the breathing circuit or ventilator tubing;
- leaks from the breathing circuit during spontaneous ventilation;
- hypotension (fall in end-tidal carbon dioxide).

Rise in end-tidal carbon dioxide indicates:

- re-breathing of the patient during ventilation;
- malignant hyperthermia.

Vapour analyser

The anaesthetist monitors the amounts of vaporising agent during anaesthesia. The vapour analyser measures the concentration of vapour over a range of gas flows and identifies the type of vaporising agent and displays the percentage on the monitoring machine.

Temperature

It is important to monitor the patient's temperature during long surgical procedures, where warming devices are being used and if the patient has a low temperature before surgery. General anaesthesia inhibits the patient's ability to maintain body temperature by depressing the thermoregulatory centre in the hypothalamus (Aitkenhead & Smith 1996).

The patient's temperature can alter with:

- a lengthy surgical procedure;
- exposure of abdominal contents during surgery;
- use of wet packs or washout during the surgical procedure.

The perioperative team has a responsibility to ensure that the temperature of the operating room is optimal for the surgical procedure. The anaesthetic practitioners prepare an intravenous infusion by attaching a blood coil to the warming machine and attaching one end to the infusion and the other to an extension tube and three-way tap; if relevant for the anaesthetic and patient's medical condition.

A warming blanket can be used to warm the patient during the surgical procedure. These come in various designs including:

- upper body;
- surgical access;
- dual-port torso;
- full body surgical.

Box 2.9   Monitoring the patient

- Be aware of the patient's base readings of the physiological observations from the ward.
- Be familiar with all equipment.
- Check monitoring machine and accessories before the commencement of anaesthesia.
- Set parameters to correct settings.
- Ensure all alarms work efficiently.
- Report any faults to appropriate personnel, locate and check replacements if necessary.
- Obtain printouts from the machine for the anaesthetist if necessary.
- Clean devices and accessories following local policies.
- Document recordings of physiological readings on the patient's care plan.
- Have all available monitoring for transfers.

The anaesthetic practitioner hands a nasopharynx temperature probe to the anaesthetist to measure the patient's temperature during the surgical procedure. The end of the probe is attached to the monitor and a reading of the patient's temperature will be displayed on the monitor.

Neuromuscular block

If the patient has been given a muscle relaxant, the anaesthetic practitioner should have a nerve stimulator available for the anaesthetist to identify muscle relaxation and paralysis. A nerve stimulator can identify the depth of the neuromuscular blockade and the amount of reversal drug required.

The role of the anaesthetic practitioner during the monitoring of the patient is summarised in Box 2.9. Monitoring equipment is illustrated in Figure 2.6.

SURGICAL EQUIPMENT

Electrosurgery (diathermy)

One of the most commonly used items of equipment within the operating room is the electrosurgery machine. Electrosurgery is a technique providing both coagulation and cutting effects by application of a high frequency alternating electric current to the tissue. Two methods of electrosurgery are commonly used in the operating room environment: these are monopolar and bipolar

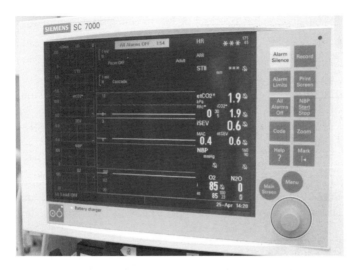

Fig. 2.6 Monitoring equipment.

electrosurgery. The method of completion of the electrical circuit is the fundamental difference between them.

Monopolar electrosurgery

Monopolar circuitry current originates in the generator, flows through the active electrode and into the patient. It is then recaptured by the return electrode (also called dispersive or patient electrode) attached to the patient's body, and finally channelled back into the generator. The patient forms the major part of the electrical circuit. An active cable from the electrical surgical unit carries current to the monopolar electrode.

The innate resistance of the tissues to the flow of current causes a rise in temperature. This resistance is related, in part, to the area of tissue involved and the power of the current. This high temperature is used to control haemorrhage by coagulation (desiccation or fulguration) or to cut the tissues by cell disruption. The relatively large surface of the return electrode results in a lower current density than is present at the active electrode, so ensuring the rise in temperature of the tissues at this point is kept to as minimum (NATN 2004).

The surgeon has two foot pedals to control the electrosurgical machine and these are colour-coded as follows:

- blue for coagulation;
- yellow for cutting.

The safety checklist for monopolar electrosurgery use is summarised in Box 2.10.

The electrosurgical machine and accessories are illustrated in Figure 2.7.

Patient return electrode positions

The preferred return electrode positions are buttock, posterior thigh, anterior thigh, mid back, lower back, upper calf and abdomen. These are illustrated in Figure 2.8.

Box 2.10   Checklist for monopolar electrosurgery use

- Check equipment for any damage or loose connections (including of electric plugs and wiring). The alarm sounds if the theatre support worker does not attach all connections into the machine or patient.
- Use the correct position of the electrosurgical patient pad for the surgical procedure.
- The patient's skin should be dry, clean and free of excess hair before applying the return electrode.
- Do not place patient return electrode over bony or scarred tissue or near metal implants. It should be as close to the operative site as is practical and should remain dry throughout surgery.
- Ensure the patient's skin is not in contact with any metal (for example operating table or supports).
- Adjust electrosurgical settings according to local policy or surgeon's preference. Alter if necessary.

The circulating practitioner will:

- Inform the scrub practitioner of the electrosurgical settings.
- Place the correct electrosurgical foot pedal or pedals in position (next to the surgeon's feet) before commencement of the surgery.
- Record pad position and state of skin after removal.

The scrub practitioner will:

- Ensure the surgeon is aware of the electrosurgical settings before they begin the surgery.
- Place the active electrosurgical handle in an insulated quiver when it is not in use to avoid any burns to the patient.

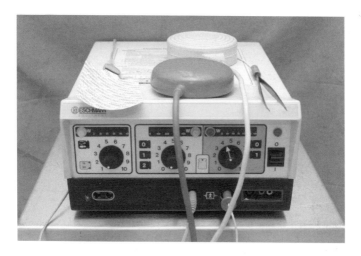

Fig. 2.7 Monopolar machine.

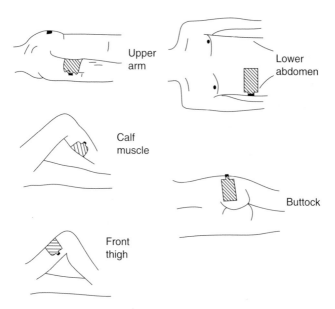

Upper arm

Lower abdomen

Calf muscle

Buttock

Front thigh

Fig. 2.8 Positions for the return electrode. (Continued on next page.)

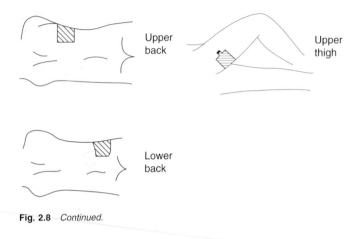

Fig. 2.8 *Continued.*

Bipolar electrosurgery

A bipolar machine has both the active and return electrodes in the one instrument. The current originates in the generator and flows down one tine of the forceps through the tissue between the forceps and back to the generator through the other tine of the forceps. Current does not flow through the patient, since it is contained within the wound, travelling between the tines of the forceps. Therefore a return electrode attached to the patient is not necessary. The machine and accessories are illustrated in Figure 2.9 and the safety checks are summarised in Box 2.11.

Considerations before the use of electrosurgery

- Ask surgeons which type of electrosurgery they will use during the surgical procedure but have all appropriate choices available.
- Communication between the scrub practitioner, the surgeon and the anaesthetist needs to be at its optimum to avoid any hazards.
- Always check the machine and attachments and identify any faulty equipment. If necessary remove it from the operating room and ask the EBME Department to check it before reuse.

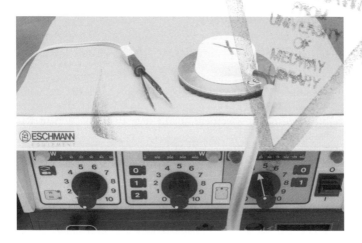

Fig. 2.9 Bipolar machine and accessories.

Box 2.11 Checklist for bipolar electrosugery use

• Check equipment for any damage or loose connections (inclusive of electric plugs and wiring). An alarm sounds if the connections are not correctly attached.

• Never switch on the machine before attaching all relevant leads and accessories.
• During laparoscopic surgery be aware of other laparoscopic instruments (clamps or clip applicator) during electrosurgery.
• Use a scratch card to clean off any debris during the surgical procedure to ensure efficiency of the electrosurgery electrode.
• Wash pedals, machine and accessories if relevant at the end of each surgical procedure and at the end of the operating list following local policy.
• Inform the anaesthetist and surgeon if the patient has a pacemaker.

Hazards of electrosurgery

Burns
Burns may occur with:

- poor contact of electrosurgical pad;
- pooling of fluids (when the surgeon prepares the patient's skin);
- breakage of the electrical circuit (e.g. disconnection of the leads or pad);
- patient contact with metal (operating table).

Electrocution
Undertake regular safety checks of wiring and plugs, according to health and safety requirements, to avoid electrocution of staff or patient.

Interference with medical equipment
- Cardiac pacemakers can interfere with monitors and video equipment.
- The anaesthetic practitioner should always inform the anaesthetist and surgeon if the patient has a pacemaker. The surgeon can use bipolar electrosurgery in this case.

Smoke inhalation of electrosurgical plume
Laser and electrosurgical devices used during surgery produce smoky emissions that may contain vapours and particulate aerosols that can have a chemical and biological impact on those exposed (Scott *et al*. 2004). These hazards and implications for perioperative staff are discussed in Chapter 5 (page 183).

Suction

Suction equipment is used during surgical procedures for removal of blood or tissue fluids from the surgical field to improve visibility (Figure 2.10). This can be achieved either by use of a portable machine or via piped access.

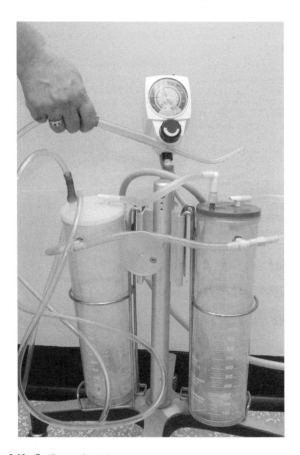

Fig. 2.10 Suction equipment.

A suitable style tip and suction tubing are used dependent on the surgery and the surgeon's preference. A Yankauer attachment is most commonly used in anaesthetics (adult and paediatric) and a Wheeler or Yankauer suction for surgery. Suction use in the recovery area is discussed in Chapter 10 (page 348). The issues to consider in suction use are summarised in Box 2.12.

Box 2.12   Issues that the practitioner should consider in the use of suction

- Use suction tubing that has an acceptable circumference to avoid blockage or collapse.
- Select the correct pressure during suction. Advise surgeons, if relevant, of the pressure and let them see the gauge and suction pressure during surgery (gynaecological surgery).
- Use a relevant filter with the suction unit.
- Use a disposable suction lining and the operating room support worker will dispose of it following local policy and standard precautions.

Pulse lavage

Surgeons can use pulse lavage which is a powered suction irrigation system. It can be used simultaneously to irrigate the wound and to remove blood and tissue fluids. The pulse switch can be used intermittently or continuously according to preference.

The surgeon can regulate the flow of irrigation and suction by controls on the disposable tip assembly. Members of the surgical team should wear masks with visors for their own safety. The machine and accessories are illustrated in Figure 2.11.

Laser

The use of laser technology in different surgical specialities and techniques decreases bloodloss, reduces operative time, post-operative complications and pain, and aids wound healing. The development of medical lasers has revolutionised surgery.

There are many types of laser and the members of the perioperative team have to consider each laser as they require different operational techniques. They will need consideration of their various features and associated hazards. It is essential that perioperative practitioners adhere to local policies and recommendations at all times (NATN 2004).

Laser is an acronym for 'light amplification by the stimulated emission of radiation' (Shields & Werder 2002). A laser is a device in which the atoms, molecules or ions in a crystal, a gas or a liquid dye, when stimulated by light, chemicals, gases, or electrical energy, emit a narrow, intense beam of energy (light). Laser light differs from ordinary light in that it is coherent, the

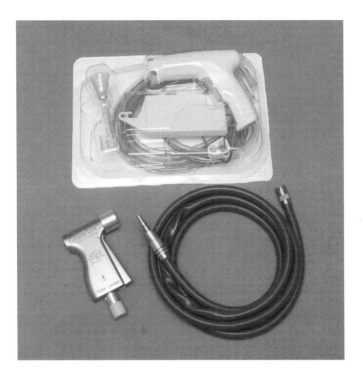

Fig. 2.11 Pulse lavage.

waves are synchronised in time and space, monochromatic (of a single colour or size) and collimated (unidirectional and non-divergent) (Gruendemann & Fernsebner 1995).

A laser beam is created by stimulating photons inside a resonating chamber. As the photons bounce back and forth, they gain energy, which is emitted through the delivery system, producing a laser beam that can be used to cut or coagulate tissue.

The components of a laser include:

- A medium to produce a laser effect of the stimulated emission. Gases, solid rods or crystals, liquid dyes and free electrons are used. Each produces a different wavelength, colour and effect.

- A power source to create population inversion by pumping energy into the lasing medium. This may be electrical, radiofrequency or an optical power.
- An amplification mechanism to change random directional movement of stimulated emissions to a parallel direction. The power density of the beam determines the laser's capacity to cut, coagulate or vaporise tissue.
- Wave guides to aim and control the direction of the laser beam.
- Backstops to stop the laser beam from penetrating beyond the expected impact site and affecting non-targeted tissue (Fortunato 2000).

There are two different types of system:

- Pulsed laser – emits its energy in short, repeating emissions that have a short duration.
- Continuous wave – produces continuous light when activated by the perioperative practitioner.

The parts of the each laser system are the same and have a combination of length, level and output of radiation emitted when operated. Power density, the irradiance is the amount of power per unit surface area during use. Power density is defined as watts per centimetre squared. The most commonly used lasers in the operating room are the carbon dioxide laser and the ND:YAG laser.

The carbon dioxide laser
The carbon dioxide laser uses molecules of carbon dioxide as the medium and may be used in many surgical specialities such as gynaecology, neurosurgery, plastic, general, and ear, nose and throat surgery. It has the ability to cut and coagulate tissues and it is used with the pulsed or continuous systems.

Different wavelengths and frequencies of the laser beam are used for cutting or coagulation of the tissue. The laser is operated through an endoscope or directly onto the tissue and different sized pieces of tissue can be removed. The beam of this laser is precise and therefore only diseased tissue is selected, which allows for decreased postoperative pain and a faster recovery.

The carbon dioxide wavelength is readily absorbed by water and, as the body's cells are 75–90% water, the carbon dioxide beam is absorbed rapidly at the surface of the tissues. The surface temperature increases and as the water temperature increases it vaporises tissue. Vaporisation is the conversion of solid tissue to smoke and gas – the plume produced should be evacuated or suctioned through a filter device for safety reasons. As the beam is so accurate the thermal effect on the surrounding tissue is minimal.

The holmium:neodymium-doped yttrium aluminium garnet (ND:YAG) laser

The laser light comes from a crystal containing the metal holmium. The surgeon can use the laser to cut tissue or coagulate blood vessels. The laser beam delivery can be through a hollow needle or through an optical fibre via an endoscope, either continuously (steady beam) or on pulse mode (emits short emissions of light) and it can be used in urological, orthopaedic, or ear, nose and throat surgery. Vaporisation occurs resulting in the removal of the tissue in a plume of vapour. The surgeon selects the laser wavelength, pulse mode and power for the procedure and the laser operator controls these.

Developments in the use of laser within the operating room have introduced extra responsibilities for the perioperative practitioner. Perioperative practitioners need to address these responsibilities, in conjunction with the EBME and risk management department, when preparing local policies and consider the potential hazards associated with lasers and the general standards to protect patients and staff. The general rules for laser use are summarised in Box 2.13.

Hazards of laser use

Eye injuries

Eye injuries can occur with accidental eye exposure during alignment of the laser beam as part of the checking procedure or during use; because of lack of eye protection or because of

---

Box 2.13 General rules for laser use

- One or more operating rooms are designated for the use of the laser.
- Store laser equipment in a locked cupboard and only allow designated personnel to have access.
- Laser warning signs or lights indicate that the laser is in use in the operating room environment (operating room and anaesthetic room doors).
- Windows in operating room door covers have opaque glass to avoid inadvertent eye injuries.
- All perioperative personnel are aware of the fire and safety procedures to be adopted during laser use.
- Keep perioperative team to a minimum during use of the laser.
- All members of the perioperative team should be aware of the fire and safety procedures during laser use.
- Ensure all perioperative personnel and the patient wear eye protection.
- In head and neck surgery the anaesthetic practitioner will cover the patient's eyes and face before surgery.
- Prevent plume inhalation by wearing relevant face masks.
- Use portable or piped suction to evacuate plume.

The laser operator undertakes the following safety checks:

- Tests the laser machine and accessories before use.
- Ensures that the laser is always on stand-by mode until required.
- Does not enable the laser unless it is directed towards the treatment site or a beam stop.
- Switches the machine off and withdraws the key from the machine if laser is not in use.
- Completes all relevant documentation.
  — The name of the laser operator.
  — Type of laser used, the use of wattage and the number of joules.
- Reports any incident to the appropriate personnel.
- The surgeon uses instruments with diffuse reflecting surfaces rather than those that give specular reflection.

---

problems with equipment. Improper handling owing to unfamiliarity with equipment and improper restoration of equipment following service can also cause possible eye injuries.

Laser light can strike the cornea of the eye causing vaporisation and possible destruction of the outer layer and it can destroy the retina (NATN 2004). The eye is most vulnerable to injury from the laser beam. The injury depends on the power and wavelength of the beam. It can be caused by a break in the laser fibre or the reflection of energy from the beam. The approved laser operator ensures all members of the periopera-

tive team wear eye protection throughout the surgical procedure when the laser machine is in use. Practitioners should
check their glasses before use to ensure that they are not faulty.
Glasses or moistened eye pads can protect the patient's eyes.

Skin preparation solutions

Surgeons should use aqueous prepping solutions and avoid
pooling of these fluids in the prepping procedure of the patient.
Alcoholic solutions are not used because of the fire hazards
associated with these solutions. The laser beam could possibly
heat the volatile fluid and ignite it.

Burns

Burns can be caused by direct or indirect emission of the laser
beam. Eye and skin burns are caused by the laser beam shining
on the body. The laser operator, surgeon and anaesthetist need
to be alert to any potential problem and take the relevant action
to reduce the possibility of any burns occurring. Surgical instruments should have a non-reflective surface and be blackened for
visible laser radiation to reduce the potential risk of reflection
of the laser beam (NATN 2004).

Fire hazard

All members of the perioperative team must observe their local
fire policy if the laser beam accidentally causes a burn and
ultimately a fire.

Laser plume

It is possible that the laser plume may be a potential risk to staff
(NATN 2004). Non-beam hazards are associated with laser
equipment. The hazardous substances are released from the
equipment and are emitted from materials exposed to laser
plumes produced during surgical procedures. The same
hazards as with electrosurgery use apply to the laser machine.
The use of smoke evacuators and efficient face masks can
minimise these hazards.

Electrical hazards

Specialised laser electrical outlets are used within identified
operating rooms for laser machines. The practitioner checks the

machine and all attachments before their use. Suitable action should be taken if any faults are identified in the pre-use check.

The legislation identified in the Health & Safety Etc. Act 1974, places a duty on the employers to maintain a working environment for employees that is as safe as is reasonably practicable. This duty extends to incorporate the environment, safe equipment, safe systems of work as well as providing necessary education, training and supervision to ensure safe working practices (NATN 2004).

TV & Camera

A visual display unit (VDU) is used to monitor and provide the primary source of information on the surgical procedure. The surgeon gathers anatomical information (state of the organs, position of blood vessels) visually by inspecting the surgical operative site via a camera which is attached to the end of a laparoscope. Surgeons are dependent on this technology for accurate visualisations of the operative field and need an efficient system that will provide the information.

A laparoscopic camera is a special lightweight attachment that fixes to the eyepiece of the laparoscope and it is able to pick up a video image of whatever the surgeon can see through the laparoscope. A cable sends the video signal to a video processing unit – an electronic box that converts the signals into a picture that the surgeon sees on a VDU. A halogen or a high performance xenon light with a fibre-optic cable transmits the light source to the telescope, which has a special attachment point for the light cable.

How to get the best from your camera system (Keymed 2005)

Laparoscopes are precision optical instruments – to ensure clear images, always check the lenses at either end of the laparoscope are clean. Most of the problems of poor illumination will be from the light cables and or cables. A camera magnifies any loss in image quality.

Examine all the light guide cables before use as any deterioration of light output will affect the overall image quality. Always consider the light cable as being an integral part of the

---

> **Box 2.14   White balance test**
>
> - With the system fully functional, wrap a clean swab around the distal end of the laparoscope, ensure it forms a cone or funnel, or use the 'white balance cap' that accompanies the system.
> - When the laparoscope is 'looking' into the funnel of white, activate the white balance function. Do not remove the swab until the white balancing process is complete.
> - A message will appear on the monitor to tell you the procedure is successful.
> (Keymed, 2005)

'system'. The quality of the image is only as good as the weakest link in the chain.

White balance
This is one of the most important functions on the camera. White balancing calibrates the camera to the colour white and it is from this baseline that it reproduces all other colours. The check for the white balance test is summarised in Box 2.14.

Laparoscopy
Laparoscopy is a surgical technique in which the abdominal cavity is distended through a medium (carbon dioxide or nitrous oxide). Carbon dioxide is usually the gas of choice used in this procedure. The surgeon inserts a laparoscope through a tiny incision just below the umbilicus into the abdominal cavity.

The laparoscope has a light source at the end and a camera that allows the surgical team to observe the contents of the abdomen under magnification and in great detail on VDUs. Video laparoscopy was introduced in the late 1970s and early 1980s.

To improve visualisation of the peritoneal cavity and ease instrument manipulation during laparoscopy the abdominal cavity is filled with an insufflating gas producing a pneumoperitoneum. This gas helps to keep the walls of the abdomen and the organs separated from each other and allows excellent exposure.

The scrub practitioner attaches gas tubing to the laparoscope and the other end attached to an insufflator machine. The gas inflates and distends the abdominal cavity (belly) through a trocar and gas tubing.

An insufflator is a machine for inflating the body cavity with the gas of choice. It delivers gas at a desired rate and measures the absolute pressure generated within the body cavity being filled. Laparoscopic insufflators are pressure-limiting gas flow regulators that make it easy to establish and maintain a pneumoperitoneum. The source of gas is a high-pressure cylinder and the pressure is stepped down by the insufflator.

Electronic insufflators are programmable and maintain an accurate intra-abdominal pressure and have warning signs and alarms. The insufflator maintains the intra-abdominal pressure at a constant pre-set level. Thus the surgeon will normally perform the procedure without having to monitor constantly the pressures and volumes.

If the gas pressure drops below the pre-set level needed to keep the body cavity inflated, then extra gas flow is necessary to re-inflate the body cavity. This requires direct operation of the insufflator by the operating room support worker on the surgeon's instructions.

An added problem is that loss of pressure often occurs slowly (e.g. via a slow leak in the skin incision). The surgeon may only realise the problem when there is a loss of vision or a loss of space restricting instrument manipulation. The scrub practitioner or surgeon will ask the operating room support worker to increase the gas flow and surgery will restart when the pressure in the abdominal cavity is re-established.

Carbon dioxide is readily absorbed, non-toxic and does not support combustion. The only serious risk is that of hypercarbia, which only develops at an absorption rate of greater than 100 ml a minute. Therefore the anaesthetist usually ventilates the patient during surgery.

The surgeon can make one to three additional incisions, 5–10 mm in length, close to the pubic bone to insert long thin instruments. These instruments are essentially extensions of the surgeon's hands and allow the surgeon to use these instruments from outside the body and perform surgery inside the abdominal cavity. Throughout the surgical procedure the surgical team need to regulate the flow of gas from the insufflator.

Within the last 10 years it has become obvious the perioperative team should use filters for the foreign gases going into the body. The filters will stop bodily fluids accidentally flowing back through the tube and into the insufflator. Insufflators are expensive units and they are difficult to clean and recondition if they become contaminated.

The roles of the scrub practitioner and operating room support worker during a laparoscopy procedure are summarised in Box 2.15.

An orthopaedic scrub practitioner and the operating room support worker will prepare for an arthroscopy procedure in a similar way as described for the laparoscopy procedure.

Infection control

Efficient cleaning of equipment should be undertaken by anaesthetic practitioners to maximise high levels of infection control. Standard precautions need to be undertaken to ensure patient

---

Box 2.15 Role of the scrub practitioner and operating room support worker during a laparoscopy procedure

Scrub practitioner
- Check and prepare all laparoscopy instruments.
- Ensure all trocar ports are closed before procedure commences.
- Pass gas tubing, light cable, suction tubing and electrosurgical cable to the operating room support worker to attach to relevant machines.
- Monitor gas flow settings during surgery and amount used.
- Ensure a filter is used with the suction machine.
- Prepare irrigation fluid and check it is flowing efficiently.
- Undertake white balance test.
- Prepare clips for clip applicator for surgeon.
- Have a bag available for gall bladder retrieval.

Operating room support worker
- Check insufflator, electrosurgery machine and TV monitors.
- Check gas pressures of insufflator machine.
- Check carbon dioxide flow and replace cylinder if empty.
- Check TV monitors for clarity of picture.
- Attach all connections from scrub practitioner and ensure all settings are correct.
- Alter settings if required by surgeon.

and staff safety. Hand washing is very important in this process and in the prevention of MRSA. Infection control and MRSA are discussed in further detail in Chapter 5.

REFERENCES

Association of Anaesthetists of Great Britain and Ireland (2004) *Checking for Anaesthetic Equipment.* AAGBI, London.

Aitkenhead, A.R. & Smith G. (1996) *Textbook of Anaesthesia.* Churchill Livingstone, Edinburgh.

Davis, P., Parbrook, G.D. & Kenny, G.N.C. (1995) *Basic Physics and Measurement in Anaesthesia,* 4th edn. Butterworth-Heinmann, Oxford.

Fortunato, R. (2000) *Operating Room Technique.* Mosby, St Louis.

Gruendemann, B.J. & Fernsebner, B. (1995) *Comprehensive Perioperative Nursing.* Jones & Bartlett, Massachusetts.

Health and Safety at Work Etc. Act (1974) HMSO London.

Illingworth, K.A. & Simpson, K.H. (1994) *Anaesthesia and Analgesia in Emergency Medicine.* Oxford University Press, New York.

Keymed Ltd (2005) *How to Get the Best Out of Your Camera System.* Keymed, Southend.

Medical Devices Agency (1997) *Code of Practice for the Safe Use of Electrical Equipment.* MDA, London.

Meyer, V.R. (1998) *Practical High Performance Liquid Chromatography,* 3rd edn. Wiley, Chichester.

Morgan, G.E. & Mikhail, M.S. (1996) *Clinical Anaesthesiology.* McGraw-Hill, New York.

Morton, N.S. (1997) *Assisting the Anaesthetist.* Oxford University Press, Oxford.

National Association of Theatre Nurses (2004) *Principles of Safe Practice in the Perioperative Environment.* NATN, Harrogate.

Shields, L. & Werder, H. (2002) *Perioperative Nursing.* Greenwich Medical Media, London.

Scott, E., Beswick, A. & Wakefield, K. (2004) Hazards of diathermy plume. *British Journal of Perioperative Nursing* **14** (9), 409–14 (part 1); **14** (10), 452–6 (part 2).

Yuill, G. & Simpson, M. (2002) An introduction to total intravenous anaesthesia. *British Journal of Anaesthesia* **2** (1), 24–9.

Perioperative Pharmacology

3

LEARNING OUTCOMES

❏ Understand the *principles of pharmacokinetics* and *pharmacodynamics*.

❏ Discuss the *routes of drug administration*.

❏ Describe the *actions of* some of the *important perioperative drugs*.

PRINCIPLES OF PHARMACOLOGY

Drug errors account for much of the litigation against the NHS. The reasons for this are obvious – the factors involved in drug administration are complex and the margins for error usually small. A minute quantity of a drug could also have a great effect on the body. Therefore, the slightest error in calculation of dosage, route of administration or wrong choice of preparation can have a fatal effect on the patient.

There are several common problems with drug administration. For example, an error in a prescription might result in the practitioner giving the wrong dose. Alteration of the distribution or elimination of the drug may cause complications in a patient with a particular condition. Failure to anticipate the side effects of drugs can lead to many unwanted results. It is possible to give the wrong drug, especially in emergency situations where mistakes can easily occur if the practitioner does not follow strict protocols. It is even possible to cause nerve damage because of wrongly sited injections. Casualties litter the fields of drug administration, so it is imperative to encourage good practice during early training into post-registration practice.

Most accidents happen because of human error. Legislation aims to reduce drug errors and increase patient safety. The main Acts involving drug use within the perioperative field include:

- the Medicines Act 1968, as amended, which regulates the manufacture, distribution, import, export, sale and supply of medical products;
- the Misuse of Drugs Act 1971, which controls the availability of drugs liable to misuse;
- the Misuse of Drugs Regulations 2001, which enables named health care professionals to possess, supply, prescribe and administer controlled drugs in the scope of their practice.

The introduction of a whole raft of government guidelines has improved drug safety. The purpose of good drugs management is to try to reduce the risk of human error and to maintain a high standard of practice. The National Prescribing Centre explored this issue and published guidelines in response to the high cost of drugs-related litigation, and the human suffering caused by drug errors (National Prescribing Centre and National Primary Care Research and Development Centre 2002). The NHS Executive (2002) also published comprehensive guidelines for managing drugs under their *Controls Assurance Standards*. While these provided useful advice, on the whole users found the Standards to be too prescriptive and complex. Therefore, from August 2004 the important elements of the standards have been incorporated into the *Standards for Better Health* (DOH 2004). This document encourages NHS organisations to bring together good risk-management practice linked to continuous quality improvement and improved patient care.

Trust drug policies, which are the mainstay of error prevention and patient safety, should incorporate and support these government guidelines, directives and legislation. Often these policies act at two levels – a Trust-wide policy and a local implementation of this policy. A good evidence-based drugs policy should contain sections on topics such as ordering, receipt and storage of drugs; procedures for administration of drugs; emergency procedures (such as cardiac arrest); and management of controlled drugs.

Safe practice during drug administration

Practitioners must know which drug to give, the quantity, when to give it and the route of administration. A suitably qualified person, in a perioperative setting normally a surgeon or anaesthetist, achieves this with a prescription. It is also becoming more common practice for suitably qualified practitioners to order drugs as required. Prescriptions are most often used outside the hospital, within the perioperative setting drugs are usually ordered either verbally or with the anaesthetic chart. The chart records the administration of the drugs. The use of the anaesthetic chart to order drugs during the postoperative period is also common practice. It is therefore essential for the practitioner to be familiar with its use as a tool for recording and administering drugs.

Accuracy in drug administration is always the mainstay of safety. The practitioner should read drug labels at least three times – before removing the drug from the shelf, before opening the container and before giving to the patient. Most institutions have a protocol for administering drugs; however, different rules often apply to the operating department. For example, it is normal practice in wards for two qualified practitioners to check drugs, however, in the operating department often only the anaesthetist will give a drug, without checking the drug with a colleague. Similarly the anaesthetist may sometimes order a drug verbally, or prepare a drug for use, but be unable to administer it. For example, during induction of anaesthesia, the anaesthetist must maintain the patient's airway and may not be able to free a hand to administer the drug. It is also possible for a member of circulating staff to prepare a drug for use by the operating team during surgery. It is therefore important to identify working policies that identify the normal scope of practice, minimum safe practice and allow the effective working of the perioperative team. This will involve developing safe working practices in areas such as:

- preparation of drugs before the operating list;
- preparation of drugs by one professional for administration by another professional;
- identification of routes of accountability for drug administration;
- defining the scope of roles for practitioners in drug administration;

- identifying the knowledge required – for example, actions, uses, side effects or dosage.

PHARMACOKINETICS AND PHARMACODYNAMICS

Pharmacokinetics is the study of how the body manages the absorption, distribution, metabolism and excretion of drugs. Pharmacodynamics is the study of the actions and effects which the drugs have on the body.

Pharmacokinetics

Absorption

The route of administration of the drug can affect the rate of absorption – this is known as bioavailability. The intravenous route gives the highest possible bioavailability of 100%. For example, an intravenous dosage of a drug will be much more quickly available to the body than a subcutaneous or oral dosage. Hence the use of intravenous analgesia throughout all areas of the operating department, where it is often preferential to use rapid-acting analgesia.

Distribution

Following absorption, drugs distribute themselves throughout the tissue of the body in various quantities. For example, a lipid-soluble drug may quickly leave the circulation and be absorbed by fat cells where it would become inactive towards its intended target. All drugs eventually leave the bloodstream and therefore patients need repeated doses to maintain a therapeutic level. The term used to describe the dose of drug required to maintain this therapeutic level is the 'maintenance dose'.

Metabolism and excretion

To maintain homeostasis, the body immediately starts to eliminate the drug from the bloodstream. It carries this out by metabolising the drug in the liver or other organs such as the lungs, and then excreting it through organs such as the kidneys, lungs or skin. The half-life of the drug is the time taken to remove half the dose given. Various factors can affect elimination of drugs from the perioperative patient, including for example cardiac failure, hypovolaemia, drug interactions and hypothermia.

Pharmacodynamics

Drugs affect the body by acting on receptors either on cell membranes or within the cells themselves. Blocking or activating receptors leads to specific cellular responses which create particular effects on the system as a whole. The drug only becomes active when it reaches its therapeutic level – too little is ineffectual, too much is toxic.

The therapeutic ratio is the ratio of the therapeutic level to the toxic level – a drug with a wide therapeutic ratio is safest. Too little of a drug will not produce the desired effect. Overdose, producing drug levels outside the therapeutic level, may produce side effects or toxicity, leading to patient harm or even death. The range between these margins is called the therapeutic margin. Some drugs, for example digoxin, have a narrow therapeutic margin, while many modern drugs have a safer, wider therapeutic margin.

Paediatric considerations

Children are not small adults and this is a particular consideration when it comes to drug dosages. Calculations of drug dosages are based on body weight or surface area. Calculating paediatric drug dosages from weight is inaccurate at best, and may even be dangerous. For example, for an overweight child, calculation of the dosage by weight does not necessarily give the correct dosage. Age factors such as the maturity of the system, the relatively large surface area of children when compared with adults, and pre-existing conditions all have a relatively greater effect on drugs in children than in on adults. These factors become increasingly important with lower age groups, such as neonates. Drug calculation is therefore often based on knowledge of drug reactions, therapeutic levels, and surface area and body weight of children. Most situations require specialist advice to manage drug treatment for paediatric patients.

Body-weight considerations

Calculation of drugs dosages in adults sometimes uses 'expected lean body weight'. This is an estimate of what the patient's body weight would be if he or she were not thin or fat.

Lean body mass depends on height and build – endomorphs (light), mesomorphs (medium) or ectomorphs (large). An obese patient, for example, would fall into one of these categories, but with extra fatty tissue. Fat is usually irrelevant in relation to drug *action* since the target is not usually fat cells. Drug dosage based on expected lean body mass therefore more closely reflects the dosage of the drug required to produce the therapeutic level. Increased distribution of drugs that are lipid soluble may occur in obese patients, requiring alteration of the frequency of the drug, even though the therapeutic level remains the same.

Considerations in elderly patients

External controllers have an increased effect on the homeostasis of elderly patients. For example, the physiological responses of organs vary with advancing age for reasons such as anatomical and physiological changes, lifestyle, and concurrent diseases and conditions. Hypothermia and declining liver and renal function lessen the rate of elimination, prolonging the effect of the drugs. Elderly patients also have a relatively low water content leading to increased drug concentrations when compared with younger people. This often means that a reduced dose of drug will produce the required therapeutic level whereas a normal dosage would produce toxic effects. Potency of drugs is also often increased because elderly less well-nourished patients have lower levels of circulating plasma protein, which normally binds drugs and makes them ineffectual. Also, elderly patients are often on various drugs because of pre-existing conditions and the chance of adverse drug interactions is thus raised.

MAJOR CHANNELS OF DRUG ADMINISTRATION

Administration of drugs is often oral. Until the twentieth century, this route was the only route available for most drugs. However, it is now possible to use almost every available tissue, tract and orifice. Available routes fall into two main channels of administration – local and systemic.

Local channels of administration

Skin

Drugs can be administered via the skin by a number of routes. Painted or sprayed drugs include iodine and other antiseptics. These produce a local effect and include several solutions and lotions. The skin is also a valuable route of administration for topical local anaesthetics such as lidocaine and tetracaine (see later in this chapter). Swabbing and painting of drugs result in direct action at the point of contact with the skin. Antibacterial skin preparation solutions such as chlorhexidine and iodine solutions used preoperatively are good examples of this route of administration. Rubbing ointments (oil based), creams (water based) and liniments (fluids) onto and into the skin, results in local action, for example, on skin lesions.

Skin lesions can also be covered with plasters, poultices or moist dressings which contain substances that act locally – although systemic effects are possible following absorption of substances into the circulation.

Mucous membranes

Mucous membranes offer a versatile and rapid route for drug administration which can lead to either local or systemic effects. Inhalations include sprays or nebulae, which are fine particles of a drug in a suspension of water. An example is a local anaesthetic spray used before intubation. Inhalations are normally effective at the point of contact with mucous membranes, but may also act systemically, for example the action of glyceryl trinitrate on the heart, or the action of inhalational anaesthetics on the central nervous system. It is also possible to use drugs in a suspension of steam (water vapour).

Aerosols are fine particles suspended in air which are drawn or forced into the respiratory tract; examples include drugs such as salbutamol or formoterol.

Cavities that communicate externally, such as the vagina, rectum, eyes or bladder can be irrigated with drugs suspended in fluids. Gargles contain drugs in fluid and are useful for conditions affecting the mouth and throat. Drugs can also be dropped directly onto mucous membranes such as the eyes (eye drops) or ears. Packs or tampons can be soaked in drugs and inserted into cavities such as the nose, ears or vagina.

Systemic channels of administration

Alimentary tract

Absorption of oral drugs occurs via the mucous membrane of either the stomach or the intestines. Specially coated drugs are absorbed selectively by the intestines and act directly on the digestive tract or are absorbed into the circulation and act systemically. Longer acting drugs tend to be absorbed via the intestines whereas short acting drugs tend to be absorbed via the stomach lining. Oral drugs come in various forms including for example, powders, tablets, capsules, pills, syrups, elixirs, spirits, emulsions or mixtures.

Sublingual drugs, such as digoxin, are usually tablets which, when placed under the tongue, are absorbed directly into the bloodstream producing a rapid systemic effect.

Suppositories are drugs that are solid at room temperature but which melt at body temperature or dissolve in body fluids. They are used either rectally or vaginally and include, for example, diclofenac (Voltarol).

Parenteral routes

A parenteral route refers to all other routes of systemic administration other than the alimentary tract. Parenteral routes are usually more complex and therefore involve more training and equipment for administration. The drugs also work much more quickly and have a shorter onset of action, they could therefore need a greater degree of care during administration and are more dangerous to administer.

Subcutaneous (SC) injection

This route involves injecting drugs into the fatty layer just underneath the skin. It can allow delivery of drugs that are low volume, cannot be used by the oral route, and when a more rapid onset than is possible orally is required. Injection of the drug is through a small gauge needle, by angling the needle in a shallow angle, just penetrating the skin into the adipose layer. It is usually possible to see a small blister of the drug fluid.

Intramuscular (IM) injection

Rapid absorption and distribution of the drug occurs with IM injection because muscle has a good blood supply. Administration of large volumes of a drug is possible because of the large muscle mass when compared with adipose tissue used for SC injection. The practitioner can give IM injections in many areas of the body, the favourite sites being upper arm (deltoid), lateral anterior side of the thigh (quadriceps) and the buttocks or gluteus muscles.

The practitioner should take special precautions when injecting into the gluteus muscles because of the proximity of the sciatic nerve. The correct site of injection into the gluteus maximus is identified by dividing the buttock into quarters and injecting into the inner angle of the upper outer quadrant. Access to the gluteus minimus is from below the outer portion of the iliac crest. The practitioner places the first two fingers of the non-dominant hand along the angle of the iliac, with the fingers following the crest, and then carefully inserts the needle.

There are two common techniques for carrying out intramuscular injections. The Z technique involves sliding the skin to one side with the fingers of the non-dominant hand, inserting the needle, drawing back to make certain that it isn't in a blood-vessel, injecting the drug and then releasing the skin. This procedure ensures that fluid cannot leak out of the injection line into the surrounding subcutaneous tissue. The pinch technique has the same effect of separating the skin from the underlying tissues. This technique involves pinching the tissue between the forefingers and injecting the bunched up tissue.

Whichever technique the practitioner uses it is essential that the drug enters the muscle, not the subcutaneous tissues. Consideration should be given to aspects such as the length of needle required and the depth of injection. Changing the site of injection for subsequent injections helps to avoid excessive damage to tissue and may prevent potential drug interactions caused by mixing of drugs within the tissues.

Intraperitoneal administration

Drugs are administered directly into the peritoneal cavity. Delivery of antibiotics using this route is common during surgical procedures on the digestive tract. Absorption is quick because of the contact with large areas of mucous tissue.

Intravenous (IV) administration

This technique involves administering a drug directly into a vein. It is possible to use many veins, with the favourite sites being the crook of the elbow, the back of the hand or other veins of the forearm such as the accessory cephalic and the median anterior brachial. In difficult cases, when it is not possible to find suitable veins, cut-down access may be required for deeper veins such as branches of the femoral, popliteal or brachial veins.

For multiple injections, venflons, butterflys or other intravenous cannulae provide semi-permanent access. Learning the technique of intravenous cannulation is relatively easy, although the outcomes of improper technique can be painful, dangerous and disturbing for the patient, especially in the perioperative setting.

An intravenous infusion is the administration of a large quantity of fluid which may or may not contain drugs. For this procedure, the practitioner attaches an intravenous giving set to the intravenous cannula; for example, to combat amoebic infections using a metronidazole infusion. Drugs can also be added to electrolyte infusions such as sodium chloride 0.9%. The drug is injected into a rubber bung close to the cannula, which then seals closed. If the cannula tip leaves the vein and enters the surrounding tissue then fluid can build up in the area around the vein causing a painful localised oedema. This extravasation or 'tissuing' can be extensive and painful at times.

Other routes of parenteral drug administration include intracardial, intrapleural and drug implants (for example some long-acting contraceptives).

DRUGS USED DURING PERIOPERATIVE INTERVENTIONS

The discovery of ether in 1846 and chloroform in 1847 heralded the age of anaesthesia and with it the ability to perform ever more extensive surgical procedures on patients, without the fear of pain, sensation and awareness. Administering ever more complex and specific anaesthetic drugs achieves the triad of anaesthesia – narcosis, analgesia and relaxation.

The range of drugs used in today's perioperative interventions is huge. Each stage of the patient's perioperative experience requires the practitioner to administer drugs to produce a therapeutic effect or to support the body systems. Surgery and anaesthesia produce a huge degree of stress on the body resulting in physiological and emotional effects which, if left untreated, may result in harm to the patient (see Chapter 1). The rest of this chapter discusses some of the common drugs used in perioperative care.

Preoperative drugs

Giving drugs weeks or months before an elective procedure helps to ensure that the patient is in the best condition possible for the impending surgery.

Anti-anaemia drugs raise haemoglobin levels in blood. Preoperative anaemia is a risk because of the oxygen-carrying capacity of blood and the dangers of hypoxia and blood loss (see Chapter 1). Anti-anaemia drugs include, for example, iron, vitamin B_{12}, folic acid and liver or stomach extracts. For less extreme cases of anaemia or general malaise vitamin complexes may improve general health.

Treatment of blood disorders, such as clotting problems, helps to reduce the risks associated with haemorrhage. Vitamin K, calcium gluconate or calcium lactate improve prothrombin times. Vitamin K is fat soluble and its absorption is dependent on the liver, especially the presence of bile. Dehydrocholic acid given with Vitamin K improves absorption in patients with liver or gall bladder disease such as cholecystitis.

Patients may need prophylactic antibiotics if they are undergoing surgical procedures that carry a high risk of infection, such as abdominal or respiratory procedures. Broad-spectrum antibiotics protect the patient against a wide range of infections; however, if the procedure points to a particular infection risk, a specific antibiotic should be given.

Admission of the patient to hospital on the day before the procedure allows the administration of various drugs. These may include, for example, sedatives, antibiotics, analgesics, or intravenous infusions such as electrolytes or blood or its derivatives. The purpose of these medicines is to increase the health of the patient's body systems in preparation for surgery. Specifically, preoperative drugs may:

- allay anxiety;
- provide a measure of amnesia;
- provide analgesia;
- reduce side effects caused by stimulation of the autonomic nervous system (mainly cardiovascular effects);
- reduce risk of nausea and vomiting;
- increase pH of gastric contents;
- reduce secretion in the airways.

The anaesthetist normally orders preoperative drugs related to the surgery since he or she is responsible for preserving the patient's condition during the procedure. Administration of a barbiturate, hypnotic or sedative (for example diazepam or temazepam) in combination with a parasympathetic depressant such as atropine before or on induction of a general anaesthetic, is common practice. Analgesia may take the form of an opiate such as morphine or fentanyl. Giving an anti-emetic, such as cyclizine or prochlorperazine, helps to oppose the side effects of opioids or to reduce nausea and vomiting caused by the effects of surgery.

Parasympathetic depressants are naturally occurring alkaloids or synthetics, and include parasympatholytics and cholinergic blocking agents. The most common naturally occurring alkaloids are atropine, from the plant *Atropa belladonna*, and hyoscine, from *Hyoscyamus niger*. Both these drugs are readily soluble in water and body fluids since they are organic esters – a combination of an acid and organic base.

All parasympathetic depressants have a similar action, only varying in degree, onset or duration of action. They act by inhibiting acetylcholine action at nerve junctions and on smooth muscle which responds to acetylcholine. They dilate pupils, relax smooth muscle, decrease secretions and increase or stabilise heart rate.

In perioperative use, the decrease in oral and upper airway secretions is useful to reduce the incidence of partial obstruction of the airway and to reduce coughing on induction and reversal of the anaesthetic. Relaxing smooth muscle may aid in some surgical procedures and the extra sedative actions of hyoscine may help in producing a preoperative calming effect.

Administration of parasympathetic depressants is by most routes, although normally in the preoperative setting intramuscular or subcutaneous injections are commonest. The preoperative dosage for atropine or hyoscine is normally between 0.3 and 0.6 mg. Combination of parasympathetic depressants in one syringe with an analgesic such as morphine can reduce the number of injections required. The most common side effects of this group of drugs are dilated pupils, blurred vision and dryness of the mouth, nose and throat. Exaggerated side effects may be early signs of toxicity and may progress to symptoms such as shallow respirations, disorientation, dizziness and tachycardia. In excessive doses, the toxic effects of these drugs can result in coma followed by respiratory and cardiac failure and death.

It is important to offer an explanation for giving the preoperative drugs – to calm the patient, reduce secretions and ease induction and maintenance of anaesthesia. This may help the patient to tolerate the dryness of the mouth, and the discomfort caused by slight tachycardia or hypotension. It is important to maintain the patient's safety, especially from injury because of falling, after giving these drugs. Similarly, because of the mild confusion or dizziness, gaining consent for surgery is good practice before their administration. With proper use, these drugs are invaluable in preparing the patient for impending surgery and anaesthesia.

ANAESTHESIA

Anaesthesia is the lack of awareness of sensation either locally or systemically resulting from drug administration. General anaesthetics affect the whole body and result in unconsciousness; local anaesthetics affect regions of the body while the patient remains conscious. Under many circumstances, anaesthesia uses a combination of the two approaches.

Anaesthesia therefore involves the use of drugs to induce the desired effects of the anaesthetic and to maintain or promote the health of the patient while protecting the body from the side effects of the anaesthetic or surgery. The most common drugs can be conveniently divided into three groups:

- drugs used during general anaesthesia;
- drugs used during local anaesthesia;
- drugs used to support body systems.

DRUGS USED DURING GENERAL ANAESTHESIA

Although general anaesthetic agents remain poorly understood, it appears that patients go through four stages of anaesthesia – analgesia, excitement, surgical anaesthesia and overdose. See Chapter 8 for a description of these stages.

On completion of surgery, the anaesthetist reverses the anaesthetic by progressively reducing the administration of drugs and allowing the patient to regain consciousness. The stages of anaesthesia reverse until the patient returns to their normal state of consciousness, which can occur either within minutes for light anaesthesia or many hours later for deep anaesthesia. Administration of reversal agents can block the effects of some of the anaesthetic drugs and speed up the reversal. Reversal agents include: parasympathetic depressants which help to stabilise pulse and blood pressure; neostigmine which reverses the effects of non-depolarising muscle relaxants; and opiate antagonists which combat the side effects of opiates.

Oxygen and nitrous oxide

Giving oxygen for 5–10 minutes before starting surgery 'pre-oxygenates' the patient, which increases alveolar oxygen concentration and therefore raises pO_2. Nitrous oxide produces light anaesthesia and some analgesia which assists in the smooth transition of the fully awake patient into the first and second stages of anaesthesia. Nitrous oxide potentiates the use of general anaesthetic agents and so its use throughout surgery reduces the need for the more toxic volatile anaesthetic agents.

General anaesthetic agents

Delivery of general anaesthetics is either by inhalation or intravenously, or a combination of both. One of the skills of the anaesthetist is to manipulate drug dosages to produce specific effects. For example, it may be desirable to provide a light anaesthetic so that the patient awakes quickly, or a deep anaesthetic which produces the best degree of muscle relaxation.

Intravenous induction agents

Administration of intravenous induction agents is usually in one bolus which then travels around the circulatory system towards their target organ, the brain. Here they depress the central nervous system. General understanding of their action is poor and varies depending on the drugs used, their overall effect however is to limit neural activity. These drugs also depress other body systems such as the cardiovascular and respiratory systems (Griffiths 2000a).

Because of the rapid onset, actions and potency of intravenous induction agents, it is essential to monitor the patient's vital signs during induction of anaesthesia. Monitoring allows for early interpretation of untoward signs and symptoms associated with cardiovascular and respiratory depression which can then be treated accordingly. As a minimum, it is normal to check ECG, SaO_2, blood pressure, CO_2 and respirations. The patient's condition and the anaesthetic may demand the use of other monitors (Simpson & Popat 2003). Table 3.1 gives some examples of intravenous induction agents.

Volatile (inhalational) anaesthetic agents

Volatile anaesthetic agents perform the same role as intravenous agents, but are inhaled and absorbed by the respiratory system. Absorption thus depends in part on the health of the patient's respiratory system, they are also unpleasant and can be irritating to patients. Inhalational agents can be used for induction (for example in paediatric patients) however, they are more often used for maintaining and deepening anaesthesia following induction using intravenous agents. Inhalational agents have the capacity to produce narcosis, relaxation and analgesia although the concurrent administration of intravenous drugs potentiates the action of these drugs and reduces the effects on the cardiovascular system.

Table 3.1 Intravenous induction agents.

Name	Usual actions of this group of drugs, plus	Doses (in a 70 kg adult) and mode of administration	Uses	Usual side effects of this group, plus
Thiopental	Very short onset and action. 5–10 minutes duration, terminated by dilution and absorption by fat cells	3–6 mg/kg IV. Mixed with water to form a 2.5% solution for injection	Commonly used IV for induction of anaesthesia. Can also be given rectally or as an infusion	Severe hypotension, respiratory depression, laryngeal/bronchial spasm. Contraindicated in patients suffering from porphyria
Methohexital	Ultra short action and duration		Useful in short anaesthetics such as dentistry. Used rarely, and in most areas has been replaced either by thiopental or propofol	Can cause excitatory symptoms such as coughing, hiccoughs and salivation
Propofol	Non-barbiturate providing a smooth induction. Metabolised in the liver. Short acting	1–2.5 mg/kg IV	Used when rapid recovery is required. Effective in total intravenous anaesthesia (TIVA) because of short action, low incidence of side effects and lack of 'hangover effects'	Few side effects apart from respiratory depression when used as an infusion
Etomidate	Rapid onset, short acting induction agent	0.2–0.5 mg/kg IV		Little effect on cardiovascular and respiratory systems
Ketamine	Short acting, rapid onset. Produces dissociative anaesthesia	1–2 mg/kg IV, 3–5 mg/kg IM	Induction of anaesthesia, short surgical procedures, burns dressings	Hallucinations and other emergence reactions. Hypertension and tachycardia. Post-anaesthesia nausea and vomiting

Cardiovascular effects include reduced heart rate, cardiac output and myocardial contractility which results in lower blood pressure. Enflurane in particular may alter cerebral blood flow. This group of drugs causes increasing respiratory depression as dosage (and progression through the stages of anaesthesia) increases.

Removal of waste anaesthetic gases from the operating room is important because of the longer term dangers of these gases to staff working there. Effects have include fatigue, nausea, headaches, increased risk of spontaneous abortion and other systemic effects on the organs of the body (Pressly 2000). Table 3.2 gives some examples of volatile anaesthetic agents.

Muscle relaxants

Delivery of these drugs is by intravenous injection and they are soluble in water and body fluids. Drugs in this group induce muscle paralysis by inhibiting neuromuscular transmission. The temporary paralysis on induction helps intubation while longer acting drugs aid ventilation during anaesthesia, and help access to body cavities, organs and body parts during surgery (Griffiths 2000b).

All these drugs act in some way by affecting acetylcholine (AcH) metabolism. Normally, stimulation of a motor nerve causes the nerve endings to release AcH which binds to receptors on the motor end-plate. Depolarisation of the muscle cells occurs and the muscle contracts. Acetylcholinesterase then metabolises the AcH to allow the muscle to repolarise and relax in preparation for the next contraction.

Muscle relaxants are either depolarising or non-depolarising. Depolarising muscle relaxants, such as suxamethonium, mimic AcH and bind to the receptors. Depolarisation occurs and the muscle contracts. However, acetylcholinesterase does not immediately metabolise the drug and so depolarisation persists, preventing the muscle from contracting a second time. The patient initially displays signs of muscle contractions (fasciculations) followed by paralysis. Eventually, after between 2 and 5 minutes, serum cholinesterase or pseudocholinesterase metabolise the drug allowing the muscle to repolarise and normal function returns. The drug has a rapid onset and short

Table 3.2 Volatile anaesthetic agents.

Name	Action: narcosis, relaxation and analgesia, plus	Uses: general anaesthesia, plus	Usual side effects of this group, plus
Sevoflurane	Widely used because it produces less irritation than other drugs of this group. Produces low levels of respiratory depression. Pleasant smell, fast induction and recovery	Induction of anaesthesia in paediatrics	Little or no nephrotoxicity
Halothane	Once the drug of choice, it is now almost entirely superceded by sevoflurane. Rapid onset. Little analgesic action. The liver metabolises around 20%		Fall in blood pressure, lowers peripheral resistance. Respiratory depression. Liver damage, especially on repeated use. Postoperative shivering ('halothane shakes')
Enflurane	Similar to halothane without hepatic metabolism (less than 3%)	Used for repeated anaesthesia, especially when liver damage is a possibility	Lowers pulse and blood pressure
Desflurane	Rapid onset and short duration of action. Irritant to inhale	Maintenance of anaesthesia in day-case surgery	Can cause a fall in blood pressure
Isoflurane	Similar to enflurane but with even less metabolism in the liver (0.3%)	As for enflurane. Also used to induce hypotension, when required, for example during some surgical procedures	Hypotension caused by peripheral vasodilation. Little effect on the heart

action and is therefore ideal for helping endotracheal intubation. The depolarising group of muscle relaxants do not need antidotes, because of their short duration of action (Gwinnutt 1996).

A decrease or absence of pseudocholinesterase can prevent or slow down the metabolism of suxamethonium leading to a prolonged paralysis commonly called 'scoline apnoea'. Metabolism of the drug eventually occurs through natural degradation after several hours or even days.

Non-depolarising muscle relaxants (such as atracurium and pancuronium) compete with acetylcholine for the receptor site on the motor end-plate. Concentration of the drug increases and it displaces the AcH from the receptor site. However, the drug does not cause depolarisation and so the muscle cannot contract and paralysis of the muscle results. Metabolism of the muscle relaxants by cholinesterase does not occur, therefore it remains bound to the receptors and paralysis persists. Eventually however, AcH levels increase displacing the muscle relaxant leading to a return to normal muscle function. These drugs have a slower onset and longer duration of action when compared with the depolarising group and are therefore often used on induction for longer procedures and during longer periods of anaesthesia. Neostigmine reverses their action by inhibiting cholinesterase production thereby allowing AcH to build up quicker than normal and speeding up the return to normal function. Table 3.3 gives some examples of muscle relaxants.

Analgesics

Analgesics are a complex group of drugs with poorly understood actions. They act by either reducing the capacity of the nerve fibres to sense pain or by reducing pain recognition by the higher centres of the brain. Anaesthesia often involves the use of other analgesics; however this chapter will only discuss the use of opiates.

Opiates

Opiates are useful drugs for reducing pain, anaesthetic and surgical stress. Their use as preoperative drugs and for intraoperative analgesia is widespread (Simpson & Popat 2002). They are

Table 3.3 Muscle relaxants.

Name	Action	Doses (in a 70 kg adult) and mode of administration	Uses: endotracheal intubation plus	Side effects
Suxamethonium	Depolarising agent with rapid onset (less than 1 minute) and short duration of action (3–5 minutes)	75–100 mg IV	To assist endotracheal intubation when short onset of action is required, e.g. rapid sequence induction	Increased intraocular pressure due to contraction of the intraocular muscles, increased serum potassium due to muscle fibre rupture, postoperative muscle pain, bradycardia
Pancuronium	Synthetic non-depolarising agent. Rapid onset (2–3 minutes) and medium duration of action (15–20 minutes)	8–10 mg with 4 mg incremental doses to maintain paralysis	Endotracheal intubation when a longer onset of action is required, e.g. elective procedures	Tachycardia, raised blood pressure
Vecuronium	Similar to pancuronium, but with a slightly longer action (20–30 minutes)	0.08–0.1 mg per kg bodyweight IV	Used for patients with unstable cardiovascular systems because of normally little effect on cardiovascular system. Suitable for TIVA	Can stimulate the vagal nerve leading to bradycardia
Rocuronium	Non-depolarising. Rapid onset and medium acting			
Atracurium	Non-depolarising. Rapid onset and medium acting. Broken down in plasma by 'Hofmann elimination' independently of liver or renal function. Minimal effects on heart and blood pressure	40 mg IV	Especially useful for patients with hepatic or renal failure	May cause bradycardia

also extensively used in recovery areas where pain management is a crucial part of the role of the recovery practitioner. (Starrit 2000). Opiates can be given via several routes, including for example, intramuscular, intravenous, topical and intrathecal (spinal and epidural).

Morphine, as one of the oldest and most effective analgesic agents, is a standard to measure opiates against. Development of new opiates aims to overcome or improve one or other of morphine's problems or actions. Morphine is a potent analgesic which also produces a characteristic euphoric effect favoured by drug addicts. Respiratory depression occurs at low dosages, and so spontaneously breathing patients usually receive only 10–15 mg IM. Morphine can also produce all the other side effects of the opiate group.

Morphine and pethidine have been the drugs of choice for many years. However, the wide therapeutic margin of modern drugs, in particular fentanyl and phenoperidine, has resulted in the use of far greater doses of analgesics. These drugs help to produce anaesthesia in total intravenous anaesthesia (TIVA) or to support the body systems against the effects of perioperative stress. A wide selection of synthetic opiates have been developed as a result of specific requirements, such as analgesia during TIVA. Opiates such as fentanyl and remifentanil have also been used purposely to produce hypotensive anaesthesia to lessen bleeding and therefore reduce the need for transfusion, to increase surgical visibility or to decrease operating times. Table 3.4 gives some example of opiates.

Opiates have various actions on the body including, for example:

- analgesia – opiates are potent analgesics and many also produce a characteristic euphoric effect;
- respiratory depression – close monitoring of all patients is essential since all opiates result in a degree of respiratory depression;
- depression of the cough reflex – this may be important to consider during the patient's recovery;
- nausea and vomiting – giving anti-emetics is common with opiates and may counteract this side effect;

- reduction of smooth muscle contraction – the bowel in particular is susceptible to this action, resulting in constipation, as is smooth muscle of the bronchus, resulting in bronchospasm and difficulty in breathing;
- cardiovascular depression – this may result in bradycardia and hypotension.

Opiate antagonists

Opiate antagonists support the patient during reversal of anaesthesia and postoperative care by combating persistent respiratory or cardiovascular depression.

Nalorphine

Nalorphine is an opiate in its own right and competes with morphine or other opiates for the receptor sites. As it produces less respiratory depression than other opiates it lessens the side effects. However, like all antagonists, it also reduces the analgesic properties of the opiates. Repeated doses of nalorphine can result in hypertension. The patient is given doses of 5–10 mg IV, IM or SC every 5 minutes as required, the maximum dose is around 40 mg.

Naloxone

Naloxone is a synthetic opiate antagonist derived from oxymorphone, with no opiate activity of its own. The patient normally receives doses of around 0.1–0.4 mg IM, which will reduce the respiratory depression, cardiovascular depression and analgesia. Its duration is between 45 and 90 minutes and therefore it may require repeat doses to antagonise higher doses of opiates or longer acting drugs such as morphine.

It is also possible to use respiratory stimulants such as doxapram to stimulate respiration while maintaining effective pain relief.

DRUGS USED DURING LOCAL ANAESTHESIA

Local anaesthetics are drugs that reversibly block nerve conduction when applied locally to nerve tissue. One of the oldest drugs used for local anaesthesia is cocaine which was first used

Table 3.4 Opiates in common perioperative use.

Name	Action	Indicative dosage (in a 70 kg adult) and mode of administration	Uses	Side effects
Morphine	Opiate analgesic, sedative, actions on cardiovascular and respiratory systems	10–15 mg IM, incremental doses for IV or intrathecal administration	Perioperative analgesia, general anaesthesia, epidural and spinal anaesthesia	Respiratory and cardiovascular depression, addiction
Diamorphine	As for morphine plus potent respiratory depression	Twice as potent an analgesic as morphine, 5–7.5 mg IM, incremental doses IV	Perioperative analgesia, postoperative ventilation (because of its action of respiratory depression). Added to bupivacaine in continuous epidural infusion	As for morphine plus increased risk of inadvertent respiratory depression
Fentanyl	As for morphine, except little action on cardiovascular system. Wide therapeutic ratio	2–20 µg/kg to produce general intraoperative analgesia and with larger doses its effects can last 2–3 hours following intravenous administration	Drug of choice during many perioperative situations. Cardiac surgery (without concurrent cardiovascular effects). High doses given in TIVA	

Cont.

Table 3.4 *Continued.*

Name	Action	Indicative dosage (in a 70 kg adult) and mode of administration	Uses	Side effects
Alfentanil	Short acting potent analgesic	Administered in doses of 6–8 µg/kg	Day surgery because of its short duration of action	Relatively low respiratory depression compared with fentanyl or morphine
Remifentanil	Rapid onset, short acting potent analgesic	Approx 50 µg/ml in a controlled infusion	TIVA and neurosurgery because it is very short acting and its effects wear off soon after administration is complete	
Phenoperidine	Synthetic derivative of pethidine. Analgesic and respiratory depression. Duration of around 2 hours when given IM, 1 hour after IV administration	Does varies. Can be given as a 1 mg bolus over 1 min with 0.5 mg supplement every 30–60 min. A 2–5 mg bolus plus 1 mg every 30–60 min is used for ventilated patients	Prolonged ventilation and analgesia, for example for patients ventilated in intensive care	

for eye surgery in 1884. Cocaine has spawned several other drugs including for example lidocaine and bupivacaine.

Most local anaesthetics have similar actions: rapid onset of action, short duration, low systemic toxicity, non-irritant, soluble in water and stable in solution (Simpson & Popat 2003). There are various routes for giving local anaesthetics:

- spinal block – useful for one-off injections during for example, gynaecological surgery;
- epidural block – injection into the epidural space which can produce blockade for surgery on the lower peripheries;
- nerve block – injection directly into a local nerve, for example femoral or ulnar nerve blocks;
- local infiltration – useful for minor surgery and for intravenous cannulation;
- intravenous regional block – for example Bier's block, which is the injection of a drug into a limb and a tourniquet applied to limit its circulation;
- topical block – applied directly onto the skin or mucous membrane, for example the throat (lidocaine spray), or before vasectomy (Duncan 1999) or cannulation (lidocaine cream), especially in children.

Local anaesthetics act by preventing the normal depolarisation and repolarisation of nerve cells. In its resting state, the inside of a nerve cell is positively charged compared with its outside. When a nerve cell is stimulated, the electrolyte balance changes, polarity reverses and the inside becomes positive relative to the outside. Depolarisation, and then repolarisation as the cell returns to its resting phase, is an implicit event in nerve impulse conduction. The local anaesthetics, somehow or other, block conduction of the electrolytes and therefore block the normal action of the nerve.

After absorption of the drugs into the systemic circulation, metabolism occurs either in the liver or in the plasma by pseudocholinesterase, and the drug then excreted by the kidneys.

Toxicity occurs if there is a release of high levels of the drug into the systemic circulation. Factors such as age, body weight and poor liver function may worsen this effect. Systemic side effects can include numbness of the tongue, dizziness, or muscular twitching progressing to convulsions. As the depressive effects on the central nervous system increase, the patient becomes unconscious followed by respiratory and cardiovascular arrest.

Treatment of toxic effects include preventing further local anaesthetic absorption, treating cardiovascular symptoms and controlling the convulsions by use of sedatives or tranquillisers.

The addition of vasoconstrictors to local anaesthetics can also cause toxicity; for example, 0.5 ml of 1:1000 adrenaline is the maximum dose that should be administered subcutaneously to a man of 70 kg. More than this may result in increasingly dangerous side effects as the dose increases.

Local anaesthetic drugs such as lidocaine also have other uses, for example:

- antiarrhythmic effects – prevention of depolarisation of the cell membranes of cardiac muscle fibres reduces excitability making ectopic beats less likely;
- reducing the pressure response of intubation – spraying the throat with lidocaine before intubation may block the reflex rise in pulse rate and blood pressure;
- an aid to minor surgery – for example vasectomy (Duncan 1999);
- extensively used in specific surgical procedures, for example, eye surgery (Carroll 2002).

Table 3.5 gives some examples of local anaesthetic agents.

DRUGS USED TO SUPPORT THE BODY SYSTEMS

Anti-emetics

Perioperative patients often suffer from nausea and vomiting, or acid reflux (Farman 2004), which are common side effects of many anaesthetic drugs. Vomiting in perioperative patients occurs because of stimulation of the vomiting centre in the brain or through direct irritation of the stomach lining. The phenothiazine group of drugs are the most common anti-emetics. These drugs all produce different levels of sedation, hypotension, vasodilation, urinary retention, blurred vision etc., as well as

Table 3.5 Local anaesthetic agents.

Name	Action	Doses (in a 70 kg adult) and mode of administration	Uses	Side effects: usual systemic side effects including depression of CNS, depression of cardiac and respiratory systems, plus
Cocaine	Local anaesthetic, excitation of the central nervous system, vasoconstriction	Max: 150 mg in a 5% solution (50 mg/ml)	Topical anaesthesia in ENT surgery	Ventricular fibrillation, convulsions
Lidocaine (lignocaine)	Local anaesthetic, local vasodilatory effect	Max: 200 mg plain, 500 mg with adrenaline	Versatile drug that can be administered via any route and is used for local analgesia and systemically as an antiarrhythmic	
Bupivacaine	Long acting local anaesthetic. Effects of 'heavy' version can last 2–3 hours	Max: 150 mg	Epidural block, plexus blocks	
Prilocaine	Local anaesthetic	Max 300 mg plain, 600 mg with adrenaline	Dentistry and Bier's block	Produces methaemoglobinaemia when given in high doses – possible effects on fetus in utero
Tetracaine (amethocaine) gel	Topical local anaesthetic	4% gel	Topical anaesthetic used before cannulation or venepuncture	Little risk of systemic side effects
Emla cream (lidocaine and prilocaine)	Topical local anaesthetic	5% cream	Topical anaesthetic used before cannulation or venepuncture	Little risk of systemic side effects

anti-emesis. Long-term anti-emetics also include anticholinergic agents (such as atropine or hyoscine), with side effects including central nervous system depression. Ondansetron is a modern anti-emetic drug which shows promise for the treatment of postoperative nausea and vomiting (PONV), although there are some concerns about its use (Cox, 1999) related to patient satisfaction and increased cost. Table 3.6 gives some example of anti-emetics.

Drugs affecting the autonomic nervous system

The autonomic nervous system controls smooth muscle, for example in the gut, bronchi and blood vessels, the endocrine glands such as the adrenal and pituitary glands, and the heart. The autonomic nervous system is divided into two systems – the sympathetic and parasympathetic nervous systems.

The role of the sympathetic nervous system is to prepare the body for 'fight or flight'. Effects include increased heart rate and blood pressure, vasoconstriction of skin, vasodilation of skeletal muscle and bronchi and dilation of the pupil of the eye. The parasympathetic nervous system essentially stimulates the opposite reactions – for example, decreased heart rate, bronchoconstriction and increased gastrointestinal activity.

The autonomic nervous system's three main transmitter substances are adrenaline, noradrenaline and acetylcholine. Adrenoreceptors are the target for the actions of adrenaline and noradrenaline. Adrenaline and noradrenaline attach to these specialised groups of cells, producing the effects of the sympathetic nervous system. Blocking of these agents reduces sympathetic activity. The actions of acetylcholine are muscarinic (acting on parasympathetic nerves) and nicotinic (acting on neuromuscular and autonomic ganglia).

Drugs affecting the autonomic nervous system therefore have the following actions:

- Cholinergic agents – enhance or mimic acetylcholine and therefore stimulate the parasympathetic nervous system.
- Anticholinergic agents – block acetylcholine and therefore block the parasympathetic nervous system.
- Adrenergic agonists – enhance the actions of noradrenaline and therefore stimulate the sympathetic nervous system.

They are also called sympathomimetics or adrenoceptor agonists.
- Adrenergic antagonists – block the actions of noradrenaline and therefore block the sympathetic nervous system. They are also called sympatholytics or adrenoceptor antagonists.

Cholinergic agents

This small group of drugs mimics the effects of acetylcholine. Carbachol, for example, mainly stimulates the parasympathetic system, leading to dilation of peripheral vessels, lower heart rate and lower blood pressure. Carbachol also treats postoperative urinary retention because of its action on increasing bladder tone.

Anticholinergic agents

Atropine blocks the effects of the parasympathetic nervous system, causing tachycardia, drying of secretions, relaxation of the gut and dilation of pupils. Other drugs in this group include hyoscine and glycopyrronium bromide (glycopyrrolate). Atropine's main perioperative uses in cardiovascular support are to reduce bradycardia caused by vagal stimulation, for example, during abdominal procedures or when caused by intubation. It also blocks the parasympathetic effects (bradycardia) of the muscle relaxant antidote neostigmine.

Adrenergic agents

This wide group of drugs has effects on the cardiovascular and respiratory systems and includes drugs such as adrenaline, noradrenaline, dopamine, isoprenaline and salbutamol. Because of their effects on the cardiovascular and respiratory systems, these drugs are often used in severely ill patients or during emergencies such a haemorrhage and cardiac arrest. During surgery, they control blood pressure and pulse, and reduce the effects of anaesthetic drugs. This group of drugs represents possibly the largest group used in perioperative care. They have a multitude of uses, displaying both local and systemic effects. The effects of adrenergic agents on adrenoceptors

Table 3.6 Anti-emetics.

Name	Action	Doses (in a 70 kg adult) and mode of administration	Uses	Side effects including: sedation, hypotension, vasodilation, urinary retention, plus:
Cyclizine (Valoid)	Powerful anti-emetic	50 mg/ml IV. Often combined with an opiate such as morphine or as a ready-made preparation (Cyclimorph)	Perioperative anti-emetic	
Prochlorperazine (Stemetil)	Anti-emetic	12.5 mg IM, 25 mg rectally	Perioperative anti-emetic	Fewer sedative properties than other drugs of this group. Antidote is atropine. Can cause constipation, dry mouth, hypotension if given IV
Metochlopramide (Maxolon)	Anti-emetic which reduces the activity of the vomiting centre and reduces the peripheral stimulation to vomiting by increasing gastric emptying	10 mg orally, or IM; 10–20 mg IV	Perioperative anti-emetic	Fewer side effects than drugs in the phenothiazine group

Table 3.7 The effects of adrenergic agents on adrenoceptors.

Adrenoreceptor	Agonist activity	Antagonist activity
α1 – cardiac and respiratory	Coronary vasoconstriction, bronchial dilation	Coronary vasodilation
α2 – peripheral circulation	Peripheral vasoconstriction, intestinal sphincter contraction, sweat production	Peripheral vasodilation
β1 – cardiac	Increases force and power of the heartbeat, increases blood pressure, coronary and peripheral vasodilation	Reduces heart rate and contractility
β2 – bronchial	Bronchodilation	Bronchoconstriction

are listed in Table 3.7. Common adrenergic agonists are listed in Table 3.8 and adrenergic antagonists in Table 3.9.

CONCLUSION

Perioperative care involves the use of a wide range of drugs, many of which have not even been touched on in this chapter. These include, for example anticoagulants, thrombolytics, diuretics, antibiotics, hormones and laxatives (Griffiths 2000). These drugs have only been omitted because of space restraints, not because of lack of importance in their role of patient support.

The role of the practitioner in drug administration is to ensure that administering drugs is safe and effective, and to be able to recognise and react to the effects and side effects of the drugs. The result of good practice should be that the patient receives the correct drug, at the correct time and by the correct route. It is therefore essential that all practitioners are fully familiar with all drugs used in their area of practice to ensure safe and effective patient care.

Table 3.8 Adrenergic agonists.

Name	Action	Doses (in a 70 kg adult) and mode of administration	Uses	Side effects as usual plus
Adrenaline (epinephrine)	Stimulates $\alpha2$, $\beta1$ and $\beta2$ receptors. Cardiac stimulant, peripheral vasoconstriction, bronchial dilation	For anaphylactic shock – 100–500 μg SC or IM, repeated as required every 20 min. 100–250 μg IV slowly. Bronchospasm –100–500 μg SC or IM. Cardiac arrest – 0.1–1 mg IV or intra-cardiac (IC)	Treatment of cardiac arrest, reduces bronchospasm, local vasoconstrictor when used with local anaesthetic, reduces allergic and hypersensitivity reactions	Tachycardia, restlessness, weakness, pallor, hypertension, palpitation, sweating, nausea, cardiac arrhythmias
Noradrenaline (norepinephrine)	Stimulates $\alpha2$ receptors. Peripheral vasoconstriction leading to increased blood pressure	4 μg/ml infusion delivered at 8–12 μg/min until patient is stable	Used in severely ill patients to increase blood pressure. Cardiac surgery	Poor renal and peripheral perfusion
Isoprenaline	Stimulates $\beta1$ receptors. Increases force and power of the heart beat, reduces bronchospasm, peripheral vasoconstrictor	0.1–0.2 mg by aerosol. 0.01–0.2 mg by slow IV	Treatment of low blood pressure, treatment of bronchospasm. Treatment of atrio-ventricular heart block	Atrial tachycardia, cardiac arrhythmias

Dopamine	β2 agonist, cardiac stimulant which increases pulse and blood pressure, renal vasodilator	200 mg added to 250 ml to give an IV infusion of 800 µg/ml. Administered at 2–5 µg/kg/min	Used to increase blood pressure and improve renal function	Peripheral vasoconstriction when used in large doses
Ephedrine	Stimulates α and β receptors to increase heart rate and myocardial contractility, and peripheral vasoconstriction. Also causes bronchodilation	15–50 mg SC, IM or slow IV	Used to reduce hypotension caused by general and local anaesthesia, especially following spinal or epidural anaesthesia	Interacts with monoamine-oxidase inhibitors
Salbutamol	β2 receptor stimulant which selectively targets bronchial muscle receptors to relieve bronchospasm	1–2 inhalations (100–200 µg) from metered dose aerosol. 500 µg SC or IM, 200–300 µg slow IV	Relief of bronchospasm in asthma, bronchitis and emphysema	Can cause cardiac stimulation and peripheral vasodilation

Table 3.9 Adrenergic antagonists.

Name	Action	Doses (in a 70 kg adult) and mode of administration	Uses	Side effects
Phentolamine	α2 receptor antagonist which produces vasodilation, resulting in falling blood pressure and lower central venous pressure (CVP). Short acting drug lasting around 30 min	5–10 mg IM or IV	Vasodilator during cardiopulmonary bypass, to antagonise the effects of noradrenaline, and as a vasodilator during cardiogenic shock	Hypovolaemia because of the larger extravascular fluid compartment results in tachycardia and hypotension. Can be treated with fluids
Propranolol	β1 receptor blocker which reduces heart rate and output. Reduces oxygen demands of myocardial muscle	20–40 mg orally. 1 mg by slow IV up to a maximum of 5–10 mg	To control ectopic beats and tachycardia, and to reduce incidence of angina	Bronchospasm because of effects on β2 receptors

REFERENCES

Carroll, C. (2002) Local anaesthetic techniques in ophthalmic surgery. *British Journal of Perioperative Nursing* **12** (2), 68–74.

Cox, F. (1999) Systematic review of Ondansetron for the prevention and treatment of postoperative nausea and vomiting in adults. *British Journal of Perioperative Nursing* **9** (12), 556–63.

Department of Health (2004) *Standards for Better Health.* HMSO, London.

Duncan, C. (1999) Pain during vasectomy: a prospective audit. *British Journal of Perioperative Nursing* **9** (2), 79–83.

Farman, J. (2004) Acid aspiration syndrome. *British Journal of Perioperative Nursing* **14** (6), 266–74.

Griffiths, R. (2000a) Back to basics: Anaesthetic drugs. *British Journal of Perioperative Nursing* **10** (5), 276–9.

Griffiths, R. (2000b) Back to Basics: Supportive pharmacology. *British Journal of Perioperative Nursing* **10** (7), 383–6.

Gwinnutt, C. (1996) *Clinical Anaesthesia.* Blackwell Science, Oxford.

National Prescribing Centre and National Primary Care Research and Development Centre (2002) *Modernising Medicines Management: A Guide to Achieving Benefits for Patients, Professionals and the NHS (Book 1).* The National Prescribing Centre and National Primary Care Research and Development Centre, London.

NHS Executive (2002) *Medicines Management (Safe and Secure Handling).* DOH, London.

Pressly, V. (2000) Waste anaesthetic gases. *British Journal of Perioperative Nursing* **13** (5), 299–304.

Simpson, P.J. & Popat, M. (2002) *Understanding Anaesthesia.* Butterworth Heinemann, London.

Starritt, T. (2000) Pain management in recovery. *British Journal of Perioperative Nursing* **10** (2), 115–19.

4 | Perioperative Communication

LEARNING OUTCOMES

❏ Understand the need for *effective communication* in relation to patient care within the operating room environment.
❏ Discuss the *different aspects of communication*.
❏ Have an understanding of the *legal issues* that affect the practice of the perioperative practitioner.
❏ Identify the different *members of the operating room team* and their roles and responsibilities.
❏ Understand the different *government agencies* that influence patient care within the operating room environment.

PATIENT COMMUNICATION

This chapter will discuss the different aspects of communication between members of the multidisciplinary team and patients, and between practitioners themselves. Communication is a key factor in:

- patient advocacy;
- patient consent;
- accountability;
- documentation;
- clinical supervision;
- information technology within the NHS;
- teamwork;
- the perioperative team;
- change management;
- clinical governance;
  — government agencies;
  — performance indicators.

Communication is the key to the quality and effectiveness of patient care within the NHS. Communication between patients and the operating room multidisciplinary team is important to allay the patients' fears. Perioperative practitioners can reassure patients and provide a friendly face when they are at their most vulnerable.

The Royal Colleges of Surgeons and Psychiatrists (1997) carried out a survey to identify the concerns of patients undergoing surgical procedures. Patients expressed the following fears:

- fear of not waking up after surgery;
- waking up during the surgery;
- anxiety because of the patient face mask;
- needle-phobia.

Leinonen *et al.* (1996) also asked patients about their fears of surgery and they discovered that patients wanted information about their perioperative journey and practitioners to have a sense of humour and be of a friendly nature. Anaesthetic practitioners can ease the patients' nerves and worries on anaesthesia and anaesthetic equipment by communicating effectively with their patients and anticipating their personal needs.

Communication is the basic element of human interactions that allows people to establish, maintain and improve contacts with others. It is a complex and multifaceted process that involves behaviours and relationships and allows individuals to associate with others and the world around them (Potter & Berry 1989). In the operating room it is important to create an environment where there is effective communication between the patient and perioperative practitioner.

Communication is the basis of accurate hearing, defining, organising, interpreting and managing exchanges with patients, the operating room multidisciplinary team, and other hospital practitioners. It can be either verbal (involving issues such as volume, quality of voice and tone rate) or non-verbal (involving eye contact, facial expression, posture, closeness and touch). The effective use of both verbal and non-verbal communication by the perioperative practitioners can establish a caring and empathetic impression with patients on their perioperative journey. Practitioners must not judge or discriminate against patients of different ages, genders and race. They should treat every patient with equal respect.

Communication is the channel by which the perioperative practitioner helps to deliver effective patient care throughout the operating room. It is a two-way process where both parties should understand each other for effective interactions to occur.

A scientific knowledge base, theory-based practice, and adroit psychomotor skills, while being fundamental elements of perioperative practice, do not by themselves enable a practitioner to provide optimum patient care. However, when the practitioner exposes these practice elements to the catalyst of astute communications technique, diligently honed and regularly exercised, their patients can receive optimal care and the practitioners may enjoy professional fulfilment (Fortunato 2000).

Listening is an important facet of communication since practitioners who do not listen to patients will not understand their needs. Some patients are anxious and this will manifest itself in some by making them talkative whereas others become more reserved. It is important that the practitioner can assess the patient's needs and be able to elicit the correct amount of information from them. Barriers can reduce the efficiency of this process and the practitioners need to analyse their own and the patients' interpretation of their conversation. They always need to listen to patients and answer any questions that arise.

Effective feedback to the communication is important to the patient and may relieve the patient's stress before anaesthesia and surgery. Breakdown in communications can intensify this stress.

It is desirable for the patient to form a trusting relationship with the practitioner at their first meeting. The initial meeting, in the reception area, is where the professional relationship between patients and practitioners begins. Patients may feel vulnerable while lying on the operating room trolley so it is important that practitioners introduce themselves to the patient in a non-intimidating way. Practitioners who can detect non-verbal signs from the patient are better able to understand the patient's needs and reduce anxiety. They need to have perception and be able to interpret the needs of the patient.

In the reception area practitioners should:

- introduce themselves to the patient respectfully;
- maintain effective eye contact, speak directly to the patient and listen to their responses;
- assess the personal needs of the patient – is the patient blind, deaf or physically disabled?
- display a reassuring and calm manner during communication with the patient.

During the preoperative check the practitioner should speak to the patient directly, using simple language to assess and confirm the patient's understanding of the questions on the checklist. It is important to arrange for the anaesthetist or surgeon to speak to the patient to allay any worries if the patient is upset and needs reassurance on specific issues. An interpreter may increase the effectiveness of the communication although usually the ward practitioners will have arranged for the interpreter to escort the patient to the reception area.

Patients differ in the extent of information they need before their surgical procedure. Practitioners need to respect this difference and treat each patient as an individual.

Patients with a hearing impairment

Patients with impaired hearing may have communication problems throughout their perioperative care. Wearing a hearing aid may help the patient understand procedures better and may also help the recovery practitioner in the postoperative care of the patient.

If it is not possible for the patient to wear a hearing aid, the anaesthetic practitioner should speak slowly in order for the patient to be able to lip-read the information. If the patient is awake in the operating room, practitioners need to remember that their face masks are an obstacle to communication.

Patients with poor eyesight or who are visually impaired

Practitioners should introduce themselves to patients, so that the patient knows who they are speaking to, and use the sense of touch to help in the communication process.

Non-English-speaking patients

Normally the ward practitioners will arrange for an interpreter to accompany the patient to the operating room environment. The practitioner needs to ensure that these patients understand, via the interpreter, all the details of their anaesthesia and surgical procedure. The interpreter may accompany the patient into the anaesthetic room to ensure that he or she understands and feel less stressed in preoperative care; and the interpreter may again be present in the recovery area for postoperative care.

Paediatric patients

For paediatric patients, one relative or carer may normally accompany the patient into the anaesthetic room if allowed by local policy.

Anxious adult patients

Local protocol may allow a relative to escort an anxious adult patient, but the anaesthetic practitioner needs to confirm this before taking the patient into the anaesthetic room.

Patients have the right to be treated with skill, consideration and dignity regardless of their age, gender, race, religion, disabilities, health and legal status (Shields & Werder 2002).

Effective communication is essential between all members of the perioperative team, ward practitioners and allied professions from other departments in order to deliver quality care to the patient throughout their perioperative journey. Perioperative practitioners maintain effective communication with their patients and the multidisciplinary team to ensure optimal patient care.

PATIENT ADVOCACY

Advocacy is 'a process of acting for on behalf of someone who is unable to do so for themselves' (Royal College of Nursing 1992). Patients are vulnerable during their perioperative journey whichever type of anaesthesia is utilised. They may be unconscious during their surgical procedure and therefore they have no control over their care or may feel too nervous to ask any questions during regional, local anaesthesia and sedation techniques.

Mallik (1997) and Baldwin (2003) identify the characteristics of advocacy as:

- promoting the patient's rights;
- being involved in decision making and informed consent;
- acting as an intermediary for patients with healthcare providers and NHS.

All perioperative practitioners are responsible for the patients' care and they will be their ears and voice during their surgical procedures. They can help patients with communication barriers, clarification of their anaesthesia and surgical procedure, and provide support during their perioperative care. Effective professional relationships within the multidisciplinary operating room team can help all operating room practitioners to discuss pertinent issues with the appropriate personnel on behalf of the patient.

The Nursing and Midwifery Council (NMC) (2002) states that nurses should:

- act always in such a manner as to promote and safeguard the interest and well-being of patients and clients (clause 1);
- work in an open and cooperative manner with patients, clients and their families, foster their independence and recognise their involvement in the planning and delivery of care (clause 5).

Seedhouse (1988) believes respecting autonomy is bedevilled with controversy. The only strong reason to not respect autonomy is when it will harm one or more people. Beyond this, the issue must be resolved by personal judgment and appropriate moral reasoning. Newly qualified practitioners can discuss autonomy with their colleagues and senior managers to enhance their knowledge and experience to ease the patient through their perioperative journey.

PATIENT CONSENT

The Department of Health (DOH) issued a range of guidance documents on consent in 2004 which set out the standards and procedures for all health professionals who undertake consent procedures. Valid consent to treatment is central to the patient's surgical procedure within the operating room. This document identifies the 12 key points of consent. The points cover the following areas:

- Points 1–4 When do health professionals need consent from patients?
- Point 5 Can children consent for themselves?
- Point 6 Who is the right person to seek consent?
- Point 7 What information should be provided?
- Point 8 Is the patient's consent voluntary?
- Point 9 Does it matter how the patient gives consent?
- Point 10 Refusal of consent.
- Points 11 and 12 Adults who are not competent to give consent.

There are four consent forms within the operating room:

- Adult.
- Paediatric – only people with parental responsibility are entitled to give consent on behalf of their children. The anaesthetic practitioner checks the confirmation of signature with the parent. Children over 16 can sign their own consent, while children under 16 can sign their own consent if deemed to be competent to do so (Gillick competence).
- Consultant – they sign for patients who do not understand the implications of the surgical procedure.
- Local anaesthetic.

Kavanagh (2004) believes that education is the key when dealing with issues of consent. All practitioners should be familiar with the current law, the guidelines from their governing bodies and local hospital policies.

All patients need comprehensive information on their surgical procedure and the implications and side effects of their surgery so they can make an informed decision to give their consent. Anaesthetic practitioners can help to answer the patient's concerns about the surgical procedure or ask the surgeon to speak to the patient before the commencement of anaesthesia. If there are any problems they should be sorted out with the appropriate practitioners before the anaesthetic practitioner escorts the patient into the anaesthetic room.

It is the anaesthetic practitioner's responsibility to check the patient's consent form in the reception area and confirm with patients that they understand and are aware of their surgical procedure. They should ensure that the surgical procedure on the consent form correlates with the details on the operating list. If the surgeon adds any further details of the surgical procedure or other procedures patients should sign again to ensure that they understand the additions.

Patients who have received a premedication cannot sign for any additions as the premedication drugs can affect their understanding of the implications of extension to the surgery and therefore the surgery reverts to what was originally agreed.

Scrub practitioners should check the consent and any allergies or medical condition before the commencement of the surgical procedure. Any discrepancies (for example, correct site for the surgical procedure) should be sorted out with the perioperative team before the anaesthetist commences anaesthesia.

Problems with consent are identified in Table 4.1.

Table 4.1 Problems with consent.

Problem with consent	Action to be taken
Consent form not signed by patient	Ask medical practitioners to undertake consent procedure with patient
Consent form signed in outpatients on a previous date	Consent confirmed and signed on day of operation by ward or perioperative practitioners
Wrong limb identified on consent form and operating list	Check patient notes to confirm correct limb. Contact surgeon to change consent form and mark the correct limb. In some operating rooms members of the perioperative team have a 'time out' to ensure all parties are happy to go ahead with the surgical procedure
Patient not aware of surgical procedure	Ask the ward nurse or surgeon to confirm patient was lucid and can understand nature of surgical procedure. If patient is confused or has symptoms of dementia, ask for consultant consent.
Patient has dementia	Ask for consultant consent

ACCOUNTABILITY

Perioperative practitioners are responsible and accountable for the patients throughout their perioperative journey. They provide a safe environment for patients and check all relevant equipment for their anaesthetic and surgical procedures. They are also accountable to their employer, manager, the operating room multidisciplinary team, their work colleagues and to themselves.

Perioperative practitioners:

- have a duty of care to their patients;
- should respect, inform and protect the patient throughout the perioperative journey;
- should be aware of current legislation and implications of the law;
- keep accurate documentation;
- have loyalty to members of the multidisciplinary team;
- maintain confidentiality and dignity of the patient;
- only undertake roles and responsibilities in which they are competent;
- are accountable for their practice.

The NMC (2004a) advises registered practitioners that they hold a position of responsibility and are accountable for their actions as well as having a contractual accountability to the employer and accountability to the law for actions undertaken. Accountability is fundamentally concerned with weighing up the interests of patients in complex situations, using professional knowledge, judgment and skills to make a decision for which the practitioner can be called to account (NATN 1998).

A lack of accountability may result in patient injury or dissatisfaction with care. Health care providers have a legal and moral obligation to identify and correct situations that threaten a patient's safety and well-being. Most incidents that could endanger the patient and lead to legal actions can be prevented. Failure of a caregiver to maintain accountability can result in negligence (Fortunato 2000).

All perioperative practitioners and members of the multidisciplinary team should be aware of the issues of accountability, vicarious liability and indemnity. The employing authority is liable for the negligence of their employees and the NHS indemnity covers their employees for negligence claims. Accountability, responsibility and legal issues should be taken very seriously as litigation costs are increasing each year. Accountability is entailed in responsibility, and anyone who is responsible is thereby accountable (Hunt 2005).

Regulation of perioperative practitioners is undertaken by the Nursing and Midwifery Council (NMC) for nurses and Health Professions Council (HPC) for ODPs and these bodies have the power to strike a professional off their registers if the practitioner is found guilty of malpractice. In this event it would be illegal for that practitioner to practise in health care in the future. Some of the main reasons for litigation include:

- ignorance;
- poor communication between health care practitioners;
- incompetence;
- lack of resources.

DOCUMENTATION

It is generally accepted that written communication is significant not only as a communication medium in nursing but also in the fulfilment of a number of other professional and legal obligations for nurses (Taylor 2003).

Patient documentation within the operating room gives a written account of the patient's care through the perioperative journey from the reception area until the handover to the ward nurse in the recovery area. It also gives postoperative instructions for care in the immediate and postoperative care on the ward or on discharge.

The perioperative practitioner completes several legally important records during the delivery of perioperative care:

- computer records;
- operation register;
- patient's care plan;
- information of surgical procedure on the operative list;
- confirmation of specimen information;
- checking of equipment, stocking up, blood and blood products.

In the event of a complaint, legal case or attendance at the Coroner's Court practitioners have to defend any missing information of care that they did not record on the patient's care plan. The accuracy of the documentation will support the practitioner's defence of the patient's care.

Verbal communication between patients and healthcare providers does not provide strong legal evidence in a court of law – it is difficult to prove because there is no permanent record of what was said. The patient's medical records are the best evidence of care received or omitted and are often relied on heavily during legal cases. Entries by practitioners and physicians in the record provide a history of the patient's clinical course and responses to treatment. Deficiencies in the record can destroy the credibility of the record and the providers (Fortunato 2000). Documentation of care is summarised in Box 4.1.

The perioperative team must complete incident reports when any accidents occur. The National Association of Theatre Nurses (1998) states that all accidents involving practitioners, equipment and buildings must be reported to the head of department and relevant paperwork completed in line with national guidelines (RIDDOR 1996). The member of staff, if necessary, should seek medical assessment if they sustain any injury. Local reporting protocols should be adhered to and all the documentation should go to an agreed central collecting point and photocopies kept within the department.

The operating room manager may launch an internal enquiry into incidents where he or she identifies a problem. Any

---

Box 4.1 Documentation of care

The practitioner should record care following local policy:

- Information should be written in a legible fashion and in black ink.
- Do not cross out, use Tippex or use abbreviations.
- Record all care given to patients, before, during and after the surgical procedure in a logical order with times if relevant.
- Only record relevant information (record facts and not opinions).
- Identify any instructions from the anaesthetist or surgeon.
- Identify patient's requests, important medical facts about patients (for example, allergies).
- Sign for delivery of care.

---

member of the perioperative team completes an incident report when there is a problem or incident during patient care. The incident report is a valuable tool in reporting a problem. All members of the perioperative team should complete this form in black ink and include all evidence of their patient care on the care plan.

CLINICAL SUPERVISION

In the 1990s a succession of major failures in the NHS added momentum to an ongoing process of review and reform. Incidents such as the Bristol heart surgery tragedy, the failures of cervical screening at Kent and Canterbury Hospital and the case of Beverley Allitt have all caused widespread public and political concern and heightened general awareness of the potential harm when health services go awry. These incidents have also engendered a period of deep reflection and critical analysis among the health professions and fostered growing support for major changes in the way quality health services are managed (Smith 1998).

The operating room can be a stressful environment and the introduction of clinical supervision can provide a support mechanism for the operating room practitioners, enable individual practitioners to highlight and meet specific training and development needs and help in the delivery of clinical excellence for patients. Issues that might be discussed within clinical supervision include:

- professional issues;
- clinical issues;
- roles;
- personal issues;
- environmental issues;
- educational issues;
- support and nurture;
- critical incidents;
- reflection.

A confidential contract will be completed at the end of the clinical supervision meeting between the clinical supervisor and supervisee. If anything is disclosed in the meeting which is illegal, which breaks the relevant code of professional conduct, which relates to potential or actual harm to a patient or colleague, or which constitutes misconduct, it should be reported to the operating room manager or relevant personnel to take the appropriate action.

Clinical supervision is a formal process of providing professional support and learning (DOH 1993). It is a way of a supervisee and supervisor discussing, exploring and examining practice in a formal meeting, which may help to enhance practice, training and competence.

Wood (2004) believes that clinical supervision supports practice, enabling practitioners to maintain and improve standards of care. To facilitate clinical supervision a culture of lifelong learning needs to be embraced as an integral part of daily working life within the NHS. Education, training and lifelong learning can support the perioperative practitioners' improvement in competence and delivery of patient care. Clinical supervision can also enhance patient care by perioperative practitioners supporting each other, discussing practice issues and improving teamwork and quality within the NHS.

INFORMATION TECHNOLOGY WITHIN THE NHS

Information and communications technology is a new component within patient healthcare to modernise the storage of patient information. All practitioners require basic computing skills as information on the patient's healthcare is input on computers by all practitioners within the NHS. Practitioners need to feel comfortable using computers and have the ability to input the relevant information.

Individual managers can arrange training for their practitioners but there is an opportunity to undertake a recognised training programme of IT skills. The European Computer Driving Licence course is a national scheme to equip all practitioners with a comprehensive practical knowledge of basic computing skills. The NHS Information Authority tracks and monitors registrations of practitioners and has access to the learning and testing materials.

Electronic storage of information is becoming more prominent within all areas of patient care and can give valuable information to all NHS agencies. It is an innovation to provide electronic health records, evidence-based decision making and valuable resources for NHS practitioners.

In the operating room, computer information can provide names of individual practitioners who undertake the different roles in each theatre discipline and time of the patient entering and leaving all areas of the operating room environment. It can also be used to record information on:

- type of anaesthesia;
- identification of laryngeal mask airway (LMA) number and the number of times it has been used during anaesthesia;
- time of commencement and completion of anaesthesia and surgical procedure;
- planned surgical procedure and details of any changes to it;
- any extra equipment necessary for the surgical procedure (for example TV and laparoscope);
- any change of ward on discharge;
- cancellation of surgical procedure with the identification of the reason.

The NHS is trying to improve clinical performance within the operating room environment and reduce cancelled surgical procedures. Effective utilisation of the operating room sessions is critical to the provision of efficient surgical procedures and to achieve full capacity and use of the operative lists. Computer information can identify an individual patient's surgical procedure cancellation and allow managers to reschedule the procedure within the specified government time limits.

The implementation of the electronic patient record systems has modernised patient information within the NHS. It allows practitioners and medical practitioners to access patient information to aid delivery of patient care, audits or incident reports. It can improve multi-agency information and minimise frustration for all.

Computer reports can provide:

- for the patient:
  — satisfaction – arrange suitable appointments, admissions and discharge;

— reduction of delays in their surgical procedures;
— reduction of cancelled surgical procedures.
- for the practitioners:
  — patient care information;
  — laboratory results, X-ray reports.

Access to computers for training purposes is becoming the norm for all operating room environments. All practitioners can access the intranet and internet services for information on patient care issues and also for their own professional development. They can prepare presentations for teaching and assessment of students and research information for university courses and enhance their own and others' knowledge of patient care issues.

TEAMWORK

A team is a small number of people with complementary skills who are committed to a common purpose, performance goals and approach for which they hold themselves mutually accountable (Katzenbach and Smith 1993).

Perioperative practitioners have complementary skills within their theatre disciplines and have a commitment to the operating room performance goals, and the delivery of quality care to their perioperative patients. Woodcock (1982) describes a team as a group of people who share common objectives and who need to work together to achieve them.

Issues to consider within a team:

- effectiveness of the leader or manager;
- size of the team;
- roles and responsibilities of each team member and their understanding of these;
- shared and agreed aims and objectives (do they have a clear, explicit and mutually agreed approach?);
- cohesiveness of the team;
- communication within the team members (from top to bottom and bottom to top);
- regular meetings to improve communication and to inform all members of team;
- motivation and interaction within the team;

- vision and development of team;
- forum for conflict and exchange of views (does the team listen to all members' views?);
- satisfaction of members;
- effective environment for the team: confidentiality, education and training, development, promotion, recruitment and retention;
- flexible working and responsiveness to changing developments within the NHS;
- support within the team.

Successful teams have a strong and effective leader. Team members have clear views, are clear about their roles and responsibilities, share objectives, discuss and resolve problems, value and respect each other and encourage development and growth of the team.

The team consists of a mix of people with individual personalities and talents who blend to work together effectively. Managers and team leaders should recognise the strengths and weaknesses of their team members and ensure that they make the best use of their resources to develop them into a cohesive team. All these issues encourage team cohesiveness and therefore encourage the delivery of effective patient care.

Team briefing enables managers to share information about the organisation with all levels of practitioners. It ensures all practitioners are aware of developments and changes within the organisation (Clarke & Jones 1998).

THE PERIOPERATIVE TEAM

The roles and responsibilities of the operating room are diverse and at times overlap within the different areas of the operating room environment (reception, anaesthetic room, operating room and recovery). Members of the operating room team have different levels of qualifications and experience but they pool these in the care of the perioperative patient.

The scrub practitioner

Nurses qualify and undertake an in-house scrub training programme on entry to the operating department before they work autonomously within this role. Operating department practitioners undertake the scrub discipline within their 3 years' training and can work autonomously immediately after qualification. Both types of practitioner are supported by their senior colleagues during the first few months of their scrub practice. Both are practitioners who prepare the equipment and surgical accessories for surgeons and are aware of their surgical preferences during the procedures.

Their roles and responsibilities are to:

- Check all relevant equipment for the different operations for the individual patients on the operative list.
- Maintain a safe operating room environment and sterile field for surgical patients.
- Ensure the theatre team position the patient safely and comfortably on the operating room table.
- Maintain the patient's dignity and ensure the rest of the operating room team observe this.
- Provide the swabs, needles, instruments and accessories for surgeons.
- Anticipate their needs to facilitate an efficient and safe surgical procedure.
- Communicate effectively with the theatre team throughout the patient's perioperative journey to provide holistic and efficient patient care.
- Check the specimens from the operative list following local policy and ensure the specimens go to the correct department for examination.
- Complete the relevant documentation following local policy.

The circulating practitioner

A qualified scrub practitioner or an operating room support worker can undertake this role. The circulating practitioner's role is important as they are the eyes and ears of the scrub practitioners. They assist them to prepare the theatre, ensure the operating room environment is clean and tidy, and stock the operating room after the operative list.

Their roles and responsibilities are to:

- Prepare the surgical gown and gloves and tie up the surgical gowns of the surgical team when relevant.
- Open the sterile instruments sets for the scrub practitioner, check the integrity and expiry dates of the sterile swabs, needles, instruments and accessories before delivering them to the scrub practitioner.
- Pour the skin preparation into the relevant galley pots. During this they maintain the sterile field and ensure that all the surgical team also observe this.
- Assist the theatre team to position the patients and maintain their dignity.
- Collect the specimen or specimens from the scrub practitioner, label the specimen container, use the correct medium and complete the specimen card following the local specimen policy.
- Communicate effectively with the operating room team. They give any messages to the surgeon or scrub practitioner in a respectful manner and at a convenient time.
- Clean the operating room table and positioning equipment, and other equipment after each patient following local infection control policies.

There are opportunities for some operating room support workers to undertake training for the scrub role. The Perioperative Care Collaborative (PCC) (2005) has issued a position statement for this role. The PCC is of the view that the minimum underpinning knowledge which the operating support worker must demonstrate to perform the scrub role should be in line with National Occupational Standards for Perioperative Care and assessed by National Qualification Frameworks. The qualified scrub practitioner will remain responsible for the overall management of the patient's care and the theatre support worker will only scrub for elective surgical procedures (PCC 2005).

Scrub practitioners will oversee the swab check, be present throughout the surgical procedure and complete the patient documentation. Operating room managers will create training programmes, in liaison with training personnel, to ensure competences and training needs are met by the operating support worker who undertakes this new role.

Pirie (2005), states that the PCC recommends a thorough risk assessment of each potential procedure that may be delegated to a support worker in the scrub role. It is advisable and essential that all practitioners are aware of their limitations with these new developments and that practitioners are not pressured to undertake more duties than those detailed in the policy.

This is a controversial issue as qualified practitioners are taking responsibility for the theatre support worker during their scrub role. All perioperative practitioners' roles (qualified and ancillary) are expanding but guidelines and policies must be in place and training and support must be given to all the support workers undertaking this new role.

The first assistant

A first assistant is a registered nurse providing skilled assistance under the direct supervision of the surgeon. At no time will the nurse undertake an activity that may be described as surgical intervention (NATN 1993).

A scrub practitioner who gains experience and competence in the scrub discipline may undertake the further role of the first assistant. He or she should never undertake the dual role of scrub practitioner and first assistant. The first assistant assists the surgeon when there is no junior doctor to help the surgeon with the surgical procedure.

Their roles and responsibilities include:

- Swab and drape the patient before the surgical procedure.
- Assist with haemostasis in order to secure and maintain a clear operating field: excluding applying haemostats, ligation and applying active electrosurgical electrodes to tissue.
- Assist with the cutting of sutures and ligatures.
- Retract tissues and/or organs.
- Handle tissue.
- Handle instruments.
- Perform skin closure by suture or clip but excluding deep tension sutures.

The National Association of Theatre Nurses (1993) states that nurses who adjust their scope of individual practice should ensure that they follow the NMC principles for their scope of practice; and should consider their competence to undertake these duties. There are university courses to achieve competence for this role but many operating rooms offer an in-house training programme. Practitioners must be aware of their local policies, legal accountability, vicarious liability and must keep up to date with clinical issues.

The first assistant course is not a new concept to (operating room) practitioners, having traditionally been within the remit of the scrub practitioner. However, with increasing awareness of legal issues and ethical implications the roles clearly need to be defined and separated from each other (PCC 2003).

The operating room support worker

There are different names for the unqualified practitioner who cares for the operating room equipment. They can be named assistant operating room practitioner, operating room technician or operating room orderly.

Their roles and responsibilities include:

- Check, prepare and monitor the relevant equipment and accessories for the surgical procedures on the operative list following manufacturer's recommendations and local policies.
- Position patients safely on the operating room table.
- Maintain the patient's dignity and ensure the patient's limbs are free from pressure and the patient is comfortable.
- Prepare and clean the theatre at the relevant times and ensure the waste bags, linen and needle sharp boxes are available following local policies of infection control, waste management and health and safety.

Operating room orderlies

Orderlies are the first members of the operating room team to meet the patient. They can help allay the patients' fear and anxieties with effective communication.

Their roles and responsibilities include:

- Collect patients from the ward and return them after their surgical procedure.
- Take the patients' specimens to the pathology department.
- Collect blood or blood products from the pathology department following local policies.
- Collect and return any relevant equipment to the hospital departments when necessary.

Reception practitioners

Qualified anaesthetic practitioners or ancillary practitioners can undertake this role.

Their roles and responsibilities include:

- Ask the porters to collect patients from the relevant wards.
- Greet patients on their arrival in the operating room reception area.
- Allay the patients' fears and anxieties with effective communication.
- Check their identification in line with the operative list.
- Check the preoperative document and request any missing information for the anaesthetic practitioner.
- Monitor the patient's physiological readings if relevant.
- Communicate with the patients while they are waiting for their surgical procedures.

Anaesthetic practitioners

Nurses qualify and undertake an in-house anaesthetic training programme on entry to the operating department before they work autonomously within this role. Operating department practitioners undertake the anaesthetic discipline during their 3 years' training and can work autonomously immediately after qualification. Both types of practitioner are supported by their senior colleagues during their first few months of practice.

Their roles and responsibilities include:

- Prepare, check and stock the anaesthetic equipment and accessories for the anaesthetist for the operative list.
- Prepare equipment for the relevant technique of anaesthesia for each patient. Preparation is the key to effective anaesthetic practice.

- Undertake the preoperative checklist and inform the anaesthetist of any patient allergies, loose teeth etc.
- Assist the anaesthetist to establish and maintain anaesthesia.
- Complete the patient documentation to identify patient care throughout the anaesthetic phase.
- Give an effective handover to the recovery practitioner.

The roles and responsibilities of the anaesthetic practitioner are further discussed in Chapter 8.

Recovery practitioners

Nurses qualify and undertake an in-house recovery training programme on entry to the operating department before they work autonomously within this role. Operating department practitioners undertake the recovery discipline within their 3 years training and can work autonomously immediately after qualification. Both types of practitioner are supported by their senior colleagues during their first few months of practice.

Their roles and responsibilities include:

- Prepare, check and stock all relevant recovery equipment before patients arrive in the recovery area.
- Check the patient's airway and maintain it throughout their stay in the recovery area.
- Monitor the patient's physiological readings, intravenous infusion, dressing, drain, catheter, stoma, oxygen therapy and any other surgical or anaesthetic intervention.
- Communicate with the anaesthetic team, patient, carer and the ward nurse.
- Complete effective documentation of the recovery care of the patient.
- Give an efficient handover, to the ward nurse, of the patient's care throughout the operating room environment and the anaesthetist's and surgeon's instructions for the patient's postoperative care.

The roles and responsibilities of the recovery practitioner are further discussed in Chapter 9.

Both anaesthetic and recovery practitioners who acquire experience and competence within their operating room disciplines may undertake further roles within their practice. They undertake all these roles following local policies.

These roles include:

- Intravenous cannulation.
- Administration of intravenous drugs.
- Administration of boluses for patient's pain management machines (patient controlled analgesia (PCA) and epidural machines).
- Programming of pain management machines: patient controlled administration machines (PCAs and epidural machines).

The non-medical anaesthetist

Several recent reports have focused on the need to improve the efficiency of operating departments (Audit Commission 2002). Due to the European Time Directive and its implications for the reduction in doctors' hours, non-medical practitioners have been considered for a role in anaesthesia, in line with the expanding roles being introduced within the operating room environment.

Within Europe nurse anaesthetists undertake the direct care of the patient, chiefly during the maintenance of anaesthesia. An anaesthetist supervises them when they establish and reverse anaesthesia.

In the United States of America there are two types of nurse anaesthetists: certified registered nurse anaesthetists (CRNAs) and anaesthetic assistants (AAs). The CRNA may undertake relatively independent anaesthetic practice under the supervision of a non-anaesthetist (surgeon or general practitioner) and the AA is supervised on a 1:2 basis as are the majority of CRNAs in large hospitals when they practise anaesthesia. An anaesthetist, again, is present when they establish and reverse anaesthesia.

Rod (2003) believes that a nurse anaesthetist is someone who 'provides or participates in the provision of specialist nursing and anaesthetic services to patients requiring anaesthesia, resuscitation or any other life sustaining interventions'.

The Royal College of Anaesthetists, in collaboration with the Changing Workforce Programme, undertook visits to several countries (Sweden, Holland and the United States of America) and their views on non-medical anaesthetists were highlighted in their report in 2003.

Pilot schemes for non-medical anaesthetists have been commenced in Salford, Northumbria, Royal Devon and Exeter, Morecambe Bay, and Birmingham. This is to support New Ways of Working in Anaesthesia (NWWA) and the term 'Anaesthetic and Critical Care Practitioner' (A&CCP) is used to distinguish the non-medical anaesthetist role from other similar roles in the United Kingdom and abroad (RCA 2003). It will be interesting to see how this role develops in the next few years.

CHANGE MANAGEMENT

Changes can be political, economic, social, technological, legislative or environmental. It is important to acknowledge and respond to changes and identify ways of communicating changes to all NHS practitioners.

Efficient change management results in the successful implementation of change by practitioners in the organisation, systems, procedures or work practices. Managers need to have commitment to the changes, integrity and effective negotiation and communication skills to ensure that practitioners adopt the changes without too many problems. Problems of acceptance of the change can be resistance to change, poor communication and possible stress to all parties.

To accept change all practitioners need to have an awareness of the reasons for the change and the benefits that it can bring them. Commitment and communication need to be effective to achieve success. Effective communication on the reasons and strategies for achieving the change can make practitioners more receptive to change. Any change in working practices or threats to job security may meet with opposition and reduce job satisfaction. Managers need support and commitment and a willingness to listen to the reasons for the change from the practitioners. Time should be allowed to secure a discussion for the timetable of potential changes; and practitioners need to own the changes and feel that they have had an input into the final implementation.

Marriner-Tomey (1996) believes that resistance to change can be reduced by informing personnel of the reasons for change, especially when the advantages of the change are stressed. Personnel can be involved by requests for their input, including feelings, suggestions, and talents; their negative as well as positive feelings should be respected. Communicating honestly about the changes, giving specific feedback, asking what assistance is needed to help them cope and recognising their contributions to the implementation of the change can further minimise resistance.

Change agents may help to introduce the change and liaise with all parties. They have an understanding for the need of the change and its ultimate success. They can help by:

- introducing reasons for the change;
- analysing how practitioners will react;
- encouraging a working environment conducive to change and for the practitioners to 'own' the change;
- creating an environment for progression of change;
- advising on communication strategies for the change;
- facilitating meetings or sessions to explain the change and strategies to overcome opposition;
- facilitating training if necessary;
- providing facilities for reviewing and developing change;
- developing performance measures to enable progress of change.

Possible management change issues that operating room practitioners may encounter:

- operating room aims and objectives;
- organisational structure – change of manager or teams;
- communication – lack of support of senior management;
- changes in practice;
- roles and responsibilities;
- operating lists, sessions and specialities;
- skill mix;
- new technology;

- retention and recruitment;
- delivery of patient care;
- reimbursement of pay.

Recent changes within the NHS are the empowerment of patients and the public, and the extension of traditional roles undertaken by all practitioners, both qualified and unqualified.

The Agenda for Change is a new pay system for all NHS practitioners and was introduced by the Government in 2004. It introduces standard arrangements for hours, annual leave and overtime. The government believes it rewards all practitioners for any new responsibilities they undertake to improve patient care.

The knowledge and skills framework (KSF) incorporated in the Agenda for Change works in conjunction with the practitioner's annual personal development review or plan (PDR or PDP), helps to identify and develop skills and knowledge, and supports lifelong learning throughout his or her career. Each practitioner has a KSF outline and has core and specific dimensions of practice to achieve. Experience and the job description determine the pay band of the individual practitioner. An annual PDR or PDP identifies the practitioner's development needs and clear objectives to progress through the gateways on their band (these are after one year in post and between the three top points on the band).

NHS practitioners are involved with the process of developing the job descriptions, KSF post-outlines and pay banding. It may be a contentious issue to many practitioners, and managers must communicate changes to their practitioners effectively.

CLINICAL GOVERNANCE

The government introduced clinical governance in the DOH White Paper, *A New NHS, Modern and Dependable* in 1997. Its aim was to introduce self-regulation and accountability of care issues for the NHS.

Clinical governance is a system through which NHS organisations are accountable for continuously improving the quality of their services and safeguarding high standards of care by creating an environment in which excellence in clinical care will flourish (Scally & Donaldson 1998).

The Commission for Health Improvement (CHI) was set up in 2001 and its aim was to improve the quality of patient care and address any unacceptable variations in care. It had four remits, to:

- assess NHS organisations, undertake clinical governance reviews and make its findings public;
- conduct investigations into serious failures within the NHS;
- check that the NHS follows national guidelines;
- advise on best practice within the NHS.

The introduction of clinical governance, assessed by CHI, aimed to ensure that patients receive the highest quality of care possible, to monitor patient services and to improve these services if necessary.

These measures should create an improvement of patient services and care, a patient-centred approach to care, a commitment to quality, the prevention of errors and a commitment for all NHS practitioners to learn from mistakes. All hospitals take responsibility for the quality of patient care and work in partnership with allied agencies of health care to achieve this. Hospital boards are accountable for their clinical performance and are audited by government agencies to ensure all practitioners and patients have an involvement in quality care for patients and their relatives.

Their commitment to the evaluation of patient care is independent and supports the continuous improvement of care. Patients' views and reports are available to all to dissect and review and to assist improvements across all specialities and hospital and community services.

Government agencies

The government created the following to ensure commitment to patient healthcare and commitment to clinical governance:

- the National Institute for Clinical Excellence;
- the Commission for Healthcare Audit and Inspection;
- the Modernisation Agency;

- the National Patient Safety Agency;
- Patient Advice and Liaison Service and user involvement groups;
- the Clinical Negligence Scheme for Trusts;
- performance indicators.

The National Institute for Clinical Excellence (NICE)(1999)

The NICE provides patients, health professionals and the public with authoritative, robust and reliable guidance on current 'best' practice.

The Commission for Healthcare Audit and Inspection (CHAI)

The Commission for Healthcare Audit and Inspection (CHAI) became the independent regulator of the NHS in 2002 in place of The Commission for Health Improvement (CHI) and is responsible for the NHS performance indicators of healthcare. The CHI was established to help in the improvement of quality of patient care by assisting the NHS in addressing unacceptable variations and to ensure a consistently high standard of patient care. Members of the CHI team inspected hospitals and their systems to evaluate patient care and report their findings to the hospital board.

The Modernisation Agency (2001)

This agency helps the NHS bring about improvements in services for patients and contributes to national and planning and performance improvement strategies.

The National Patient Safety Agency (NPSA) (2001)

The NPSA collects and analyses information on adverse events in the NHS, assimilates safety information from elsewhere, provides feedback to the NHS on lessons learnt, produces solutions, sets national goals and establishes mechanisms to track progress. The National Clinical Assessment Authority (2001) provides a support service to health authorities and hospital and community trusts that are faced with concerns over the performance of an individual doctor. This agency subsequently merged into NPSA.

Patient Advice and Liaison Service (PALS) and user involvement groups (2004)

PALS acts on behalf of their service users when handling patient and family concerns. PALS staff liaise with staff, managers and, where appropriate, other relevant organisations to negotiate speedy solutions and to help bring about changes to the way services are delivered.

User involvement groups include: equality and diversity, disability and discrimination, community relations, complaints, and patient and public involvement groups, which all report their views on all issues of patient care and hospital services to improve present and future patient care.

The Clinical Negligence Scheme for Trusts (1996)

This scheme handles claims and indemnifies NHS bodies in respect of both clinical negligence and non-clinical risks. They also have risk management programmes in place against which NHS Trusts are assessed. All these agencies are accountable to central government and provide effective strategies, regulate and audit patient care.

Performance Indicators

The Department of Health performance indicators are part of an intensive process of publishing information on the performance of NHS organisations in order to provide comparisons and improve performance over all NHS Trust Hospitals and Primary Care Trusts (PCTs). These indicators were first introduced in 1997.

The publication of the Kennedy Inquiry Report on the Bristol Royal Infirmary has reinforced the need to make more information on NHS performance available in more easily accessible formats (DOH 2005). Performance indicators focus on the issues that matter most to patients and the public, and are there to

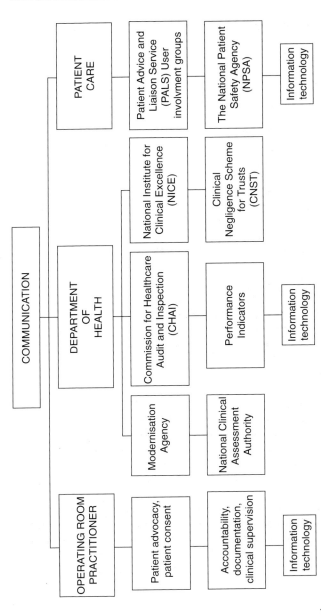

Fig. 4.1 Organisations and agencies involved in clinical governance.

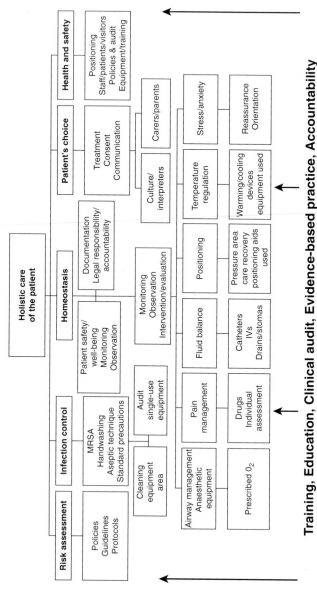

Training, Education, Clinical audit, Evidence-based practice, Accountability

Fig. 4.2 Clinical governance and effective patient care.

encourage an open and honest debate about the state of the NHS.

Perioperative practitioners deliver quality care (clinical governance strategies) to the patient with the consideration of:

- risk assessment strategies;
- incident reporting;
- evidence-based practice;
- clinical effectiveness;
- education and training and professional development;
- clinical supervision;
- effective communication;
- collaboration between allied professions.

Government policy concerned with the modernisation of the NHS has urged nurses and others working in the health services to become more collaborative, adopt a flexible approach to role boundaries and establish clear lines of accountability for the quality of clinical care. However the government's clinical governance agenda gives little recognition to the ways in which health care professions have been hierarchically ordered in the past and how these historical relationships may continue to shape multidisciplinary working in the modernised NHS (Savage & Moore 2004).

Figures 4.1 and 4.2 are examples of clinical governance and effective patient care.

CONCLUSION

Effective communication between the patient, operating room practitioner, anaesthetist and surgeon, all allied professions and NHS agencies will enhance patients', their relatives' and carers' concerns of the care delivered to them within the operating room. Patient involvement, choice and views can help the NHS to develop and shape ongoing clinical practice.

REFERENCES
Audit Commission (2002) *District Audit – Operating Theatres. A Bulletin for Health Bodies.* Audit Commission, London.

Baldwin, M. (2003) Patient advocacy: A concept analysis. *Nursing Standard* **17** (21), 33–9.

Clarke, P. & Jones, J. (1998) Organisation and management. In: Clarke, P. & Jones, J. (eds) *Brigdens Operating Department Practice.* Churchill Livingstone, Edinburgh.

Clinical Negligence Scheme for Trusts (1996) www.legislation.hmso.gov/uk.

Collins, J. (ed.) (2001) Bristol and Kennedy: The take-home messages for physicians. *Clinical Medicine* **1** (September/October), 341–3.

Commission for Health Improvement (1999) www.chi.nhs.uk.

Cummings, T.G. (1981) Designing effective work groups. Cited in: Nystrom, P.C. & Starbuck, W.H. (eds) *Handbook of Organisational Design.* Oxford University Press, Oxford.

Department of Health (1993) *A Vision for the Future. Report of the Chief Nursing Officer.* DOH, London.

Department of Health (2004) *Consent.* DOH, London.

Department of Health (2005) *NHS Performance Indicators Health Authorities.* NHS, London.

Fortunato, R. (2000) *Operating Room Technique.* Mosby, St Louis.

Hunt, G. (2005) www.freedomtocare.org/page15.htm.

Katzenbach, J. & Smith, D. (1993) *The Magic of Teams.* Harvard Business School Press, Boston.

Kavanagh, R. (2004) Consent and confusion. *British Journal of Perioperative Nursing* **14** (11), 489–91.

Leinonen, T., Leino-Kilpi, H. & Jouko, K. (1996) The quality of intraoperative nursing care: The patient's perspective. *Journal of Advanced Nursing* **24** (4), 843–52.

Mallik, M. (1997) Advocacy in nursing: A review of the literature. *Journal of Advanced Nursing* **25** (1), 130–8.

Marriner-Tomey, A. (1996) *Nursing Management and Leadership*, 5th edn. Mosby, St Louis.

Modernisation Agency (2001) www.modern.nhs.uk.

National Association of Theatre Nurses (1993) *The Role of the First Assistant.* NATN, Harrogate.

National Association of Theatre Nurses (NATN) (1998) *Principles of Safe Practice in the Perioperative Environment.* NATN, Harrogate.

National Clinical Assessment Authority (2001) www.ncaa.nhs.uk.

National Institute for Clinical Excellence (1999) www.nice.org.uk.

National Patient Safety Agency (2001) www.npsa.nhs.uk.

Nursing Midwifery Council (2002) *Code of Professional Conduct.* NMC, London.

Nursing Midwifery Council (2004a) *Accountability.* NMC, London.

Nursing Midwifery Council (2004b) *Code of Professional Conduct.* NMC, London.

Patients Advice and Liaison Services and User Involvement Groups (2004) www.equip.nhs.uk/services/pals.html.

Perioperative Care Collaborative (2003) Position statement. *British Journal of Nursing* **13** (9), Supplement PCC.

Perioperative Care Collaborative (2005) *Delegation: The Support Worker in the Scrub Role.* Harrogate PCC 2004. Optimising the Contribution of the Perioperative Support Worker. Position Statement. NATN, Harrogate.

Pirie, S. (2005) Support workers and the scrub role. *British Journal of Perioperative Nursing* **15** (1), 22–6.

Potter, P.A. & Berry, A.G. (1989) *Fundamentals of Nursing.* Mosby, St Louis.

Reporting of Injuries, Diseases and Dangerous Occurrences (RIDDOR) (1996) www.riddor.gov.uk/infocontent.html-29k.

Rod, P. (2003) Nurse Anaesthesia: Implications for the UK. Presentation given at the NATN. Managing Modernisation Conference, Olympia, London. 16–17 May.

Royal College of Anaesthetists (2003) *The Role of Non-Medical Practitioners in the Delivery of Anaesthesia Services.* R.C.A. London.

Royal College of Nursing (1992) *Guidelines on Patient Advocacy.* RCN, London.

Royal College of Nursing (2002) *Guidelines on Accountability.* RCN, London.

Royal College of Surgeons of England and Royal College of Psychiatrists (1997) *Report on the Working Party of Psychological Care of Surgical Patients.* (CR55). R.C.S. & R.C.P., London.

Smith, R. (1998) All changed, changed utterly. British medicine will be transformed by the Bristol case. *British Medical Journal* **316** (7149), 1917–18 (editorial).

Savage, J. & Moore, L. (2004) *Clinical Governance and Nursing.* Kings Fund, London.

Scally, G. & Donaldson, L. (1998) Clinical Governance and the drive for quality improvement in the new NHS in England. *British Medical Journal* **317**, 61–5.

Seedhouse, D. (1988) *The Heart of Health Care.* J. Wiley, New York.

Shields, L. & Werder, H. (2002) *Perioperative Nursing.* Greenwich Medical Media, London.

Taylor, H. (2003) An exploration of the factors that affect nurses' record keeping. *British Journal of Nursing* **12** (12), 751–4, 756–8.

Wood, J. (2004) Clinical supervision. *British Journal of Perioperative Nursing* **14** (4), 151–6.

Woodcock, M. (1982) *Team Development Manual.* Gower, Aldershot.

5 | Managing Perioperative Risks

LEARNING OUTCOMES

❏ Understand the principles of *risk assessment strategies* within the operating room.

❏ Understand the different *types of hazard* involved in risk assessment.

❏ Identify the *strategies for effective patient care* and the implications of poor practice in the following areas:
  - maintenance and use of equipment and manual handling;
  - temperature management;
  - pressure area care;
  - anaesthetic agents;
  - latex allergy;
  - smoke inhalation;
  - infection control;
  - methicillin resistant *Staphylcoccus aureus* (MRSA);
  - deep vein thrombosis (DVT).

❏ Be aware of the principles of *infection control* and the implications for the NHS if these are not observed.

RISK ASSESSMENT

Perioperative personnel like any other healthcare professionals, are personally accountable and, therefore, have a duty to do a risk assessment of all situations that may potentially cause harm to patients, or indeed, practitioners. In order to minimise any risk to patients it is essential that there is a control mechanism for authorisation of people visiting the operating department (Beesley 2005).

In the modern, highly technical operating room environment there is a need for perioperative practitioners to undertake risk management strategies to assess, monitor, control and prevent risks within their workplace. This will help retain quality practitioners, ensure patient safety and limit litigation costs in this complex and technical area. Risk assessment has an increasingly greater importance in the NHS as it grows more technical in nature. Strategies can identify danger or problems to healthcare practitioners, patients and visitors and reduce financial loss to hospitals by reducing accidents.

Mosby (2002) believes risk management is a function of the administration of a hospital or health facility. Risk management directs people to consider identification, evaluation and correction of potential risks that could lead to injury to patients, practitioners, or visitors and result in property loss or damage.

The European Commission (1996) defines the following terms:

- **Hazard** – the intrinsic property or ability of something (for example, work materials, equipment, work methods and practices) with the potential to cause harm.
- **Risk** – the likelihood that the potential for harm will be attained under the conditions of use and or exposure and the possible extent of the harm.
- **Risk assessment** – the process of evaluating risk to the health and safety of workers while at work arising from the circumstances of the occurrence of a hazard in the workplace.

The key to effective risk management strategies for all perioperative practitioners is to be able to identify, evaluate, lessen, manage and treat any potential risks within the operating room. There is a Risk Management or Health and Safety Department within each hospital to guide all employees on safe patient and healthcare practice. Each Trust devises policies that aim to prevent risks or to keep them to a minimum. Education and training are necessary to inform all practitioners of their roles and responsibilities. Perioperative practitioners should keep themselves up to date with safe practices within the operating room environment.

A risk assessment evaluates whether harm can occur because of hazards in the workplace. Health and Safety Departments in the hospitals can assess hazards and potential risks following these five steps:

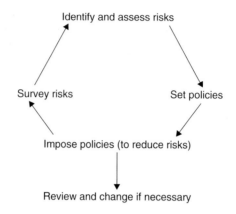

Fig. 5.1 Procedure for risk assessment.

(1) Identify the hazard and assess the harm that may occur (to practitioners, patients, carers and visitors to the operating room).
(2) Evaluate the risks.
(3) Assess existing precautions and the need for new ones.
(4) Identify risks as high, medium and low and record the results.
(5) Review and revise the assessment, if necessary, annually or whenever relevant.

Figure 5.1 provides a flowchart of this assessment process.

Managers and all members of the perioperative team have a responsibility to identify risks. Managers should:

- Encourage the perioperative team to identify and analyse potential risks in their department.
- Clarify risks and achieve better risk management strategies and results.
- Write and revise, if necessary, protocols and policies for the perioperative team to follow.
- Identify training that is necessary to ensure safe patient practices.

The effective management of risks can prevent problems from occurring and, in turn, produce efficient and cost-effective care.

Risk assessment strategies recommend procedures for technical and professional perioperative practices. The health and safety of the perioperative multidisciplinary team and patients is a responsibility of employers.

Managers should:

- Develop recommendations and guidelines, local policies and procedures, to prevent occupational hazards which might occur.
- Recommend and produce policies and guidelines for all practitioners on equipment, medical devices and holistic patient practices to deliver optimal care. These recommend and impose achievable practices and guidelines for the safety of patients and help to identify potential hazards in perioperative practice settings.

Hazards are classified under the following headings as illustrated in Box 5.1.

Preventive measures

It is important for all the perioperative team to be aware of the potential hazards within the perioperative environment. They should have knowledge of the risks, preventive measures to avoid them and the procedures to follow if an incident occurs.

Safe work practices are developed within the framework of risk identification, risk assessment and risk control. Storage and ventilation of hazardous substances is a priority and all practitioners should be aware of these issues. All members of the perioperative team should adhere to protective measures that minimise risks to and from patients and equipment. Perioperative practitioners face a wide range of occupational hazards that can create risk to themselves and to their patients.

ACCIDENTAL HAZARDS

Protective clothing and safety equipment should be available for all members of the perioperative team. The aim of the principles of standard precautions is to limit the exposure of the perioperative team to blood-borne infections and spillages of blood and bodily fluids. The transmission of viruses (hepatitis B and C, and human immunodeficiency virus (HIV)) can occur

---

Box 5.1 Classification of hazards within the operating room environment

Accidental hazards

- Needle-stick injuries from sharps: blades and needles
- Falls and slips on wet floors
- Electrical shock from equipment
- Injuries from moving patients and equipment

Physical hazards

- Exposure to radiation. X-ray machine
- Temperature control

Chemical hazards

- Anaesthetic agents
- Cleansing agents
- Chronic poisoning due to anaesthetic gases and cleansing agents chemicals
- Latex allergy – exposure to latex gloves and latex-containing devices

Biological hazards

- Exposure to blood-borne products – blood, body tissue leading to possible hepatitis B, C and HIV
- Needle-stick injury from syringe and needle – infectious hepatitis, syphilis, malaria
- Possibility of contacting palm and finger herpes (herpes whitlow)
- Increased hazard of spontaneous miscarriage

Organisational factors

- Stress

---

in several ways: by the penetration of the skin by contaminated needles, by splashing into the eye or through cuts and grazes.

These precautions recommend safe practices to protect the perioperative team and patients. Practitioners adopt these practices for each individual patient regardless of diagnosis. If practitioners observe these precautions within their practice they can reduce the risk of transmission of blood-borne diseases such as hepatitis B and C and HIV between patients and members of the perioperative team.

Hepatitis B (HepB) is a viral hepatitis caused by the virus HBV. It is transmitted by: blood or blood products, by sexual contact with an infected person or by the use of contaminated needles and instruments. Severe infection can cause prolonged illness, destruction of liver cells, cirrhosis, and increased risk of liver cancer or death. A HepB immunoglobulin, a passive immunising agent, can be prescribed for exposure to the HepB virus.

Hepatitis C (HepC) is a type of hepatitis transmitted most commonly by blood transfusion or percutaneous inoculation (sharing of needles by drug users or when they share straws for nasal inhalation of cocaine). It is transmitted less commonly by sexual intercourse. The disease progresses to chronic hepatitis in up to 80% of patients acutely infected. Human immunodeficiency virus (HIV) is a retrovirus that causes acquired immunodeficiency syndrome (AIDS). HIV is transmitted through contact with an infected individual's blood, semen, breast milk, cervical secretions, cerebrospinal fluid or synovial fluid (Mosby 2002).

Perioperative practitioners should regard all patients as potentially infectious and should adopt standard precautions in their care. The surgeon and anaesthetist will schedule patients who are known to have an infectious disease at the end of the operating list to ensure effective management of their care.

Guidelines include:

- Use of protective clothing including gowns, gloves, eye protection (goggles, glasses with side shields, face masks with visors) aprons and shoes. These all protect the perioperative team from hazardous substances and exposure to bloodborne products.
- Wash hands before and after contact with individual patients and before putting on and removing gloves.
- The surgeon should adopt double gloving if applicable.
- Cover all cuts and grazes.
- Wear gloves and other protective clothing when handling swabs, instruments and specimens.
- Clean up any spillages of blood or bodily fluids. Dispose of wipes into the clinical waste bag.
- Take care when filling the specimen containers with formalin as this can be hazardous. Practitioners should report any

accidents or spillages and take the appropriate action to ensure their health. (Normal saline should be available as an eyewash.)

- Observe safe practices with sharps, blades and needles. It is the responsibility of the individual members of the perioperative team to dispose of their own sharps.
- Use a 'hands-free' technique when handing scalpel blades or syringes and needles to the surgeon. Place them in a receiver from which the surgeon can take them and replace them after use. When two surgeons are operating each must have their own receiver.
- Rinse off excessive blood from the surgical instruments before sending the instrument sets to the Hospital Sterilisation and Decontamination Unit (HSDU).
- Dispose of all protective wear in the clinical waste bin and linen bag. Each patient has an individual bag or bags and the perioperative practitioner can identify the clinical waste bag by an individual number which matches the patient's linen bag.

To prevent exposure to blood and bodily fluids and needle-stick injuries from sharps (blades and needles) all perioperative practitioners should follow their 'local sharps policy.' Members of the perioperative team should handle, remove or dispose of any sharps safely in a sharps container. They should:

- Avoid sharps use where possible.
- Place the sharps bin near the point of use if possible (anaesthetists undertaking venous and arterial cannulation).
- Take responsibility when using sharps and during their disposal into the sharps bin. If other practitioners dispose of the sharps or needles they should inform the user of their disposal.
- Not resheathe, bend or break needles before disposal.
- Change the sharps bin when it is three-quarters full and replace it. No member of the perioperative team should ever put their hands in the sharps bin to recover any item.

If perioperative practitioners suffer a needle-stick injury they must follow their local policy. They have to gain the patient's consent to take a sample of their blood for testing. If the patient undergoes a general anaesthetic it is important to wait several hours until the patient is fully awake and *compos mentis* before a member of the perioperative team informs the patient of the incident. The patient has the right to refuse. The practitioner also informs the Occupational Health Department and completes an incident report to the operating room manager.

It is essential that there is effective communication between all relevant departments. If there is a positive exposure to an infectious virus of a member of the perioperative team, professional counselling and follow-up services should be available.

Standard precautions are summarised in Box 5.2.

Box 5.2   Standard precautions

Gown, apron, shoes

- Wear these when necessary to protect yourself from blood and bodily fluids.
- Dispose of them in the clinical waste bag after use.

Gloves

- Wear gloves before handling blood or bodily fluids.
- **Do not** go from one care intervention to another on the same patient wearing the same gloves.
- Dispose of the gloves in the clinical waste bag after use.

Eye protection

- Wear a face mask with visor, goggles, and glasses with side shields to protect you from any splashes of blood or bodily fluids.
- Dispose of them in the clinical waste bag after use.

Cuts and grazes

- Cover all cuts and grazes.
- Protect your skin from any infection.
- Wear gloves if relevant.
- After use wash your hands.

Sharps: blades or needles

- Dispose of sharps in a sharps bin according to local policy.
- Wear gloves if relevant.
- After use wash your hands.

Waste and linen

- Dispose of clinical waste following local policy.
- Dispose of linen in a red alginate bag (water soluble) and a laundry bag.

Cont.

> **Box 5.2** *Continued.*
>
> - Wear gloves if appropriate.
> - After use wash your hands.
>
> *Equipment*
>
> - Wear gloves and appropriate clothing when cleaning equipment.
>
> *Cleaning the theatre*
>
> - Clean the operating table and any relevant equipment between operations.
> - Use mops for floors. Clean them following local policies.
> - Use warning signs to advise the perioperative team of wet floors.
>
> *Specimens*
>
> - Wear appropriate clothing when handling specimens and specimen containers.
>
> WASH HANDS:
>
> - Before and after individual patient care.
> - Before setting up a trolley using an aseptic technique.
> - After contact with blood or bodily fluids.
> - Before handling food.
> - After personal contact (blowing your nose or visiting the toilet).

MAINTENANCE OF EQUIPMENT

Perioperative practitioners use, clean and store all medical equipment following the manufacturer's instructions and receive training on how to operate it and care for it. Any faults are reported to the appropriate practitioner and they ensure that the Medical Electronic Department check it before reuse. Appropriate documentation is completed to ensure effective tracking of faulty equipment following local policies. The management provide service agreements for all equipment.

Perioperative practitioners should report any faults in electrical equipment to avoid the hazard of electrical shock. All practitioners must be aware of the location and use of emergency equipment. They must attend annual mandatory lectures on resuscitation, fire and manual handling.

MANUAL HANDLING

It is the employer's responsibility to ensure that all their employees are not exposed to a foreseeable risk of injury from manual handling as set out in the Health and Safety at Work

Etc. Act, 1974 and the Manual Handling Operations Regulations, 1992 (HSE 1992). Employer's measures to minimise risks for practitioners are to:

- implement a local policy;
- induct all new practitioners;
- provide annual mandatory manual handling tutorials and training on new equipment;
- identify personnel's health problems and injuries from manual handling.

Employee's responsibilities are to:

- take reasonable care with own and patient safety during manual handling;
- use equipment in accordance with local policy;
- have sufficient personnel present when transferring patients;
- report any incidents involving patients or perioperative personnel;
- attend an annual mandatory lecture on manual handling.

Factors that predispose practitioners to injury during patient handling:

- lifting patients;
- working in an awkward, unstable or crouched position including bending toward, sideways or twisting the body;
- lifting with a starting (or finishing) position near the floor, or overhead or at arm's length;
- handling an uncooperative patient or falling patient (RCN 1996).

The perioperative team coordinates the transfer of the patient from the operating trolley to the operating room table and vice versa following their local policy. The aim of patient positioning is to provide optimal exposure of the surgical operative site and also to prevent any complications to the patient caused by nerve or tissue damage.

There should always be a sufficient number of the team available to transfer the patient to ensure their safety and that of the perioperative team. Practitioners should not move the patient until this is achievable. They should consult their operating room coordinator or person-in-charge. All members of the operating room team have individual and collective responsibility for patient well-being (Wilson 1995).

Burden (1993) states that proper positioning ensures correct anatomical alignment and avoids any circulatory or nerve impairment and there should be no pressure on bony prominences or nerves and little on skin. The following points ensure patient safety:

- Arms are not hyper-extended past 90° to prevent brachial plexus injury.
- No body parts extend over the edge of the operating room table or trolley.
- Unprotected body parts are not touching metal or unpadded surfaces.
- Patient's legs in supine position remain uncrossed.
- Place pillow between patient's legs in lateral position.
- Patient's legs are moved into lithotomy poles simultaneously by two people.
- Use a patient-moving device. Never pull or push an unconscious patient.

The transfer

- There should be effective communication with patients:
  - if they are awake, sedated under regional anaesthesia to inform them of the transfer procedure;
  - between the perioperative team for general anaesthetic patients.
- The patient trolley should be as near to the operating room table as possible and in the correct position for the identified patient position.
- Anaesthetists should coordinate the transfer as they are in charge of the patient's airway and have an overall view of the patient in the transfer.
- The team should be aware of any intravenous infusions, catheters, arterial and or central venous pressure lines etc., medical problems or injuries (unstable limb fractures, arthritis etc.) of the patient before surgery and they should take these into consideration during the transfer.

- Practitioners should use appropriate aids to relieve pressure on the patient's nerves and tissues.

Whichever transfer equipment the perioperative team uses during transfer they must ensure they support the patient's head and feet and do not drag the patient across from the operating room patient trolley to the operating room table. Effective moving and handling of patients has a role to play in the prevention of pressure areas for perioperative patients. Uncoordinated or ineffective transfer can result in patient discomfort, tissue damage or formation of pressure sores.

PRESSURE AREAS

Pressure sores are an unwanted complication of in-patient care. All surgical patients are at risk during their ward stay and perioperative journey. There is the possibility of reduced mobility as a result of circulatory and metabolic changes from anaesthesia and surgery. Pressure sores may result from compromised circulation over bony prominences, nerves or other pressure points when the practitioner and operating room team position the patient.

Pressure sores can adversely affect the recovery of patients postoperatively and can have cost implications for the hospital and patients, causing stress to themselves and their families. Caring for patients with pressure sores costs the NHS in excess of £250 million each year. There is a great personal cost to the individual in the form of pain, discomfort, a reduction in the quality of life and the potential threat to life (Arblaster 1998).

Forest (2001) suggests the NHS spends an estimated £45 million per year on equipment directly related to the prevention and management of pressure ulcers. Tissue viability nurses are helping to develop policies, protocols and guidelines for healthcare practitioners to prevent the development of pressure sores and ulcers; to manage patient care; and in the use of relevant pressure relieving equipment.

Extrinsic factors

Three factors that can influence the development of pressure sores are pressure, shearing and friction.

Pressure

Pritchard & Mallett (1993), state the blood pressure at the arterial end of the capillaries is approximately 30 mmHg while at the venous end this drops to 10 mmHg (the average mean capillary pressure equals about 17 mmHg (Guyton 1984)). Any external pressure exceeding this will cause capillary obstruction so that tissues depending on these capillaries are deprived of their blood supply. Eventually the ischaemic tissues will die (Waterlow 1985; David 1986; Department of Infection Control, Memorial Hospital 1989; Johnson 1989). However research has demonstrated that with constant pressure a critical period of 1–2 hours exists before pathological changes occur (Kosiak 1958; 1976).

Shearing

Shearing can occur when the operating room team have to adjust the patient's position on the operating table, for example, if they drag the patient up the table instead of lifting shearing can occur. Pritchard & Mallett (1993) believe as the skeleton moves over the underlying tissue the microcirculation is destroyed and the tissues die of anoxia. In more serious cases lymphatic vessels and muscle fibres may also become torn, resulting in a deep pressure ulcer (Waterlow 1985; Department of Infection Control, Memorial Hospital 1989; Johnson 1989).

Friction

Pritchard and Mallett (1993) believe that friction is a component of shearing which causes stripping of the stratum corneum leading to superficial ulceration (Waterlow 1985; Johnson 1989).

Intrinsic factors

Intrinsic factors that affect the development of pressure sores in the perioperative patient include: age, level of consciousness, immobility, medical conditions (e.g. vascular disease and diabetes) malnutrition, previous pressure damage, chronic or terminal illness, smoking, alcohol abuse, neurological disease, impaired circulation and moisture. Regional anaesthesia and anaesthetic drugs may also be contributing factors.

Peritoneal washout may cause the patient's canvas to be damp postoperatively and the perioperative team should either change the canvas or remove it (and dry the patient's skin) before the transfer of the patient into the recovery area.

Bliss & Simini (1999) believe that pressure sores should be viewed as the result of yet another organ failure – that of peripheral circulation which can cause tissue damage. They assert that the prevention and management of peripheral circulatory failure, both inside and outside the operating room should become part of doctors' training or else pressure injuries will continue to torture patients and keep their carers busy when it is too late.

Despite surgical patients' vulnerability, they do not all develop pressure sores during their perioperative journey. Waterlow (1985) states the operating room is, however, sometimes seen as the cause of any pressure sores that a surgical patient might develop. Underweight and overweight patients undergoing lengthy surgical procedures may be more at risk. It is practitioners' responsibility to minimise this risk. The NMC (2004) Code of Professional Conduct states that a registered nurse must act always in such a manner as to promote and safeguard the interests and well-being of patients and clients and maintain and improve professional knowledge and competence. The Association of Operating Department Practitioners' Code of Conduct (2003), superseded by the Health Professions Council, states that an ODP must at all times let no action or omission place at risk the care afforded to any patient.

The preoperative checklist should identify the patient's vulnerability to pressure sores. An assessment of the patient's skin is essential on arrival in the operating room. Anaesthetic practitioners should assess the patient's skin integrity (heels, sacrum, elbows, shoulders, toes and any other area of the body where protection is necessary to prevent pressure occurring. They should document any problems on the patient's care plan before the surgical procedure begins. They maintain the patient's dignity and privacy during transfer to the operating room table and inspect the patient's skin for any redness, discoloration, oedema, local indurations or pressure ulcer formation already present. If they use any pressure relieving equipment they will record its use in conjunction with the recognised pressure-sore scale. If patients are wearing anti-embolism stockings practitioners will check that they fit properly and no pressure is placed on their skin. Stockings should be removed if necessary.

The perioperative team will position patients to avoid pressure, shearing or friction and any damage to their limbs or nerves. The operating room table should have a pressure-relieving mattress. All operating room table accessories should be made of suitable padding material to alleviate any pressure on the patient's body: heels, arms or head or relevant area. Practitioners should follow local policies and manufacturer's recommendations in the use, cleaning and storage of these accessories.

Prevention of pressure sores involves moving the patient frequently to relieve pressure on the limbs and circulation. Practitioners cannot alter the patient's position once the surgical procedure commences unless for access for the surgeon. Therefore it is essential to position the patient correctly before surgery.

The perioperative team will inspect and assess the patient's skin for any deterioration during the surgical procedure. Practitioners will then record the results on the patient's care plan and hand over this information to the recovery practitioner.

Flanagan (1995) states that the identification of risk factors has helped the healthcare professional understand in more detail the complex aetiology of pressure sore formation. Pressure sore risk assessment scales represent an attempt to determine an individual's risk status by quantifying a range of the most commonly recognised risk factors affecting the patient at a given time. There are many risk assessment scales for practitioners to use: Norton *et al*. 1962; Gosnell 1973; The Pressure Sore Prediction Scale 1975; Waterlow 1985; and Braden & Bergstrom 1989.

The Waterlow Score remains the most widely used risk assessment tool in the United Kingdom as it has raised awareness of pressure sore prevention and offers practical guidelines for the management of patients. It was developed as a result of a pressure sore audit and its design offers guidelines on the selection and use of preventative equipment and dressings. It includes a pressure sore classification model which can help to improve consistency when grading and auditing tissue breakdown. The Gosnell and Braden Scales are incorporated in the assessing and preventing of pressure sores (Flanagan 1995).

Perioperative practitioners should attend mandatory annual manual handling lectures and be able to position patients correctly following hospital local policies and guidelines. There should be relevant training in pressure sore or ulcer assessment and prevention, which identifies the risk factors, skin assessment and care, the use of pressure-relieving equipment and documentation of care. The prevention and management of pressure sores remains a high priority for all healthcare workers. In the operating room all members of the operating room team aim to reduce patients' vulnerability to pressure area formation. Pressure relieving equipment plays an important role in the prevention and treatment of pressure sores.

RADIATION HAZARDS

To protect ovaries, testes or thyroid all members of the perioperative team use protective x-ray shields for themselves or the patient when radiological procedures are in progress. They handle, clean and replace the shields following local policy to ensure their maximum efficiency. The x-ray technician should never take an x-ray if any member of the perioperative team is not wearing a shield. Pregnant practitioners should not be present in the operating room when the patient undergoes x-rays.

If it is necessary to use x-ray equipment in the recovery room it is essential that protective shields are worn by all recovery practitioners and patients, if appropriate. No other patient should be in the recovery room during this procedure.

NATN (1998) states that only authorised personnel who are trained and assessed may use x-ray equipment. It is their responsibility to ensure a safe environment for all patients and practitioners present.

TEMPERATURE CONTROL

Patients need to maintain their normal temperature at 37°C to ensure their organs function efficiently. The induction of anaesthesia can alter this temperature, either by raising it (malignant hyperthermia), or by lowering it (hypothermia).

Malignant hyperthermia

The use of volatile anaesthetic agents or muscle relaxants can trigger malignant hyperthermia (MH). Allmann & Wilson (2001) identify that MH can be triggered by the use of suxamethonium combined with anaesthetic vapours.

The symptoms can cause muscle rigidity, tachycardia, unstable blood pressure and a rapidly increasing temperature. In order to combat this, anaesthetists discontinue the use of the anaesthetic agents and muscle relaxant and oxygenate (100% oxygen) the patient. They intubate the patient if necessary; administer dantrolene sodium to reduce the rapidly increasing temperature; use ice packs to help to reduce the temperature; and monitor this during treatment.

Hypothermia

All surgical patients are vulnerable, during the intraoperative phase, to hypothermia, which is a recognised complication of anaesthesia (Sessler 1997), when normal thermoregulation is inhibited. There is strong research that patient outcomes will improve if the anaesthetic team prevents hypothermia. Over 70% of surgical patients experience postoperative hypothermia every year (Augustine 1990).

Hypothermia can be a result of impaired thermoregulation. The patient's temperature can decrease because anaesthesia inhibits the protective reflexes that generate heat (shivering). It also depresses the thermoregulating centre in the hypothalamus, decreases the basal metabolic rate and increases vasodilatation for heat loss by radiation and conduction. The exposure to the operating room environment (temperature and humidity) when the perioperative team open and close the operating room doors, movement of personnel, the surgical excision and skin preparation products can all help to decrease the patient's core temperature.

Hypothermia can cause cardiovascular problems. Accurate recording of the patient's temperature is, therefore, essential to detect this problem. Anaesthetists recognise inadvertent or unintended hypothermia as a complication of anaesthesia. It is not usual for core temperatures to drop to less than 35°C. All surgical patients are at risk of intraoperative hypothermia and anaesthetists estimate that, if no preventative action is taken, 70% of all patients suffer from its effects during the immediate postoperative periods (Augustine 1990), although this figure may be as high as 85% (Richards 1989). Scott & Buckland (2004) identify that it is clear that patients having the abdominal cavity opened or undergoing fluid irrigation or infusion, are at risk of intraoperative hypothermia if no preventative action is taken.

Anaesthetists and anaesthetic practitioners usually measure the patient's temperature with a probe which they position in the patient's nasopharynx or oesophagus. Recovery practitioners may also use tympanic temperature monitors. To minimise and help to prevent hypothermia the practitioner can begin care in the reception area and continue it throughout the anaesthetic room, theatre and recovery area. This is illustrated in Box 5.3.

Box 5.3   Temperature management by the perioperative practitioner

Reception

- Correct temperature of room
- The use of blankets to ensure the patient is warm

Anaesthetic room

- Blankets
- Warmed intravenous fluids

Theatre

- Correct temperature and humidity
- Remove patient covers only before surgical procedure
- Limit exposure to surgical site only
- Warm irrigating fluids
- Warmed intravenous fluids
- Forced air skin surface warmer, e.g. Bair Hugger
- Full monitoring including body temperature

Recovery

- Warmed intravenous fluids
- Forced air skin surface warmer, e.g. Bair Hugger
- Full monitoring including body temperature

Patients who are hypothermic on admission to the recovery area may have a prolonged recovery and elderly patients can be at high risk of this anaesthetic and surgical complication. It is one of most important roles of anaesthetic practitioners to maintain the patients' temperature regulation throughout their perioperative journey. They have a responsibility to be aware of all the complications that can occur, and the correct treatment of hypothermia.

CHEMICAL HAZARDS

The Health and Safety Executive (HSE) (2002) states that the law requires employers to control exposure to hazardous substances in order to prevent ill health. They have to protect both employees and others who may be exposed by complying with The Control of Substances Hazardous to Health (COSHH) Regulations (2002). All members of the perioperative team should adhere to COSHH Regulations, which were introduced in 1988 and revised in 2002 by the HSE.

Dimond (2002) believes that all healthcare workers have responsibilities under these regulations. The practitioner has a responsibility to be aware of the hazards and to take care in their use; and if negligent is liable for prosecution. Also any injury caused as a result of failure by the employer can result in a civil action and compensation can ensue.

The HSE (1999) issued guidance on the implementation of the regulations and recommended a seven-stage assessment guide for hazardous substances:

- Identify hazardous substances in the work area and assess the risks to the employees' health.
- Decide the precautions to take with their use.
- Prevent exposure if possible or control the exposure.
- Follow safe practices with their use.
- Monitor their use and exposure to employees.
- Carry out health surveillance where necessary.
- Ensure all employees are aware of the hazards and safe use of the identified substances.

In the operating room environment practitioners will identify all hazardous substances and make an assessment to identify potential risks and preventive measures to limit these. Regular monitoring and documentation are necessary and named members of the perioperative team are responsible for this. They identify the hazardous substances in the operating room, which include anaesthetic vaporising agents and gases, cleansing agents, disinfectants and sterilants, and tissue preservatives.

To ensure safe practice all perioperative practitioners should store and use these products in the correct manner following local policies, wear protective attire if appropriate (standard precautions), and take care in their use. They will follow local policies if any spillages of anaesthetic agents occur. They will take care when they change any gas cylinders following local policies and manufacturer's instructions.

Anaesthetic gases and agents

There has been considerable controversy regarding the risk to practitioners of atmospheric pollution by anaesthetic gases and vapours. Earlier investigations suggested that perioperative practitioners are more likely than other hospital personnel to suffer from hepatic and neurological symptoms and for their children to have an increased risk of congenital abnormality. However none of these problems has been substantiated. There was more convincing evidence from earlier studies that female practitioners who worked in the operating department during the early months of pregnancy suffered an increased incidence of spontaneous abortion. However, the most recent comprehensive and randomised prospective investigation of practitioners failed to demonstrate any increased health risk (Aitkenhead & Smith 1996).

Perioperative practitioners must ensure that the scavenging system is working effectively. Female practitioners may have the choice to work in another area in the hospital in their first trimester if they have any concerns with their pregnancy.

LATEX ALLERGY

Latex is a natural substance which occurs in the sap of the rubber tree (*Hevea brasiliensis*). A water-soluble protein in natural latex contains an antigen that can cause a potentially fatal allergic response. Latex allergy is an allergic reaction to one or more of the components of natural rubber latex products. There are three reactions: irritation, delayed sensitivity (type IV) and immediate hypersensitivity (type I).

Irritation
Irritation is a non-allergic reaction which is usually reversible. A dry and itchy rash may occur after wearing gloves that contain natural rubber latex. Symptoms disappear or fade after discontinuation of use.

Delayed hypersensitivity
The accelerating agents used in the glove manufacturing process can cause contact dermatitis on the hands after glove use. This can appear after several hours and last for 24–48 hours. Further exposure can cause a further a rash that extends beyond the glove area.

Immediate hypersensitivity
This is a response to the protein in the natural rubber latex. It can produce a reaction after 5–30 minutes of latex exposure. The reaction will decrease after discontinuation of the latex contact. Local oedema can occur and, if the natural rubber latex comes in contact with mucous membranes, respiratory difficulties and anaphylactic shock can occur. Repetitive contact with latex can cause sensitisation. The signs and symptoms of the anaphylactic shock are hypotension, tachycardia, bronchospasm and generalised erythema.

Latex allergy and healthcare
Most of the surgical sterile gloves that the surgical scrub team wear are of natural rubber latex. All members of the multidisciplinary perioperative team may show signs of sensitivity to latex with frequent glove use. There is a risk of airborne exposure to latex allergens during the donning of gloves procedure with prepowdered gloves. Practitioners should be aware of this possibility through inhalation and direct contact with the glove powder.

Latex allergy can be a serious occupational hazard for people working in healthcare settings because they are repeatedly exposed to products containing latex. Since so many clinical products contain latex, patients who are sensitised to latex or are predisposed to developing a latex allergy are also at risk. For practitioners, latex allergy can lead to chronic ill health, early retirement and, in extreme cases, death. Employers must bear the cost of increased sick leave, the loss of skilled practitioners and possibly the costs of injury benefit and personal injury litigation (Royal College of Nursing 1999).

The Medical Device Agency in response to concern regarding the emergence of latex allergy issued a bulletin: *Latex Sensitisation in the Health Care Setting* (MDA 1996). The aims of this bulletin were to advise all healthcare practitioners of the increase in reports of the incidence of latex allergy, emphasise the importance of the identification of latex sensitisation, provide information on latex and other gloves used in the healthcare settings, and advise on the implementation of local policies to address this issue.

Under Health and Safety Law (Health and Safety at Work Etc. Act 1974) employers have a responsibility to reduce or remove risk as far as is reasonably practicable to establish and maintain a natural rubber latex safe environment. For this reason the NHS providers and Trust hospitals have taken this health risk seriously and local policies are in place to minimise the risk to both patients and practitioners. Measures introduced into local policy to minimise this risk are:

Practitioners:

- To have a protocol and policy for latex allergy.
- To increase the awareness of the health risks of latex.
- To educate all practitioners of these risks.
- To reduce the use of powdered latex gloves and have non-latex gloves for latex allergy patients. The awareness of healthcare practitioners of the potential risks of glove use and the introduction of local policies will assist in the control and decrease the prevalence of latex sensitisation and allergy.
- To purchase non-latex equipment. To identify within the operating room items of equipment (surgical and anaesthetic) that are latex-free.

- To support and testing of practitioners in liaison with Occupational Health departments.
- To advise management and practitioners of any adjustments to their perioperative practice.
- To arrange mandatory resuscitation lectures and guidelines for anaphylactic reactions.

Patients:

- Preoperative patient assessment by anaesthetists. This will identify patients who have a latex allergy.
- Preparation of the theatre for the latex allergy patient following local policy.
- Effective communication of the multidisciplinary perioperative team.
- Resuscitation equipment available.

Preparation for a latex allergy patient

- All equipment containing latex is removed from the operating room.
- Instrument sets assessed by the HSDU and identified as latex-free.
- Non-latex gloves provided for the perioperative scrub team.
- Resuscitation drugs are available.
- Effective communication between the perioperative team – all are aware of the status of the patient.
- The patient is recovered within the operating room.

The National Association of Theatre Nurses (NATN) has published a resource *Understanding Latex in the Perioperative Setting* and this acts as a reference source for all perioperative practitioners.

BIOLOGICAL HAZARDS

The risks to healthcare workers of occupational exposure to blood-borne pathogens from sharps injury have been documented since 1984, following the first reported occupational exposure to the human immunodeficiency virus (HIV). Consequently universal or standard precautions were implemented (Trim *et al.* 2003).

Herpes whitlow

The herpes simplex virus type 1 (HSV-1) causes infections of the lips, mouth and face. It is the most common herpes simplex virus. Contact with saliva or the herpes sore can cause the perioperative practitioner to develop a herpes whitlow.

A whitlow is an inflammation or an abscess on the end of the finger that causes suppuration (Mosby 2002). The wearing of gloves during intubation and extubation of the patient will help the practitioner to avoid this infection.

Inhalation of electrosurgical plume

The perioperative team and medical electrical departments have concerns with the use of electrosurgical equipment and the generation of smoke or plume. The thermal destruction of tissue creates a smoke by-product. This smoke may cause ocular or upper respiratory tract irritation in healthcare personnel.

Surgical smoke is the smoke produced when tissues are cut or coagulated during electrosurgery. There are three concerns that make plume and inhalation a problem:

- odour;
- particulate matter size;
- potential viability of the actual smoke.

When tissue is vaporised biological contaminants are released into the atmosphere. This can include carbonised tissue, blood or potentially infectious diseases and bacteria (Biggins 2002). Kokosa & Eugene (1989) and Ott (1994), suggest that over 80 chemicals have been identified in surgical smoke and many are known carcinogens.

Surgeons and scrub practitioners wear face masks to protect the patient and themselves. Masks were originally designed to protect patients from the droplets expired by healthcare professionals, but today the focus of protection has shifted to how surgical masks can be used as a safeguard for the perioperative practitioners (Crook *et al.* 1996). In the future these practitioners may wear a special design of face mask to protect them, if necessary, after more research into this issue. The use of suction machines for the evacuation of the surgical smoke produced during invasive and laparoscopic surgery will also be a high priority for the safety of the perioperative practitioners.

Surgical smoke produced by an electrosurgical unit is not routinely evacuated because of factors that go beyond current guidelines and standards, and available equipment for the purpose (Dyke 1999). Local policies will define practice for the disposal of surgical smoke and plume in the future. Specialised filters may be incorporated into electrosurgery and suction machines to ensure safety for all operating room personnel.

ORGANISATIONAL HAZARDS

Stress

There are many reasons for stress within the operating room environment, including:

- lack of control over workload;
- time pressures;
- poor understanding of roles and competencies;
- management support;
- ineffective teams.

Recognising the signs and symptoms, and strategies to relieve stress can all help the practitioner and their colleagues to lessen or overcome stress levels. Stress can impact on employees and patient care in the operating room environment. Support from the operating room manager and a culture of trust among work colleagues are necessary to achieve optimal patient care.

Some of these issues have been addressed with the introduction of the *Improving Working Lives* document (DOH 2000). It is a blueprint by which NHS employers and staff can measure the management of human resources. Organisations are kitemarked against their ability to demonstrate a commitment to improving the lives of their employees.

The introduction of clinical supervision and reflective practice can help to alleviate stress. It can empower and support perioperative practitioners in their patient care, clarify their worries and concerns and also help them to develop a theoretical knowledge base from practical experiences. Butterworth & Faugier (1992) describe clinical supervision as an exchange between practising professionals to enable the development of practice skills.

INFECTION CONTROL

Infection is one of the most frequent adverse events associated with healthcare interventions and is compounded by the ever-increasing threat from multi-drug resistant organisms. Hospital acquired infection (HAI) increases the hospital stay of a patient by 7–11 days. The cost to the NHS has been estimated at £1 billion and 30% of the current HAIs are preventable. Every year there are 320,000 healthcare associated infections and at any one time 9% of hospital inpatients are suffering from an infection which they acquired following admission to hospital (National Audit Report 2000).

Although sometimes unavoidable, a significant proportion of healthcare-associated infections could be prevented by better quality clinical practice. All healthcare practitioners are responsible for ensuring that they consistently deliver high quality clinically effective care and that they protect patients from the risk of infection (Pratt 2004).

The primary objective of infection control is to prevent the spread of infection by practitioners and patients. Practitioners have the responsibility to uphold high personal standards of infection control and to ensure that their colleagues also adhere to these. Practitioners should follow local policies and guidelines and may develop further knowledge by attending lectures to ensure optimal patient care within the perioperative environment.

The human body is remarkable in its ability to protect itself by intact barriers, membranes and bacteriostatic secretions (Fortunato 2000). The body deters infecting organisms by its defence mechanisms. The first defence is by the skin, eyes, reflexes, mucous membranes, cilia, secretions and muscular closures. The second defence incorporates inflammatory response, antibody production and temperature elevation. The third defence is by passive and active immunity. Infections can pass from patient to patient or from patient to practitioner or vice versa by direct (touch) or indirect contact (from equipment, linen or waste) or by droplet infection (sneezing, talking, dust).

The management strategies for infection control are to control, minimise, prevent and isolate any infection or infectious substances for all patients. Practitioners undertake interventions to prevent the infection; these include a high standard of personal hygiene, correct cleaning of the operating room, application of standard precautions, and the use of anaesthetic filters with patients' breathing systems. Practitioners also maintain a clean operating room environment, set at the correct temperature and humidity. Aitkenhead *et al.* (2001) state that temperatures of 22–24°C are usually acceptable in the operating room with a relative humidity of 50–60%, but a higher environmental temperature is required during surgery on the neonate or infant.

All perioperative practitioners maintain effective principles of aseptic technique, sterile field and patient care. They should wear relevant operating room clothing and shoes and look after their own health. The length of the surgical procedure, skin preparation, the use of drains and catheters during the surgical procedure and care interventions such as the preoperative shave can all increase the risk of postoperative infection.

Perioperative practitioners can be at risk from infections and it is important that they ensure their own skin integrity and cover any cuts and grazes. Exposure to infection from blood, blood-borne products and bodily fluids within the operating room environment is always a possibility. Therefore, all members of the perioperative team need to follow local infection control policies and recognise that they hope to minimise the sources of infection, interrupt their transmission and increase patient resistance. It is important that perioperative practitioners apply standard precautions to prevent contamination by any blood or blood products within their patient care.

Methicillin resistant *Staphylococcus aureus* (MRSA)

In the last few years MRSA has become one of the major threats to in-patient care. *Staphylococcus aureus* bacteria are found naturally on the skin and in the nose. Sometimes these bacteria can cause an infection and in the past methicillin was given to treat these infections. Over the years resistance to this antibiotic has grown and hence it is more difficult to treat these infections now. These infections can cause skin, bone and severe blood infections and, if the postoperative patients are susceptible, the problem can be severe.

The control of MRSA in hospitals currently presents one of the most challenging aspects of infection control principles for all healthcare practitioners. It is an expensive problem for the NHS and, for the patient, the cause of skin and bloodstream infections. There is no risk to healthy people but young, old and immunocompromised patients undergoing invasive and surgical procedures are susceptible. The spread of infection is by close contact and it is transmitted between practitioners and patients by hands and also through contact with equipment, medical devices, bedlinen and work surfaces.

Practitioners undertake optimal principles of infection control to prevent or limit the infection by:

- The MRSA patient's surgical procedure is last on the operating room list. The practitioner recovers the patient in the operating room and not in recovery, following local policy.
- Simple precautions, universal or standard, are the key to prevent the spread of MRSA.
- Effective communication is established between the perioperative team and ward practitioners.
- A clean operating room environment is provided.
- Practitioners are aware of local policies and guidelines.

Data collection on MRSA cases in NHS Acute Trusts is undertaken by the DOH's MRSA Surveillance Scheme and results are available for the public, patients and healthcare practitioners to read.

DEEP VEIN THROMBOSIS (DVT)

A major risk to patients undergoing a surgical procedure is deep vein thrombosis. Deep vein thrombosis is thrombo-occlusive disease of the peripheral veins. It occurs in the lower extremities and results from the reduction of venous flow due to the patient's positioning during surgical procedure. If these clots travel to the heart, lungs or brain they can become life threatening. A pulmonary embolism occurs when a clot travels through the heart and blocks the pulmonary arteries, and a cerebral embolism is when the brain arteries become blocked.

Aitkenhead *et al.* (2000) state that a higher incidence of DVT has been reported in patients with extensive trauma, infection, heart failure, blood dyscrasias, malignancy and metabolic disorders. It is more common after hip, pelvic and abdominal surgery but there is also an association with oestrogen and the risk increases during a surgical procedure.

The incidence of DVT has been shown to be as high as 80% in major general, gynaecological, urological and orthopaedic surgery. Of all pulmonary emboli (PE) 90–95% arise from lower extremity DVT. Pulmonary emboli account for 1% of hospital admissions (Thrift II 1998). In 2000/2001 this equated to over 110 000 hospital admissions in the United Kingdom alone. The annual cost of DVT and PE to the NHS is thought to be in excess of £220 million. If all high-risk patients received prophylaxis the NHS could save up to £80 million, which is equivalent to an additional 30 000 hip operations. Proximal vein thrombosis increases a hospital stay by 5 days (DOH 2001). DVT is often asymptomatic. Only 25% of patients with DVT will demonstrate clinical symptoms (Hull *et al.* 2000).

The alarmingly high incidence of DVT and the potentially serious consequences of the condition, coupled with the fact that the majority of cases will go undetected, indicate the urgent need for DVT prophylaxis. DVT poses a threat to many hospitalised patients resulting in increased hospital stays and higher patient costs. In addition, those who have suffered with the condition often have to live with a lifetime of complications, such as recurrent venous thrombosis, post-thrombotic syndrome and leg ulcers, at a high cost to themselves as well as to healthcare resources (Milne & Ruckley 1994).

Preventive strategies

Ward assessment
Ward nurses assess the DVT score of the patient and the perioperative practitioner observes this score on the perioperative patient checklist. The anaesthetist may prescribe preoperative, intraoperative or postoperative heparin to the patient.

During the surgical procedure anaesthetic practitioners should observe the patient's physiological recordings and the suction machine for signs of bleeding (Drinkwater 1989).

Positioning

The patient should be positioned using padded operating table accessories and ensuring the patient is comfortable (limbs and nerves) in the identified position.

Anti-embolism stockings

Patients wear support stockings (knee or thigh) through their perioperative journey and postoperatively. It is important for the patient to wear the correct size and have no pressure from ruffled stockings at the top of the knee or thigh. Static compression on the legs helps to promote venous flow and reduce venous stasis. Drinkwater (1989) suggests that thigh stockings (seamless and contoured to the limbs) be worn because the velocity of the flow is increased not only in the legs but in the pelvic veins and inferior vena cava, and they provide a graduated compression from the ankle to the mid-thigh.

TED anti-embolism stockings are designed to prevent blood from pooling in the veins of the leg, which may contribute to blood clot formation. These stockings are intended for use during the patient's hospital stay only. They can increase blood velocity, reduce the incidence of venous stasis, DVT and pulmonary embolisms. They can be knee high or thigh length. They should fit the patient and not cause any restriction to blood flow.

Intermittent pneumatic compression systems

Patients wear inflatable woven leg wraps or boots during their surgical procedure. The tubing from these devices attaches to a pump which delivers compression and relaxation to the legs or feet at pressures that vary between devices. The garment inflates and deflates intermittently and has adjustable cycle times and pressures. The anaesthetic practitioner should ensure that the patient is not lying on the device tubing, as this could cause a pressure sore.

Huntleigh Healthcare offers a comprehensive range of intermittent pneumatic compression (IPC) systems for the prevention of DVT. The products are safe and help to reduce the incidence of DVT (Ginzburg *et al.* 2003). The lightweight garments (calf or thigh length garments, foot system or air-walk system) are made of soft, breathable fabric and have been shown to reduce oedema and postoperative pain, enhance circulation, provide a drier postoperative field, and reduce wound haematoma (Huntleigh Healthcare 2005).

Training

The perioperative practitioner should undertake training in the use of compression devices to ensure effective care of the patient. Then they will be aware of the indications, recommendations and contraindications of their single use and report any faults to the relevant personnel. They should also attend regular updates on DVT and the appliances available to reduce this disease.

REFERENCES

Aitkenhead, A.R. & Smith, G. (1996) *Textbook of Anaesthesia,* 3rd edn. Churchill Livingstone. Edinburgh.

Aitkenhead, A.R., Rowbotham, D.J. & Smith, G. (2001) *Textbook of Anaesthesia.* Churchill Livingstone. Edinburgh.

Allmann, K.G. & Wilson, I.H. (2001) *Oxford Handbook of Anaesthesia.* Oxford University Press. Oxford.

Arblaster, G. (1998) Pressure sore incidence: A strategy for reduction. *Nursing Standard* **12** (28), 49–54.

Association of Operating Department Practitioners (2003) *Code of Conduct.* www.aodp.org

Augustine, S.D. (1990) Hypothermia therapy in the postanesthesia care unit: A review. *Journal of Postanaestheia Nursing* **5** (4), 254–63.

Beesley, J. (2005) Minimising the risk to patients. *Nurse 2 Nurse Magazine* **4** (1). www.n2nmagazine.co.uk/print.asp?ArticleID=297

Bliss, M. & Simini, B. (1999) When are the seeds of postoperative pressure sores sown? *British Medical Journal* **319**, 863–4. www.bmj.bmjjournals.com/cgi/content/full/319/7214/863

Biggins, J. (2002) The hazards of surgical smoke – Not to be sniffed at. *British Journal of Perioperative Nursing* **12**, 136–8, 141–3.

Braden, B.J. & Bergstrom, N. (1989) Clinical utility of Braden scale for predicting pressure sore risk. *Decubitus* **2** (3), 44–6, 50–1.

Burden, N. (1993) *Ambulatory Surgical Nursing.* W.B. Saunders. Philadelphia.

Butterworth, T. & Faugier, J. (1992) *Clinical Supervision & Mentorship in Nursing.* Chapman & Hall. London.

Crook, B., Brown, R.C., Wake, D. & Redmayne, A.C. (1996) *Final Report to HSE. Efficiency of Respiratory Protective Equipment against Microbiological Aerosols.* HSL Report, Sheffield.

David, J.A. (1986) *Wound Management: A Comprehensive Guide to Dressing and Healing.* Martin Dunitz. Cited in: Pritchett A.P. & Mallett J.M. (1993) *The Royal Marsden Hospital Manual of Clinical Nursing Procedures,* 3rd edn. Blackwell Science, Oxford.

Department of Health (2000) *Improving Working Lives.* DOH, London.

Department of Health (2001) *Hospital In-patient Data Based on Hospital Episode Statistics (HSE) 2000/2001 Key Facts and Figures.* www.doh.gov.uk/hes/beginners/001_key_facts_and_figures/index.html

Department of Infection Control. Memorial Hospital (1989) *Blueprint for the Prevention and Management of Pressure Sores.* Convatec Ltd, England. Cited in: Flanagan, M. (1995) Pressure sore risk assessment. *Educational Leaflet* **3** (4), Smith & Nephew Healthcare.

Dimond, B. (2002) *Legal Aspects of Nursing,* 3rd edn. Prentice Hall, London.

Drinkwater, K. (1989) Management of deep vein thrombosis. *Surgical Nurse* **2**, 224–6.

European Commission (1996) *Guidance on Risk Assessment at Work.* Office for Official Publications of the European Communities, Germany.

Dyke, C.N. (1999) Is it safe to allow smoke in the operating room? *Today's Surgical Nurse* March/April, 15–21.

Flanagan, M. (1995) Pressure sore risk assessment. *Educational Leaflet.* **3** (4), Smith & Nephew Healthcare.

Forest, S. (2001) Research to inform the strategic management of supply in pressure area care. *Journal of Tissue Viability* **11** (1), 20–5.

Fortunato, R. (2000) *Operating Room Technique.* Mosby, St Louis.

Ginsburg, E., Cohn, S., Lopez, J., Jackowski, J., Brown, M. & Hameed, S.M. – Miami DVT Study Group. (2003) Randomised clinical trial of intermittent pneumatic compression and low molecular weight heparin in trauma. *British Journal of Surgery* **90**, 1338–44. Cited in: Huntleigh Healthcare Ltd (2005) *Flowtron DVT Prophylactic Systems.* Huntleigh Healthcare, Luton.

Gosnell, D.J. (1973) An assessment tool to identify pressure sores. *Nursing Research* **22** (1), 55–9. Cited in Flanagan M. (1995) Pressure sore risk assessment. *Educational Leaflet* **3** (4), Smith & Nephew Healthcare.

Guyton, A.C. (1984) *Physiology of the Human Body,* 6th edn. CBS College Publishing, USA. Cited in: Pritchett, A.P. & Mallett, J.M. (1993) *The Royal Marsden Hospital Manual of Clinical Nursing Procedures,* 3rd edn. Blackwell Science Oxford.

Health and Safety at Work Etc. Act (1974) HMSO, London.

Health and Safety Executive (1992) *Manual Handling Operations Regulations.* HMSO, London.

Health and Safety Executive (1999) *Control of Hazardous Substances Hazardous to Health.* HMSO, London.

Health and Safety Executive (2002) *Control of Substances Hazardous to Health Regulations.* HSE, Suffolk.

Hull, R.D., Pineo, G.F., Francis, C., Bergquist, D., Fellenius, C., Soderburg, K., Holmqvist, A., Mant, M., Dear, R., Baylis, B., Mah, A. & Brant, R. (2000) Low-molecular-weight heparin prophylaxis using dalteparin in close proximity to surgery vs warfarin in hip arthroplasty patients: a double-blind, randomized comparison. The North American Fragmin Trial. *Archives of Internal Medicine* **160** (14), 2199–207.

Huntleigh Healthcare Ltd (2005) *Flowtron DVT Prophylactic Systems.* Huntleigh Healthcare. Luton.

Johnson, A. (1989) Granuflex wafers as a prophylactic pressure sore dressing. *Care – Science and Practice* **7** (2), 86–8. Cited in: Pritchett, A.P. & Mallett, J.M. (1993) *The Royal Marsden Hospital Manual of Clinical Nursing Procedures* 3rd edn. Blackwell Science, Oxford.

Kokosa, J. & Eugene, J. (1989) Chemical composition of laser-tissue interaction of smoke plume. *Journal of Laser Applications* July, 59–63.

Kosiak, M. (1958) Evaluation of pressure as a factor in the production of ischial ulcers. *Archives of Physical Medicine and Rehabilitation* **40**, 62–9. Cited in: Pritchett, A. & Mallett, J.M. (1993) *The Royal Marsden Hospital Manual of Clinical Nursing Procedures,* 3rd edn. Blackwell Science, Oxford.

Kosiak, M. (1976) A mechanical resting surface: Its effects on pressure distribution. *Archives of Physical Medicine and Rehabilitation* **57**, 481–3. Cited in: Pritchett, A.P. & Mallett, J.M. (1993) *The Royal Marsden Hospital Manual of Clinical Nursing Procedures,* 3rd edn. Blackwell Science, Oxford.

Medical Devices Agency (1996) *Latex Sensitisation in the Health Care Setting. (MDA DB 9601).* MDA, London.

Milne, A.A. & Ruckley, C.V. (1994) Venous insufficiency following deep vein thrombosis. *Vascular Medical Review* **5**, 241–8.

Mosby (2002) *Medical, Nursing and Allied Health Dictionary.* Elsevier Science, St Louis.

National Association of Theatre Nurses (1998) *Principles of Safe Practice in the Perioperative Environment.* NATN, Harrogate.

National Audit Report (2000) *The Management and Control of Hospital Acquired Infection in Acute NHS Trusts in England.* National Audit Office. HMSO, London.

Norton, D., McLaren, R. & Exton-Smith, A.N. (1962) *An Investigation of Geriatric Nursing Problems in Hospitals.* National Corporation for the Care of Old People, London. Cited in: Flanagan, M. (1995) Pressure sore risk assessment. *Educational Leaflet* **3** (4), Smith & Nephew Healthcare.

Nursing Midwifery Council (2004) *Code of Professional Conduct for the Nurse, Midwife and Health Visitor.* NMC, London.

Ott, D. (1994) Smoke production and smoke reduction in laparoscopic surgery procedures. *Surgical Services Management* **3** (3), 11–13.

Pratt, R.J. (2004) An evidence-based approach to preventing healthcare associated infections in the elderly – The epic initiative in England. *Journal of the Royal College of Physicians of Edinburgh* **34** (1), 11–15.

Pressure Sore Prediction Scale (1975) Cited in: Flanagan, M. (1995) Pressure sore risk assessment. *Educational Leaflet* **3** (4), Smith & Nephew Healthcare.

Pritchett, A.P. & Mallett, J.M. (1993) *The Royal Marsden Hospital Manual of Clinical Nursing Procedures*, 3rd edn. Blackwell Science, Oxford.

Richards, R.H. (1989) Perioperative nursing research. Part IV: Postoperative phase. *AORN Journal.* **50** (1) 95–97.

Royal College of Nursing (1996) *A Guide to Manual Handling of Patients* 4th edn. RCN, London.

Royal College of Nursing (1999) *Latex Allergy Campaign. Briefing Document for Practitioners and Safety Representatives.* RCN, London.

Scott, E.M. & Buckland, R. (2004) The importance of temperature management in surgical patients. *Nurse 2 Nurse Magazine* **4** (4). www.n2nmagazine.co.uk/articleDetails.asp?ArticleID=295

Sessler, D.I. (1997) Current concepts:mild perioperative hypothermia. *New England Journal of Medicine* **336** (24), 1730–7.

Thrift II – Second Thromboemboltic Risk Factors Consensus Group (1998) Risk of prophylaxis for venous thromboembolism in hospital patients. *Phlebology* **13**,87–97.

Trim, J.C., Adams, D. & Elliott, T.S. (2003) Healthcare workers' knowledge of inoculation injuries and glove use. *British Journal of Nursing* **12** (4), 215–21.

Waterlow, J. (1985) A risk assessment card. *Nursing Times* **81** (49), 49–55.

Wilson, J. (1995) Clinical risk management in theatres. Professional practice. Are you a team player? *British Journal of Theatre Nursing* **4** (11), 5–7.

Section 2

Perioperative Care

6 | A Route to Enhanced Competence in Perioperative Care

NES Perioperative Working Party

LEARNING OUTCOMES
❏ Discuss the *developing role of the perioperative practitioner*.
❏ *Identify the competencies* displayed by the experienced perioperative practitioner.

INTRODUCTION
Perhaps the greatest change in the perioperative environment has been in the roles of perioperative practitioners, who have now developed into integrated and autonomous members of the multidisciplinary team. The aim of this chapter is to discuss the competencies displayed by qualified perioperative practitioners following an initial period of consolidation, but before developing specialist practice.

The work carried out by an NHS Education Scotland working party (2001–2002) in developing perioperative competencies provides the basis to this chapter. This work resulted in a portfolio which guides professional development in the early years of practice as a foundation to a specialist practice programme. The full portfolio can be downloaded from the NHS Education web site (www.nes.scot.nhs.uk/publications/qacpd/portfolios/periop.html).

THE ROLE OF THE PERIOPERATIVE PRACTITIONER
The role of the perioperative practitioner begins even before the patient enters the operating department. Chapter 7 of this book discusses the advantages of preoperative visiting by a practitioner. The main aims of this visit are to gain information which

will help to plan the patient's care in the operating department. The visit can also help to educate the patient, which may help relieve anxiety. Chapters 4, 8, 9 and 10 explore aspects of the role of the perioperative practitioner in depth.

The role of the perioperative practitioner, when used to its full extent, can involve a huge range of influence extending well beyond the traditional boundaries of the 'theatre doors'. Figure 6.1 shows the wide range of areas where perioperative practitioners work.

The developing role of the perioperative practitioner

The two main groups of registered professionals who perform the role of perioperative practitioner are nurses and operating department practitioners (ODPs). The ODP Diploma programme lasts either 2 or 3 years and provides the individual with a qualification tailored specifically to the perioperative environment. The courses are patient centred, evidence based, reflective and encourage autonomous practice. They focus specifically on the care of the patient undergoing surgery or anaesthesia.

Nurses enter perioperative care with a Diploma in Nursing and with a broad range of experience which can include perioperative experience. Preregistration training equips nurses

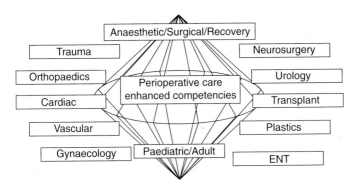

Fig. 6.1 The scope of the perioperative practitioner's experience.

with transferable skills adaptable to various areas, including perioperative care; for example airway maintenance, drug administration and pressure area care. However, practitioners need to develop specific skills (for example scrubbing and circulating) following registration while working in the area. The similarity between ODP diplomas and nursing diplomas, especially in the early modules, leads to greater opportunities for shared learning between the professions than was possible with the previous NVQ-based ODP courses.

Various postregistration courses are available for nurses and ODPs, none of which is essential for entry into the area although most are required for career progression. Postregistration courses available in the UK include, for example, degrees, postgraduate diplomas and masters in perioperative care. ODPs have had limited access to these courses in the past, mostly because their vocational background did not provide the necessary entry qualifications for higher education. However, with increasing access to preregistration education in higher education institutions and a greater familiarity with higher education principles of teaching and learning, such access is likely to increase (Wicker & Strachan 2001).

One of the greatest effects of this harmonisation of training will be a greater understanding of each profession's ethics of practice. Many barriers between the professions will dissolve because of the greater understanding of the approaches to patient care and the increased career opportunities that result.

In common with many other clinical specialities, the role of the perioperative practitioner has come under increasing scrutiny. During the 1970s and 1980s it appeared as though the nurse as a member of the perioperative team might disappear altogether. This occurred because there was a general devaluing of what many saw as caring for an unconscious patient. Questions were being asked: 'Why is there a nurse in theatre?' and 'What is the nursing role?'. The nurse's professional body, the National Association of Theatre Nurses (NATN), responded to this challenge and led the way in justifying the role of the nurse in theatre. These questions were answered in full and even the authors of reports such as the Bevan report, which looked at the staffing and utilisation of theatres, eventually admitted there was a place for nurses in the perioperative team (Bevan 1989; 1994).

Concurrently, Operating Department Assistants found themselves at a disadvantage because they were viewed as technical staff rather than professional practitioners. However, the increasing focus on the patient as the centre of approaches to care encouraged the move from theatre technicians, to assistants in the operating department, and finally to registered practitioners in their own right. The modern training for ODPs provides a patient-centred approach to patient care which encourages harmony between these two professions. The Association of Operating Department Practitioners was vital in leading ODPs towards full professional registration.

The overlap in the roles and education of the two professional bodies has continued to increase in recent years. The NATN has been proactive in this change in the perioperative team and increasingly turned to looking at the role of the practitioner in perioperative care, rather than limiting itself to the role of nurses. This led to a change in name to the Association for Perioperative Practice and redefining its membership to include nurses and ODPs.

Practitioners now accept that the unconscious patient deserves at least as much care as the conscious patient. Perioperative practitioners, with their knowledge of the patient's preoperative and postoperative episodes of treatment and their holistic approach to patient care, are ideally placed to provide that care (Johnson 1991; West 1993). Now the question that needs to be answered is 'what can registered perioperative practitioners do?' The answer can be found in the increasing number of roles that practitioners are now adopting. These include, for example, the role of first assistant, the surgeon's assistant, non-medical anaesthetist and a myriad of role improvements such as cannulation, intubation, extubation and 12-lead ECG recording.

Practitioners have adopted the role of first assistant in ever increasing numbers and in fact many view this as an integral part of a scrub practitioner's role. For example, practitioners have for many years routinely prepared patients' skin with skin disinfectants, draped limbs and parts of bodies with surgical drapes, cut sutures, retracted tissues and applied dressings and bandages. These skills are all medically delegated and in the past would normally have been developed and integrated into the practitioner's role on an improvised basis. The problem with this approach is that there is no boundary to this practice and there is often no recognition, or remuneration, for the role. Recognising that the role exists is the first step to providing education and a job description. This is essential both for the safety of the patient and the well-being of the practitioner.

The non-medical first assistant only helps the surgeon, and does not operate on the patient. However, surgical assistants perform surgery on the patient. There is normally a consultant surgeon available to help if necessary, possibly in another part of the hospital, but essentially the practitioner takes responsibility for undertaking the surgery alone. Well-established surgical assistants posts include cardiac surgeon's assistant, urology specialists who undertake cystoscopy lists and surgical practitioners who run minor plastic surgery lists using local anaesthesia.

Non-medical anaesthetists are not a new idea and have been in place in the USA and several European countries for many years. There is now a move to introduce anaesthetic assistant roles through direct entry to degree and master level programmes, without the need to go through nurse or ODP training.

The future of the perioperative team is complex. The two main groups of professionals now have the opportunity for developing closer links by harmonising their training. Into this arena also comes the generic health care worker, currently at NVQ Level 3, but also developing diploma and degree level courses. The push towards patient-centred care is also obvious in this group, and developments in their training seem certain as the government strives to maintain the perioperative workforce across the country.

In response to these challenges, the main perioperative professional bodies – the Association for Perioperative Practice, the Association of Operating Department Practitioners, the National Association of Assistants in Surgical Practice and the British Association of Anaesthetic and Recovery Nurses, among others, have combined in a group called the 'Perioperative Collaborative'. The purpose of this group is to provide a voice to represent the perioperative workforce and to provide greater harmonisation of the workforce in the way that they work. Professional boundaries are fading fast – the emphasis must be on the roles that are provided and the care the patient needs.

ENHANCED PERIOPERATIVE COMPETENCIES

Developing the diverse and complex competencies required of an experienced perioperative practitioner starts with entry-level competence through nursing and operating department practice programmes of learning. However, it is only through experience and continuing professional development that the practitioner can develop and enhance such competencies. The experienced perioperative practitioner therefore has the potential to develop specialist knowledge and a complex portfolio of skills.

The difficulties with identifying competence within the complexities of perioperative practice resulted in robust discussion within the Working Party. This Working Party first identified the competence which they were aspiring to define. Figure 6.2 shows how the competencies of these experienced practitioners could match education and career progression.

The group recognised the need for providing clear descriptors of enhanced competencies for the delivery of high-quality perioperative care. This work developed in the form of a portfolio which is discussed in this chapter. It provides the framework to support a route to enhanced competence in perioperative care which uses the 17 enhanced competencies identified by the group. Box 6.1 describes the key steps in portfolio development.

The features of the portfolio are that it:

- meets the needs of perioperative practitioners from novice to experienced practitioner level;
- will have application for preparing in-house clinical courses as well as having a place in informing curricula developed by higher education providers either in partnership with NHS Trusts or independently;

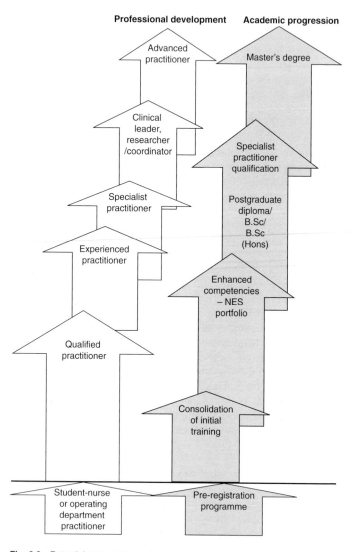

Fig. 6.2 Potential career progression framework for perioperative practitioners.

Box 6.1   Essential steps for building a portfolio

Step 1: Review your experience and practise identifying any perioperative knowledge and skills that you have.

Step 2: Appraise your competence and identify strengths and any areas that need to be developed.

Step 3: Agree with your senior manager, in-house continuing professional development staff and/or higher educational institution a training programme which meets your learning needs.

Step 4: Set goals and devise an action plan to achieve the stated perioperative competencies in partnership with your named facilitator.

Step 5: Provide evidence of competence through your portfolio.

- can be achieved as a work-based programme through rotational placements in identified, educationally audited, practice placements;
- supports programmes of preparation for qualifications in specialist practice;
- provides a bank of evidence of enhanced competence which could be presented for Accreditation of Prior Learning (AP(E)L) for specialist qualifications in perioperative care.

This portfolio can be completed with the NES (NHS Education Scotland) 2002. It encourages reflection on past experience and learning to record enhanced clinical competence in perioperative care. It will help the individual practitioner to identify sources of learning and evidence of good practice for providing high-quality care. An electronic version of the NES Portfolio Route to Enhanced Competence can be downloaded from the NES Education Website (www.nes.scot.nhs.uk/publications/qacpd/home.html).

Perioperative competencies

Figure 6.3 shows the five key areas of perioperative practice the group identified and subdivided into their individual competencies. Box 6.2 describes the terminology of the framework.

The indicators are samples of skills and knowledge that practitioners can use to show achievement of the competencies. The area of 'Professional attitudes underpins the approach to perioperative practice and therefore applies to all the areas equally

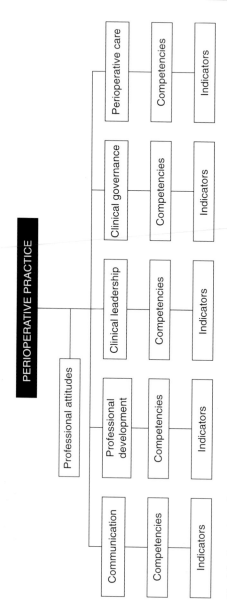

Fig. 6.3 Competency framework.

> **Box 6.2   Terminology of the perioperative competencies framework**
>
> **Key areas** are identified categories of perioperative practice.
>
> **Competencies** are broad statements of intent which identify the component parts of the key areas.
>
> **Indicators** are measurable markers of the achievement of the competencies. They are included here for guidance and must be adapted or expanded to reflect local environments.

(Box 6.3). The five key areas of perioperative practice (Figure 6.3) are:

- communication;
- professional development;
- clinical leadership;
- clinical governance;
- perioperative care.

The competencies identified within the first four areas of perioperative practice were common to all the perioperative areas. It was only in the 'Perioperative care' section where the group identified areas of competence specific to each clinical area of anaesthetics, theatre and recovery.

Subdividing the main areas of practice into broad competency statements helps to define the competencies that the practitioner should achieve. Each competence is then further defined by indicators. Indicators are areas of skill and knowledge that a practitioner working at this level of competence should achieve or display.

The portfolio includes examples of indicators. Each NHS Trust, hospital or operating department using this portfolio should also identify specific indicators for their own area using this portfolio as guidance. This model allows for flexibility and recognises that each area will have specific needs which practitioners can translate into indicators. For example, a unit specialising in respiratory surgery will have different indicators of knowledge and skills than a day surgery unit, although the competencies remain the same.

The rest of this chapter is made up as follows:

- **perioperative competencies** (Box 6.4) – displays a compact list of the competencies associated with the five areas of perioperative practice;
- **perioperative competencies and indicators** (Box 6.5) – displays the list of competencies and their associated sample indicators.

Box 6.3 Professional attitudes

The perioperative practitioner will display the following attitudes and approaches towards his or her role in the perioperative environment:

- Self-aware of own professional development needs
- Committed to learning and continual professional development
- Encourages others to develop clinical practice
- Open to constructive criticism and change
- Knows when to ask others for advice
- Aware of own strengths and limitations
- Develops personal professional standards of conduct and attitude
- Shows respect for patients' dignity in the perioperative environment
- Shows concern for patients' perioperative needs
- Shows empathy for their patients' perioperative experience
- Open to suggestions and concerns of other team members
- Aware of and upholds standards and quality in perioperative practice
- Actively seeks an evidence base for research and developments in perioperative practice
- Promotes the speciality of perioperative practice

CONCLUSION

This chapter has introduced the full range of competencies – knowledge, skills and attitudes – that the experienced perioperative practitioner requires. The role of the practitioner is multifaceted – a diverse and challenging one which requires years of experience to develop fully. The following four chapters further develop some of the specific aspects of knowledge, skills and attitudes associated with the roles of anaesthetic, surgical and recovery practitioners.

ACKNOWLEDGEMENT

The authors of this book would like to acknowledge the support of NHS Education Scotland in giving permission for the use of their material in this chapter.

Box 6.4   Perioperative competencies

Key areas	**Enhanced perioperative competences**
Communication	• Applies effective communication skills to promote clinically effective perioperative patient care • Establishes and maintains effective relationships with patients, carers and the members of the perioperative team • Applies the principles of good communication which bring about trust and confidence in perioperative services
Professional development in the perioperative environment	• Demonstrates personal accountability for their own continuing professional development in perioperative practice • Contributes to the continuing professional development needs of the multidisciplinary team • Contributes to developing an environment which supports continuing professional development
Clinical leadership	• Demonstrates leadership skills to enhance patient care • Manages and motivates members of the perioperative team within a specific area of responsibility • Supports and promotes clinical effectiveness by developing an evidence-based approach to perioperative practice
Clinical governance	• Identifies and effectively manages perioperative risks and hazards associated with the patient and the perioperative environment • Participates and contributes to a perioperative quality assurance strategy • Demonstrates and promotes professional, ethical and legal approaches to perioperative practice • Demonstrates personal and professional accountability in the role of a perioperative practitioner
Perioperative care	• Provides an optimum environment for the care and treatment of the perioperative patient • Provides evidence-based individualised perioperative care • Applies knowledge of pharmacology within perioperative care

Cont.

Box 6.4 *Continued.*

- Demonstrates competence in the use of medical devices which support the care of perioperative patients
- Demonstrates competence in the following roles:
  — anaesthetic practitioner
  — scrub and circulatory practitioner
  — recovery practitioner

Box 6.5 Competencies and indicators

(a) Communication

Competencies	Indicators
Applies effective communication skills to promote clinically effective perioperative patient care	• Understands and applies principles of good communication
	• Communicates significant information to the appropriate member of the perioperative team
	• Informs patients and colleagues by providing accurate and concise verbal and written information related to the care and treatment of the perioperative patient
	• Maintains effective formal and informal channels of communication within and outside the perioperative team
	• Demonstrates keyboard and data management skills
	• Utilises available information technology
Establishes and maintains effective relationships with patients, carers and the members of the perioperative team	• Demonstrates a knowledge of teamwork strategies related to the perioperative environment
	• Displays skills in managing interpersonal issues within the perioperative team
	• Establishes and maintains clarity of role within the perioperative team
Applies the principles of good communication which engenders trust and confidence in perioperative services	• Uses appropriate listening and responding skills in developing relationships with patients, carers and the perioperative team
	• Educates and informs patients and carers about the perioperative experience
	• Provides accurate and comprehensive records
	• Demonstrates the effective use of perioperative records

Box 6.5 *Continued.*

- Contributes to developing local and national policies and protocols for record keeping
- Contributes to recruiting and retaining staff by promoting the perioperative role

---

(b) Professional development in the perioperative environment

Competencies	**Indicators**
Demonstrates personal accountability for their own continuing professional development in perioperative practice	• Identifies their own professional development needs • Maximises opportunities for personal professional development • Recognises own limits in professional practice • Demonstrates personal accountability for ensuring own clinical competence • Develops a personal development plan • Develops a professional portfolio • Utilises appropriate development resources • Uses reflection to develop own skills and knowledge
Contributes to the continuing professional development needs of the multidisciplinary team	• Provides clinical supervision of others as appropriate • Promotes clinically effective practice in self and others • Contributes to perioperative teaching and learning programmes • Supports and assesses learners
Contributes to developing an environment which supports continuing professional development	• Delivers teaching using methods appropriate to the perioperative environment • Develops teaching strategies appropriate to the perioperative environment • Participates in performance appraisal programmes • Contributes to developing and maintaining learning resources • Able to access learning resources, for example a clinical skills laboratory

---

(c) Clinical leadership

Competencies	**Indicators**
Demonstrates leadership skills to enhance patient care	• Develops confidence, skills and techniques in managing people and resources • Makes effective clinical decisions

Cont.

Box 6.5 *Continued.*

	• Effectively manages resources
	• Develops autonomy in own role within personal sphere of responsibility
	• Establishes external professional networks and relationships
Manages and motivates members of the perioperative team within a specific area of responsibility	• Is aware of and applies management techniques in perioperative teamwork
	• Participates in management projects
	• Participates in managing change to bring about advances in perioperative practice
	• Demonstrates an ability to respond to a changing environment
Supports and promotes clinical effectiveness by developing an evidence-based approach to perioperative practice	• Shows evidence of research awareness
	• Develops clinical practice based on research findings
	• Motivates and supports others in developing evidence-based clinical practice

(d) Clinical governance

Competencies	**Indicators**
Identifies and effectively manages perioperative risks and hazards associated with the patient and the perioperative environment	• Understands the principles, issues and factors associated with risk management in the perioperative setting
	• Utilises risk assessment to draw up action plan to remove or reduce identified perioperative risks and hazards
	• Understands and displays safe management of clinical waste
	• Uses knowledge of risk management in the care of perioperative patients
	• Participates in evaluation of risk management strategies
Participates and contributes to a perioperative quality assurance strategy	• Utilises knowledge of quality assurance techniques to review the quality of practice
	• Actively takes part in quality, audit and peer review projects
	• Is aware of the work of the Quality Standards Board in relation to perioperative practice

Box 6.5 *Continued.*

Demonstrates and promotes professional, ethical and legal approaches to perioperative practice	• Critically analyses perioperative policies and protocols in the light of legal and ethical issues • Ensures perioperative documentation follows recommended national and local directives • Maintains confidentiality of perioperative documentation • Develops an ethical approach to perioperative practice • Discusses and applies the principles of ethical, legal and professional issues that may affect patient care, for example advocacy, legislation, data protection, health and safety, mental health, dignity, consent, negligence and discrimination, bias, religious and cultural diversity
Demonstrates personal and professional accountability in the role of a perioperative practitioner	• Applies the principles of accountability to perioperative practice • Practises within the limits of own scope of practice • Recognises limits of competence when exposed to new procedures or situations and where appropriate seeks the guidance and support of colleagues • Demonstrates an awareness of Health and Safety policy • Implements protocols to ensure the safety and well-being of patients and staff • Uses equipment correctly and effectively to reduce risk of harm • Develops an evidence-based approach to practice which reduces the risk of harm to patients and theatre users

(e) Perioperative care

Competencies	**Indicators**
Provides an optimum environment for the care and treatment of the perioperative patient	• Identifies the requirements of an optimal physical environment, for example: — ventilation systems — temperature control — humidity control — traffic — lighting — active gas scavanging

Cont.

Box 6.5 *Continued.*

	• Complies with local and national directives on decontamination of surgical instruments, tracking and traceabilty
	• Demonstrates skill in selecting appropriate clothing and equipment for specific procedures
	• Adheres to national and local policies for the safe collection and processing of clinical specimens
	• Shows competence in managing the progress of operating lists
	• Shows competence in providing an appropriate skills mix
Provides evidence-based individualised perioperative care	• Plans, delivers and evaluates perioperative patient care, for example:
	— appraises the patient's condition and responds fittingly to changes
	— applies a knowledge of the use of wound management techniques
	— manages pain relief for perioperative patients
	— positions patients safely and effectively for procedures and situations
	— uses techniques to ensure acceptable levels of tissue perfusion and nerve damage
	• Utilises knowledge of impact of anaesthesia and surgery on homeostasis to develop approaches to the effective care and management of the perioperative patient
	• Identifies changes in patient's condition and initiates appropriate action to restore homeostasis
	• Develops an understanding of the rationale behind medically delegated treatment
	• Applies knowledge of homeostasis to aid understanding of surgical procedures
	• Integrates and applies knowledge of homeostasis of wound healing: for example, suture materials, wound dressing techniques
Applies knowledge of pharmacology within perioperative care	• Applies knowledge of pharmacology of drugs within perioperative care, taking notice of pre-existing medical conditions
	• Demonstrates an understanding of groupings of drugs used in perioperative care

	• Utilises knowledge of potential adverse reactions of drugs in the perioperative care
Demonstrates competence in the use of medical devices which support the care of perioperative patients	• Is aware of the issues involved in the introduction and use of medical devices, for example: — legislation and professional guidance — introducing new medical devices — management of speciality specific equipment such as electrosurgery, tourniquets
	• Understands the role of manufacturers and uses their resources in training and education • Competent in: — preparation and checking of medical devices — safe and effective use of medical devices — supporting the introduction of new equipment into the area with teaching and education
Demonstrates competence in anaesthetic practitioner role	• Utilises an evidence-based approach to the care of the patient undergoing anaesthesia • Prepares and supports the patient for and during anaesthetic procedures • Is familiar with local and national guidelines for anaesthetic care • Prepares a safe environment considering and implementing risk assessment strategies specific to anaesthesia • Prepares and uses anaesthetic equipment, for example anaesthetic machines, ventilators, monitors and infusion devices • Undertakes basic airway management • Recognises and responds appropriately to specific adverse anaesthetic conditions • Adheres to local and national guidelines on drug administration • Recognises and responds appropriately to anaesthetic emergencies • Demonstrates safe and skilled support for anaesthetist • Develops clinical skills in line with role of anaesthetic practitioner
Demonstrates competence in scrub and circulatory practitioner role	• Utilises an evidence-based approach to the care of the patient undergoing an invasive procedure • Prepares and supports the patient for and during surgical recovery procedures

Cont.

Box 6.5 *Continued.*

- Is familiar with local and national guidelines for anaesthetic care
- Establishes and maintains integrity of a sterile field
- Maintains a safe intraoperative environment
- Prepares the operating room to receive the patient
- Anticipates the needs of the surgical team
- Safely handles the process and transport of clinical specimens
- Provides assistance to the operating surgeon within the role of scrub and circulatory practitioner
- Maintains accurate status of identified accountable items
- Participates effectively during all phases of the surgical procedure, for example:
  — Utilises knowledge of an applied anatomy and physiology during surgery procedures
  — Applies understanding of operative procedures to prepare and use equipment and medical devices
  — Works effectively as part of the perioperative team during operative procedures
  — Develops clinical skills in line with role of scrub practitioner
  — Develops clinical skills in line with role of circulating practitioner
  — Develops skills in preparing and draping the operative site

Demonstrates competence in the recovery practitioner role

- Utilises an evidence-based approach to the care of the patient in recovery
- Plans, delivers and evaluates postoperative patient care
- Debates issues of accountability in postoperative care
- Utilises knowledge of an applied anatomy and physiology during recovery procedures
- Applies an understanding of core principles of immediate postoperative care, for example:
  — Anxiety
  — Dignity
  — Pain management
  — Resuscitation

Box 6.5 *Continued.*

- Prepares the recovery environment for the patient
- Undertakes early postoperative assessment of perioperative patients
- Is competent in airway management and ventilation techniques for the postoperative patient
- Competently monitors and assesses the patient's vital signs: invasive and non-invasive
- Manages information about the patient such as handover and discharge criteria
- Recognises and responds appropriately to adverse conditions in postoperative recovery:
  — Haemorrhages
  — Hypotension
  — Desaturation
  — Respiratory obstruction
- Applies discharge criteria before discharging the patient to the care of the ward nurse
- Develops clinical skills in line with role of recovery practitioner

Authors' Note: The NES Perioperative Competencies have also recently been used during the revision of the core curriculum for the Diploma of Higher Education in Operating Department Practice, led by the Association of Operating Department Practice (AODP).

NES PERIOPERATIVE WORKING PARTY
Paul Wicker – Working Party Facilitator and Lead Author
Garry Bodsworth – Working Party Facilitator
Liz Gillies – NES Professional Officer

Group Members:

Jill Ferbrache	Ann Molloy
Claire Lewsey	Jackie McHage
Jackie Leslie	Linda Dunion
Steve McIntosh	Christine Hughes
Christine Allan	Sue Johnston
Caroline McDonald	Liz Wood
Raymond Rose	Agnes Lafferty

Rosanne Robinson   Jackie McKendrick
                       Sue Johnstone

REFERENCES

Bevan, P. (1989) *Report on the Management and Utilisation of Operating Departments.* DHSS, London.

Bevan, P. (1994) Bevan on Bevan. *British Journal of Theatre Nursing* **4** (8), 5–6.

National Health Service Education Scotland (NES) (2002) *A Route to Enhanced Competence in Perioperative Practice.* NES, Scotland.

West, B. (1993) Caring – The essence of theatre nursing. *British Journal of Theatre Nursing* **3** (9), 16–22.

Wicker, P. & Strachan, R. (2001) Advancing perioperative care. *British Journal of Perioperative Nursing* **11** (1) 28–33.

Johnson, G. (1991) Non-nursing duties in theatre. *British Journal of Theatre Nursing* **1** (3), 24–25.

FURTHER READING AND RESOURCES

Books

Clancy, J. McVicar, A.J. & Baird, N. (2002) *Perioperative Practice: Fundamentals of Homeostasis.* Routledge, London.

Gruendemann, B. & Fernsebner, B. (1995) *Comprehensive Perioperative Nursing (Vols. 1 and 2).* Jones and Bartlett Publishers, London.

Hind, M. & Wicker, P. (eds) (2000) *Principles of Perioperative Practice.* Churchill Livingstone, Edinburgh.

Nightingale, K. (ed.) 1999 *Understanding Perioperative Nursing.* Arnold, London.

Palmer, R., Burns, S. & Bulman, C. (1994) *Reflective Practice in Nursing: The Growth of the Professional Practitioner.* Blackwell Scientific, Oxford.

Schober, J.E. & Hinchliff, S.M. (1995) *Towards Advanced Nursing Practice: Key Concepts for Health Care.* Edward Arnold, London.

Smith, C.M. & Reynard, A.M. (1995) *Essentials of Pharmacology.* WB Saunders, Philadelphia.

Walsh, M. 1991 *Models in Clinical Nursing – The Way Forward.* Baillière Tindall, London.

Journals

AORN Journal

British Journal of Perioperative Nursing

Journal of Advanced Perioperative Care

Nursing Times

The Journal of Operating Department Practice

Professional guidelines

Association of Operating Department Practitioners (1999) *A Curriculum Framework for Operating Department Practice*. AODP, London.

National Association of Theatre Nurses (1993) *The Role of the Practitioner as First Assistant in the Operating Department*. NATN, Harrogate.

National Association of Theatre Nurses (1994) *The Practitioner as Surgeon's Assistant*. NATN, Harrogate.

National Association of Theatre Nurses (1997) *Developing New Roles for Non-Medical Staff within Perioperative Care*. NATN, Harrogate.

National Association of Theatre Nurses (1998) *Quality Assurance Document*. NATN, Harrogate.

National Association of Theatre Nurses (1998) *Risk Assessment Guide*. NATN, Harrogate.

National Association of Theatre Nurses (2000) *Principles of Safe Practice in the Perioperative Environment*. NATN, Harrogate.

Scottish Society of Anaesthetic and Recovery Nurses (May 1996) *Special Report: The Future Role of Nurses in Anaesthetics and Recovery*.

Government documents

Bevan. P. (1989) *Report on the Management and Utilisation of Operating Departments*. DHSS.

Clinical Governance: In the New NHS (HSC 065/1999)

Review of the NHS Workforce Planning (HSC 216/1999)

A First Class Service: Quality in the New NHS (HSC 139/1999)

Modernising Regulation – The New Health Professions Council: A Consultation Document (NHSE Aug 2000)

The NHS Plan: A Plan for Investment, A Plan for Reform (CM4818-1 July 2000)

A Health Service of all the Talents: Developing the NHS Workforce (NHSE 2000)

www.hsedirect.com/ Health and safety web site

www.ukonline.gov.uk Public face for various online government information

www.doh.gov.uk/ Department of Health web site

www.hse.gov.uk Health and Safety web site
www.doh.gov.uk/cjd/riskassessmentsi.htm
   Risk assessment of CJD and surgical instruments
www.official-documents.co.uk/ A database of official government documents
www.doh.gov.uk/nhs.htm Department of Health NHS site
www.doh.gov.uk/riskman.htm Controls assurance website

Web sites

www.bioserve.latrobe.edu.au/vcebiol/cat1/aos2/u3aos21.html
   Introduction to homeostasis
www.nmap.ac.uk Guide to quality internet resources in nursing, midwifery and the allied health professions
www.baoms.org.uk/links.html Links and resources to educational web sites
www.watchtower.org/ The official site for Jehovah's Witnesses
www.linacre.org/ A Catholic healthcare ethics site
www.healthcentre.org.uk/hc/pages/ethics.htm
   A directory of healthcare ethics sites
www.nhsdirect.nhs.uk/ NHS Direct online
www.nhs.uk/ NHS home page
www.rhpeo.org/ Health promotion web site
www.eddesign.com/electrosafety/index.htm
   CONMED online education website for electrosurgery
www.uchsc.edu/sm/chs/ Interactive human simulation website
www.rnceus.com/index.html Online education and testing
www.ethicon.com Ethicon web site
www.regent.com Regent website
www.cochrane.org/ The Cochrane Library
www.chi.nhs.uk Commission for Health Improvement
www.hqs.org.uk Health Quality Service
www.kingsfund.org.uk The Kings Fund
www.gasnet.med.yale.edu GASNet
www.rah.sa.gov.au/periops/room.htm The recovery room
www.bads.co.uk The British Association of Day Surgery
www.baccn.org.uk The British Association of Critical Care Nurses

www.show.scot.nhs.uk/SIGN/index.html The Scottish Inter-
collegiate Guidelines Network

Professional associations

Association for Periperative Practice www.afpp.org.uk
Association of Operating Department Practitioners
www.aodp.org
Association of Anaesthetists www.aagbi.org/
Royal College of Anaesthetists www.rcoa.ac.uk
Scottish Society of Anaesthetists and Recovery Nurses

1 Preoperative Preparation of Perioperative Patients

LEARNING OUTCOMES

❏ Discuss the role of the practitioner in the *preoperative preparation* of patients.
❏ Discuss *preoperative assessment* and *care planning*.
❏ Identify ways to *reduce postoperative complications* through preoperative preparation.

INTRODUCTION

Good preparation of surgical patients improves their experience of surgery and anaesthesia and leads to positive outcomes. Perioperative practitioners are in a unique position to play a part in patient preparation because of their understanding of the perioperative environment and their ability to assess the individual needs of a patient for what is likely to be one of the most significant events of their life.

Although preoperative visiting is a useful tool for achieving this aim, practitioners do not routinely adopt it for all patients (Wolfer & Davis 1970; Booth 1991). Perhaps the hierarchical and segmented roles that practitioners adopt in anaesthetics, surgery and recovery do not fully align with the holistic needs of the patient. Further research may identify reasons for the lack of uptake of this role on a wide scale.

Some may argue, however, that it is possible to provide safe care to patients without any preoperative assessment by practitioners other than that gained in the few moments available in the anaesthetic room before induction. The routine delivery of care to patients, developed over years through experience, is often enough to ensure that suitable equipment is available and that practitioners follow the correct procedures and give the correct care. Situations such as this occur in every operating department, every day.

Practitioners should be aware that surgeons, anaesthetists and other members of the perioperative team do not necessarily share the same priorities. For example, a surgeon may not see the need for a delay in the anaesthetic room while practitioners readjust the environment to the patient's individual needs. Members of the team should understand the implications of their own knowledge of the patient and share information useful for planning patient care. For example, sharing information about the patient's inability to extend an arm or their wish to keep dentures in position until the last possible minute may help with the overall preoperative preparation for surgery or anaesthesia.

Planned preoperative visiting is important because lack of prior knowledge of the patient means that perioperative practitioners can only react to the patient's needs, rather than proactively prepare for them (Crawford 1999). There is little a practitioner can do in the confines of an anaesthetic room for a patient who suddenly tells them of a fear of needles or who voices worries about their dignity during surgery.

The patient is subject to many stressors that provoke anxiety, including for example:

- threats to their sense of identity;
- fear of dying;
- fear of not awakening following anaesthesia;
- threat to body image caused by scars or deformation;
- fear of an unknown environment;
- financial worries (Fyffe, 1999).

The patient's anxiety could also increase because of problems such as a delay in surgery, change of anaesthetists, mistakes in documentation or lack of coordination of information. The practitioner is able to address some of these problems because of their involvement with the preoperative and postoperative care of the patient; and training in communication and interpersonal relationship issues.

Practitioners within the day surgery setting often carry out preoperative assessment and visiting as a necessary part of all patients' treatment. In this area, preassessment clinics enable the multidisciplinary team to find out which preoperative medical and nursing assessments need to be undertaken.

This chapter is about taking the time to make the patient's experience safer, more comfortable and better informed than it would be otherwise. It includes a discussion of preoperative education, preoperative assessment, diagnostic screening and preoperative planning to prevent perioperative complications. In today's environment of increased accountability and increased awareness of patients' rights, it could be argued that preoperative preparation of patients is a fundamental role for the practitioner, and a fundamental right for the patient.

PREOPERATIVE PREPARATION

Preoperative education

Communication with perioperative patients is one of the essential skills that practitioners must develop. Research has long shown that informed patients are better prepared for surgery, experience the best outcomes from surgery and anaesthesia, and recover faster (Boore 1975; Hayward 1978; Fyffe 1999).

Skills involved in communication with patients are many and varied, and often only develop after years of experience. The roots of communication are in interpersonal experiences and relationships. Communication is open to many influences which can either improve or block it (Brown & Duxbury 1997). An anxious patient is much less likely to voice their worries or share information about themselves, than a relaxed patient. Most patients are not, of course, relaxed about their forthcoming surgery. It is therefore, a challenge to practitioners to identify and overcome the patient's normal reticence to share information. The patient's capacity to learn limits the information that he or she can absorb. Noise, discomfort, high levels of activities or other distractions affecting the surrounding environment can also reduce the information a patient absorbs (Dyke 2000). See Chapter 4 for further discussion about perioperative communication.

Practitioners can employ various teaching strategies to maximise patient education. For example, Schrecengost (2001) conducted a study to discover whether the use of humour in preoperative instruction affects patients' recall of this instruction. The study involving 50 patients compared the use of cartoons in a teaching booklet used to teach patients about three postoperative pulmonary exercises. The results of this study were inconclusive, however, they implied that humour at worst was better than no education at all, and potentially could improve it. Humorous teaching strategies may promote open, flexible communication and allow patients to ask questions they otherwise may not ask and hear instructions they otherwise may not hear (Bellert 1989). Despite being inconclusive, this study supports the argument that patient information handed over in an informal and accessible way by perioperative practitioners may help this learning.

The traditional view of preoperative visiting in the ward on the day before surgery is not the only technique available for preoperative visiting (Hathaway 1986). In fact, research shows that patients hold information better when given two or three weeks before their surgery (Nelson 1995). Practitioners achieve this in day surgery through preassessment clinics, or through specially arranged preoperative education sessions similar to antenatal classes provided by midwives.

Information leaflets are a useful and effective method of providing written information (Lowery 1995; Fyffe 1999). Leaflets can be especially useful when giving specific information to the patient, for example about patient-controlled analgesia or postoperative exercises.

Gaining information for intraoperative use

Another main aim for preoperative visiting is so that the practitioner can gain valuable information about the patient which he or she uses to help plan care. This role is important for various reasons. For example, the operating list gives little information about the patient's physical and mental status. If the medical notes are not available until the patient arrives in the operating department, the practitioner may obtain some information too late to be of use in planning care. For example, patients with Creutzfeldt–Jacob disease (CJD) need special precautions which practitioners can only fully carry out with correct planning and organisation of resources (McNeil 2004).

Also, elderly patients often present with various issues that may need special attention in both patient assessment and discharge planning – including for example, lack of home support, non-compliance with drug regimes and concurrent medical conditions (Tappen *et al.* 2001). The practitioner can only carry out activities such as team briefings, preparation of disposable equipment and materials, and informing staff if there is enough time to do so. The alternative is a sudden flurry of activity as practitioners take emergency measures to try to ensure patient and staff safety – hardly reassuring for the patient or staff.

In emergencies, for example when preparing for trauma patients, preoperative visiting is a low priority because of time restraints and the patient's immediate needs. However, a trip to the accident and emergency department before the patient's arrival in the operating department may provide essential information about issues such as the patient's physical status, degree and location of injuries and mental status. Practitioners can use this information to prepare the right equipment and resources for the patient's admission to the operating department. This is important because quick and efficient treatment of trauma patients is one of the major factors involved in successful recovery from major injuries (Clevenger & Tepas 1997).

The development of a relationship between the practitioner and the patient has to occur in a much shorter time-frame during emergencies. Practitioners need to identify problems and decide on solutions in a small space of time; these are skills that practitioners develop through years of experience of emergency situations.

Informed consent

One of the major reasons that preoperative communication is so important is to support informed consent. The practitioner's role in this varies between NHS Trusts, but in all situations the patient's right to a choice in their treatment is sacrosanct.

All actions carried out on the patient need his or her consent, otherwise the patient could claim to have been assaulted. Patients usually give consent either by implication, for example when a patient raises an arm to receive an injection, or verbally, for example when a patient agrees to receive a drug. However, some procedures are so dangerous, or the choices for the patient so complex, that it is necessary to record the act of consent. Most anaesthetic and surgical procedures fall into this category. The role of the practitioner is to ensure that the surgeon, anaesthetist, or the practitioner undertaking that particular task has obtained the informed consent. The practitioner is not usually responsible for obtaining consent, only ensuring that it has been obtained. The policies and procedures of the hospital, underpinned by legal practices, guide the practitioner's role in ensuring patient safety. See Chapter 4 for further discussion on informed consent.

Informed consent concerns the rights of the patient to be told of all the implications of the planned procedure and any possible alternatives. To be valid, consent has to be informed and voluntary and come from a legally competent source.

Discharge planning

Perioperative practitioners often carry out discharge planning, especially in day surgery units. In general surgical wards it is more often the responsibility of the surgical ward staff. Practitioners may forget that patients have a life outside hospital and the practitioner may overlook preparation for discharge during the early stages of the patient's treatment. If discharge planning is considered later it may be difficult to make the necessary arrangements. With the increased use and sophistication of technology, the time patients stay in hospital has become much reduced. The need for discharge planning has therefore increased. Discharge planning should cover such areas as:

- postoperative drugs regimes;
- mobilisation exercises;
- pain relief;
- identifying and managing complications;
- dressing changes.

Community agencies, such as social services, district nurses, intermediate care teams, occupational therapists and community-based physiotherapists can provide support for such procedures.

PREOPERATIVE ASSESSMENT

Care planning

Practitioners have generally accepted the problem-solving approach as a suitable way of approaching the care of patients. This has been defined as 'the nursing process' and involves the following stages:

- assessment;
- diagnosis;
- goal setting;
- intervention;
- evaluation.

Care planning involves all these phases, and the literature explores various approaches to care planning.

Several models of care have been proposed as frameworks for developing approaches to patient care. The purpose of these models is to place the many different approaches to patient care within a more or less logical framework, which can help practitioners systematically deliver the care required. Each model of care focuses on a particular view of the patient's needs. For example, Roper Logan and Tierney stress the daily activities of living and their importance to normal patient life patterns, whereas Roy's model focuses on the patients' adaptation to their perioperative experiences (Roy 1976; Roy & McLeod 1981).

Practitioners can use an appropriate model of nursing to develop approaches to the delivery of the care that their patients need. These are usually formulated into care plans, which can then be used to plan and record individualised care. Perioperative care plans are usually standard documents which are individually completed for each patient. Accuracy and completeness of documentation is important for continuity of care and patient safety. The rest of this section will focus on assessing patients' needs as the root of all care planning.

The following areas of assessment were drawn from the stages of Roy's adaptation model:

- physiological assessment;
- psychosocial assessment:

— self-concept,
— role function,
— interdependence,
— contributing stimuli.

Assessment

Physiological assessment

Physiological assessment, according to Roy's model, looks at areas such as oxygenation, nutrition, elimination, activity and rest, protection, the senses, fluids and electrolytes, neurological and endocrine function.

Physiological assessment may involve areas of perioperative patient care such as monitoring and assessing airways, intravenous fluids, mobilisation or pain. These areas are especially important for the perioperative practitioner in the recovery area. In the anaesthetic and operating rooms, these assessments are often within the role of the anaesthetist or surgeon. However, understanding the underlying physiological needs of the patient helps the practitioner to interpret the results from the various patient monitoring devices and to react proactively to changes in the patient's condition.

Psychosocial assessment

Assessment of the patient's psychosocial needs at this level involves the patient's self-concept, role function and interdependence. Practitioners often give the reason of 'lack of time' as a reason for not assessing the patient's psychosocial needs. However, experienced practitioners are often adept at assessing these needs during their other duties, so all is not lost even if the assessment doesn't happen during the preoperative care-planning stage. In other words, practitioners often see this area as being important and they may need to adopt innovative ways of assessing these needs during the patient's surgery or anaesthesia. Preoperative visiting allows the practitioner to undertake this assessment before the patient's arrival in the operating department, therefore reducing the need for immediate assessment of needs at a difficult time.

Roy's model identifies the following areas for assessment:

- self-concept;
- role function;
- interdependence;
- contributing stimuli.

Assessing self-concept focuses on how the patients view themselves and their self-esteem. This includes the physical self (such as appearance) and the personal self (such as characteristics, opinions, values and worth). During preoperative assessment, this information is worth gathering to be able to plan preoperative teaching or information giving. For example, the feelings that patients experience when facing the challenges of facial surgery affect the way they perceive surgery and their behaviour in the anaesthetic room. Addressing this area is important because the patient's cooperation and understanding are important during their surgery.

This mode also includes an assessment of the patient's spiritual needs. Many people are spiritual, and some choose to express this through their religion. A patient relates their spirituality to the way they view the world, their place in it, their self-worth or value to themselves and others, their views on life and death, and their relationships within society. The perioperative experience affects spirituality, and its impact varies from patient to patient. A practitioner must therefore be aware of how patients express their various spiritual needs, either through religion, personal beliefs or behaviours. In particular, knowledge of religions can make the patient's perioperative experience more effective and may help the practitioner to deliver effective patient-focused care.

Assessing the patient's role can help provide care later. Role function includes primary roles such as gender and age, secondary roles such as family and work roles, and tertiary roles such as interests and activities. Understanding these roles helps to avoid seeing the patient just as a 'patient' rather than as a holistic being with a life outside their current position. How often do practitioners get a surprise when they suddenly find out that their patient is a doctor, operating department practitioner (ODP) or nurse; or discover too late that a partner died the previous year of the same condition?

Assessing interdependence involves exploring the patient's relationships with his family and friends, support networks, and his relationship with the surgeon, anaesthetist and practitioners. There are various situations where this information may be important for planning and delivering care, for example:

• when considering discharge arrangements;
• family support in the anaesthetic room;
• informing family of the patient's return to recovery;
• support from partners during surgery – for example during caesarean section, or during local procedures.

The final area of assessment in Roy's model identifies the stimuli that produce normal or abnormal behaviours. Roy describes these as focal (the immediate or provoking factors), contextual (other stimuli affecting the patient's life) and residual (underlying stimuli which are not obvious). Such stimuli could include:

• concurrent illness;
• fear of surgery;
• impact of surgery on appearance;
• impact of surgery on role in society;
• change in physical abilities following surgery;
• anticipated positive changes;
• fear of anaesthesia;
• absence from work;
• family care worries;
• pet care worries;
• fear of needles;
• previous unvoiced unsatisfactory perioperative experiences.

CARE PATHWAYS

Care pathways have been in use for some years for surgical patients. The focus by all team members on the perioperative patient, and shared common aims and outcomes, can help identify an expected pathway for patient-care requirements within a cost-effective and efficient environment (Johnson 1994).

A care pathway is a multidisciplinary approach to planning the patient's journey from admission to discharge. This plan guides and coordinates the patient's entire experience. It is especially effective in the more predictable situations, for example during minor surgery in otherwise healthy patients. Therefore, practitioners in day surgery find it especially useful.

Care pathways are potentially able to lessen duplication of care, and can also help to encourage cross-boundary inter-professional cooperation and communication. The use of these pathways does not reduce the need for individual care, however, since variations to the expected pathway occur in almost every patient. Patient care pathways should always therefore be flexible enough to allow the judgement of individual practitioners to come into play.

DIAGNOSTIC SCREENING

Diagnostic screening sets a baseline for assessment of changes to these measurements taken during anaesthesia or surgery and to ensure the patient receives the correct treatment. Recording of these measurements is common during surgery and so practitioners need to be familiar with normal levels so they can recognise deviations as they occur. Deviations from normal levels often require medical intervention or changes to therapy.

Observations range from standard tests and observations, such as blood pressure and pulse, to more specific and interventional tests such as blood tests and ECGs. Practitioners are often involved in the initial and continuing measurement of these observations.

Baseline observations

Chapter 1 discusses the physiological changes endured by the perioperative patient. Measuring these changes gives essential information which guides medical therapy. For example, there is often a preoperative rise in blood pressure because of stress, and a drop later because of the effects of anaesthetic drugs, hypovolaemia or surgery itself. Preoperative baseline observations normally include pulse, blood pressure, respiration and temperature. Practitioners often carry out routine urinalysis on patients because this simple test can help to identify many important conditions, such as diabetes and renal disease. During preoperative visits, the practitioner can ensure that patients have given consent for these procedures, understand the need for the tests, and that they have informed of any results, especially if abnormal.

Laboratory tests

Perioperative patients routinely undergo several blood tests. A full blood count (FBC) is carried out to exclude conditions such as anaemia. Patients always have their blood crossmatched before major procedures, in case blood transfusion is required later. Patients undergoing minor procedures, such as day surgery patients, normally have their blood grouped and saved, but not crossmatched. Measuring blood urea and electrolyte levels (commonly known as U&Es) helps to exclude organ disease, for example diabetes or renal disease.

PREOPERATIVE INVESTIGATIONS

Patients usually undergo several preoperative investigations. They are all designed to identify conditions that affect the patient perioperatively or to identify the need for surgery or other therapies. These investigations can guide the treatment required and help to plan the surgery and anaesthesia with greater accuracy and precision.

Radio-opaque dyes are used in various situations to outline the body passages or tubes and the flow of fluids through them.

Patients requiring surgery on the cardiovascular system or on the vascular system of organs such as the brain or renal system often undergo arteriograms and venograms. Blood vessels injected with a radio-opaque dye are viewed by X-ray or image intensifier to assess blood flow, blockages or abnormalities in vessel walls.

A barium swallow or enema allows the gastrointestinal tract to be viewed on an X-ray monitor in real-time and the images are then recorded for later use. An endoscopic retrograde pyelogram outlines the passages of the renal system while endoscopic retrograde cholangiopancreatography outlines the gall bladder and bile ducts. These tests can help to identify abnormalities in the bile ducts and tubes and the presence of renal or gallstones.

Diagnostic imaging involves investigations such as X-ray, ultrasound, computerised tomography (CT) and magnetic

). Development of the latter three
...ed a more accurate and detailed view
...can provide. CT, MRI and ultrasound
...ensional views of the body and highlight
... invisible to X-rays. These imaging tech-
...ul to identify conditions such as cancer or
...s.

...ndergo many more investigations and it is
impo... ...re aware of their purpose and the results. This
will help to c... ...ure compliance with the investigations and will
also serve to contribute to the patient's understanding of the
need for further interventions. Knowledge of the surgery and
the possible perioperative implications of medical interventions
will help the practitioner to work with medical staff to help the
patient to understand the implications and possible alternatives
to their surgery.

REDUCING POSTOPERATIVE COMPLICATIONS

Effective preoperative assessment, planning and patient preparation can help to prevent postoperative complications. This is
achieved most effectively by involving the whole multidisciplinary team so that all are aware of the purpose of the various
activities. Good teamwork such as this helps to address all
aspects of patient care and avoids duplication of effort.

Respiratory care

Careful respiratory assessment can reduce the risk of postoperative chest infection. Common risk factors associated with
postoperative chest infection include smoking and respiratory
disease, especially in the elderly (Litwack 1995). To give effective care in relation to breathing, the practitioner will need to
consider assessment in areas such as:

- baseline observations, including temperature;
- sputum and secretions;
- cardiovascular status;
- blood results;
- pulse oximetry;
- chest drains.

Stopping smoking preoperatively is usually of benefit, although it is usually too late to consider after admission to the hospital. However, under the right circumstances patients with respiratory problems may still benefit from education to alter future habits. Drug therapy for respiratory conditions will normally be started preoperatively – for example antibiotics or bronchial dilators. It is important that the patient understands the need to continue taking these drugs even during the immediate preoperative period. Preoperative respiratory care also involves educating the patient about the importance of postoperative coughing and breathing exercises and the need for good positioning when in bed.

A multidisciplinary approach to airway assessment and management is important because no technique of airway assessment has been proven to be 100% effective (Aitkenhead & Smith 1996), therefore a team approach may help to identify all the predisposing factors. Neacsu (2002) proposes that preassessment practitioners are involved in airway assessment for difficult intubation and can support anaesthetists in this role. Neacsu states that an extensive airway assessment would reduce the risk of airway problems, achieve best airway management, release anaesthetists for more complex tasks, and record information for audit. Important factors to consider include presence of thyroid disease, jaw protrusion, state of dentition, and head and neck distension.

Joint stiffness

Patients with stiff joints will need particular care during surgery. For example, a stiff neck will make intubation difficult and may call for the use of flexible laryngoscopes. It will be difficult to place the patient in lithotomy position if he or she has a stiff hip. Unintentionally forcing the patient's leg into an abnormal position could lead to further damage. A stiff arm may also be compromised by placing on an arm board or at too obtuse an angle – placing strain on the brachial plexus. Assessment of joint stiffness is therefore important and preoperative exercises, as arranged by physiotherapists, may help to prepare the patient for surgery.

Urinary problems

Urinary tract infection is one of the most common infections for postoperative patients (Gould 1994) and can lead to discomfort, complications and prolonged postoperative recovery times. Pre-operatively, good catheter care is essential to prevent colonisation postoperatively. This will include educating the patient about self-care and stressing the need to maintain good fluid intake and following medical orders on fluid balance. Practitioners should follow normal sterile techniques during catheterisation in the operating department. The practitioner often inserts the urinary catheter following intubation to reduce the patient's discomfort. However, consent is still required and the patient should be informed of this procedure and consent acquired preoperatively. Care should also be taken postoperatively while the patient is recovering from anaesthesia since a confused patient could easily damage the urinary tract trying to remove the catheter forcibly. Maintaining postoperative fluid intake is important to prevent further urinary and renal problems, especially following surgery on the urinary tract.

Pressure sores

A pressure sore is an area of necrosis caused by excessive and prolonged pressure. The damage to the skin is initially caused by failure of the blood supply resulting in tissue hypoxia. Shearing forces or friction can then cause further mechanical damage to the weakened skin. The skin then blisters, breaks into open sores or develops areas of necrosis. Chapter 5 looks at a risk assessment approach to prevention and treatment of pressure sores.

Pressure sores result in extended stays and distress to patients (Starritt & Ewing 1999). Although they are potentially preventable they remain a problem, therefore early assessment of patients is essential to reduce their incidence.

Patients at risk include the elderly and those undergoing long surgical procedures, other factors include the presence of concurrent illness, those with reduced preoperative mobility and patients with poor general health and nutrition.

Pressure sores can occur anywhere the skin has pressure applied. They are therefore not only confined to common areas such as the sacrum or heels, but can also occur because of pressure caused by ill-fitting casts, table fittings pressing on the patient, and poorly placed equipment. The operating table itself has also been blamed for avoidable pressure damage (Waterlow 1996; Scott 2000) because of the firm design of the mattress. The patient therefore requires constant vigilance to prevent harm.

The risk of developing pressure sores can be assessed using scales such as Waterlow (Waterlow 1985) or Norton (Norton *et al.* 1962). Scales such as these assess the risk factors for developing pressure sores, including age, gender, smoking history, nutritional status, mobility, build, medication, incontinence, existing vascular diseases and proposed duration of the surgical procedure. A high score is an indicator of the high potential for skin damage, therefore practitioners can carry out suitable preventive measures to protect the patient. The use of risk-assessment scales targets resources at patients who need them, and helps to prevent the overuse of resources where they are not required.

There is a vast array of pressure relieving devices available to patients and various techniques that practitioners should employ to reduce pressure sore development. Therefore, individual assessment of the patient is essential. For example, a patient at risk from pressure sores may need frequent changes of position during surgery. This may not be possible unless the practitioner raises awareness of the problem with the surgical team and special measures are taken before and during the surgical procedure. If moving the patient is not possible because of anaesthetic or surgical constraints, then the patient should be protected by using gel pads, careful positioning to prevent hotspots developing or by using low-pressure mattresses. Again, multidisciplinary involvement in the use of these devices is essential to gain the support of all members of the perioperative team.

Deep venous thrombosis (DVT)

Preoperative assessment can help to reduce the incidence of DVT: blood clots developing in the venous circulation of the legs as a result of clotting abnormalities. DVT is common, affecting 10–80% of perioperative patients (Davis 1999). The result of

DVT can be potentially fatal if it results in a pulmonary embolism. Three main contributing factors include endothelial damage to blood vessels; long periods of immobility which lead to venous stagnation; and concurrent medication which affects clotting mechanisms, for example the contraceptive pill. Other contributing factors also play a part in this condition, for example dehydration, pregnancy and nephritic syndrome (Arnold 2002a).

The more complex prophylactic treatments (for example anticoagulant therapy or intermittent pneumatic compression therapy (IPCT), e.g. Flowtron boots) should be aimed at patients at high risk from this condition. Therefore, risk assessment to identify high-risk patients is an important skill for perioperative practitioners to develop (Arnold 2002a). Preassessment or preoperative visiting provides the ideal time for DVT risks assessment.

DVT risks scales such as Autar (1996) improve risk assessment. The Autar assessment tool scores the patient for seven risk factors: age, build/body mass, mobility, trauma risk, disease, special risk and type of surgical intervention. One study (Quantrill 2001) places patients into low, medium or high-risk categories with treatment given accordingly:

- low risk – graduated compression stockings (GCS);
- moderate risk – GCS plus low dose heparin;
- high-risk – GCS, adjusted dose of heparin and IPCT.

In view of the effects of DVT, it would be wise to apply some basic precautions to all patients until good research can more clearly identify ways to assess the risk of DVT developing. In all patients, education about early mobilisation is important to help prevent postoperative DVT. It also appears that GCS may be the best way to provide generalised prophylaxis according to a recent Cochrane review (Amaragiri & Lees 2001). However, this study did point out that GCS worked best when used with other prophylaxis measures, and made no mention of problems that can occur when ill-fitting stockings are used. GCS may also not be appropriate for all patients, for example if ulcers are present. Most units now have protocols in place for DVT prophylaxis to help protect patients from this condition.

Preoperative assessment for DVT can also alert practitioner during the intraoperative period to high-risk patients (Arnold 2002a). The perioperative practitioner can use methods to decrease the factors contributing to DVT development and minimise the risk to the patient during surgery. For example:

- Reduce endothelial damage by:
  — avoiding abnormal leg positioning;
  — avoiding extreme degrees of internal and external leg rotation (for example during orthopaedic surgery).
- Increase venous return by:
  — performing passive limb exercises on the patient during long surgery;
  — being aware of the need to avoid excessive tourniquet pressures and extended periods of inflation;
  — preferentially placing the patient in a leg-up position wherever possible to encourage venous drainage (10% leg raise produces 30% better venous drainage (Thomas 1999));
  — avoiding placing the patient in a limb-down positioning to reduce the risk of oedema developing in the lower limbs which could lead to venous stagnation and endothelial damage;
  — developing good techniques for applying and using GCS or IPCT.
- Decrease hypercoagulability by educating patients about the benefits of complying with drug regimes involving:
  — heparin and warfarin or other anticoagulants;
  — antiplatelet drugs such as aspirin or dextran (Arnold 2002b).

Chapter 5 looks at a risk assessment approach to prevention and treament of DVT.

Nausea and vomiting

Postoperative nausea and vomiting (PONV) is distressing for patients at best. At worst it could result in further illness such as aspiration of stomach contents into the lungs leading to respiratory complications, damage to wound sites caused by straining, and electrolyte imbalances caused by the loss of

ϽNV occurs in around 20–30% of surgical
ι 2002c).

treatment of PONV is based on the use of anti-
ιtagonise the various neurotransmitter systems
ʒea and vomiting. These include drugs such as
ιιᴄ   , ondansetron, metochlopramide and cyclizine.
Anti-emιᴄ cs are discussed in detail in Chapter 3. However, the
variety of anti-emetics available implies that no one of them is
particularly good at its job (Arnold 2002c). The lack of a 'perfect'
anti-emetic means the role of the practitioner in assessing
PONV and the use of non-medical approaches to treating
PONV are especially important.

Various scoring tools are available to assess the patient's risk
of developing PONV. Again, none of these are particularly accurate, however, they may prove useful in some situations.

Patients who are predisposed to PONV can be identified
during preoperative assessment (Jolley 1999). For example a
previous episode of PONV can highlight the need to include an
anti-emetic with the premed or preoperative drug regime. Other
risk factors include extreme anxiety and a history of seasickness.
During preoperative assessment, patients can be informed of
the possibility of PONV and the advantages of anti-emetic
therapy. Patient education is important as many patients believe
that nausea and vomiting are inevitably associated with anaesthesia and don't necessarily know that it can be prevented.

Anxiety could be a contributory cause of PONV, although
this is not certain. Common sense suggests however, that
patient education about the incidence of PONV and how it
can be prevented or treated can only help the patient during
their postoperative care by reducing anxiety about this
condition. Preoperative fasting may also affect PONV, this may
be especially important to consider during emergency surgery
when there may not have been time to prepare the patient
properly.

Careful assessment of established PONV will also help ensure
the patient receives prompt and effective treatment (Arnold
2002c) – once again patient education plays a part in this
process. The practitioner could also play a part in prevention of
PONV by exploring the incidence of this condition during post-

operative care, in order to identify predisposing factors, efficacy of drug regimes or particular successful coping strategies by the patient.

Pain

The preoperative assessment of pain and education of patients in the use of preventive analgesia can help to reduce post-operative pain and associated problems (Mackrodt 2001). For example, many patients' perception of pain has been affected by previous experience or information from parents or friends. Some patients may therefore expect pain as a part of the surgical procedure and without education, may think that it is unavoidable. Misconception about addiction from using opiate analgesics may also prevent patients from taking full advantage of drug therapy available. Preoperative education of what to expect, the different approaches to pain treatment and the support available for the patient may therefore help to prepare the patient for managing their postoperative pain. Chapter 10 discusses postoperative pain relief.

Some hospitals have developed an acute pain service (APS). The main aim of this service is to educate patients and practitioners in all aspects of pain management (Mackrodt 2001). This service is normally led by anaesthetists with practitioners specialising in treating pain. The service often offers support for the preoperative and postoperative care of patients and can include help with patient-controlled analgesia, epidural infusions and other specialised areas of pain relief.

Patient-controlled analgesia (PCA) is a common method of giving analgesia and controlling pain. The technique involves the use of an analgesic infusion which is controlled by the patient using a hand-operated device. Because it involves patient involvement, the patient must be informed of its uses, advantages and disadvantages. It is a valuable way of controlling pain which involves patients in their own recovery, helping to support the patient to a full recovery. However, PCA may not work effectively if the patient is poorly educated and trained in its use.

See Chapter 3 for further discussion on the pharmacology of analgesia.

Wound infection

Wound infection is a common complication and therefore it is important the practitioner takes any preoperative measures that help to reduce the risk of this condition. (See Chapter 5 for a risk assessment approach to infection control.)

Preoperative education about basic hygiene and cleanliness often points the way to good practice. For example, it may be necessary to bring beds into theatre, but if they are, it would make sense to ensure they are as clean as possible. The use of clean linen may also reduce the numbers of dead skin particles brought into theatre.

The need for preoperative skin preparation should be assessed preoperatively. For example, the patient may need occlusive dressings on open skin lesions. Patients with excess hair close to operative sites may need it removed using depilatory creams or shaving. Although this practice has come under much discussion in the literature, the need for shaving or hair removal is still open to question. The perioperative practitioner may have information about the site of surgery and access points for anaesthetic infusions and invasive monitors which may help to inform ward staff of the need for shaving.

CONCLUSION

Preoperative assessment and preparation is a necessary link in the chain for delivering holistic patient care. Practitioners can act as the patient's advocate and communicate relevant information to the rest of the perioperative team, helping to provide continuity of care.

Perioperative practitioners can be instrumental in providing patients with safe, positive surgical experiences and outcomes by focusing on patients as whole beings and not merely on their operative procedures, diseases or injuries. Effective patient education and preoperative assessment helps to prepare the patient effectively for their surgery and anaesthesia. Practitioners must use the small amount of time available preoperatively, to spend quality time interacting with patients so they are safe and feel cared for and secure during their perioperative experience.

REFERENCES

Aitkenhead, A. & Smith, G. (1996) *Textbook of Anaesthesia*, 3rd edn. Churchill Livingstone, Edinburgh.

Amaragiri, S.V. & Lees, T.A. (2001) Elastic compression stockings for the prevention of deep vein thrombosis (Cochrane Review). In: *The Cochrane Library*, Issue 4. Update Software, Oxford.

Arnold, A. (2002a) DVT prophylaxis in the perioperative setting. Part 1. *British Journal of Perioperative Nursing* **12** (8), 294–7.

Arnold, A. (2002b) DVT prophylaxis in the perioperative setting. Part 2. *British Journal of Perioperative Nursing* **12** (9), 326–32.

Arnold, A. (2002c) Postoperative nausea and vomiting in the perioperative setting. *British Journal of Perioperative Nursing* **12** (1), 24–32.

Autar, R. (1996) Nursing assessment of clients at risk of deep venous thrombosis: the Autur DVT scale. *Journal of Advanced Nursing* **23** (4), 763–70.

Bellert, J.L. (1989) Humor: A therapeutic approach in oncology nursing. *Cancer Nursing* **12** (April), 65–70.

Boore, J. (1975) *Prescription for Recovery*. RCN, London.

Booth, K. (1991) Preoperative visiting. *British Journal of Theatre Nursing* **1** (7), 31.

Brown, A. & Duxbury, J. (1997) Day surgery – Communication and interviewing skills. *British Journal of Theatre Nursing* **7** (4), 10–14.

Clevenger, F. & Tepas III, J. (1997) Preoperative management of patients with major trauma injuries. *AORN Journal* **65** (3), 583–4, 587–94.

Crawford, B. (1999) Highlighting the role of the perioperative nurse: Is preoperative assessment necessary? *British Journal of Theatre Nursing* **9** (7), 309–12.

Davis, P. (1999) The hidden threat: deep venous thrombosis. *Journal of Orthopaedic Nursing* **Supplement 1** (3), 28–34.

Dyke, M. (2000) Perioperative communication. In: Hind, M. and Wicker, P. *Principles of Perioperative Practice*. Churchill Livingstone, Edinburgh.

Fyffe, A. (1999) Anxiety and the preoperative patient. *British Journal of Theatre Nursing* **9** (10), 452–4.

Gould, D. (1994) Keeping on tract. *Nursing Times* **90** (40), 58–64.

Hathaway, D. (1986) Cited in: Burridge, L. (1993) Challenging the traditional view of preoperative visiting. *British Journal of Theatre Nursing* **3** (4), 12–14.

Hayward, J. (1978) Information: A prescription against pain. *Royal College of Nursing Research Society Newsletter* Series **2** (5), 36–50.

Johnson, S. (1994) Patient focused care without the upheaval. *Nursing Standard* **8** (29), 20–2.

Jolley, S. (1999) Let's get positive about postoperative nausea and vomiting. *British Journal of Theatre Nursing* **9** (10), 450–1.

Litwack, K. (1995) *Post Anaesthesia Care Nursing*, 2nd edn. Mosby Year-Book. Mosby, St Louis, Missouri.

Lowery, M. (1995) Knowledge that reduces anxiety: creating patient information leaflets. *Professional Nurse* **10** (5), 318–20.

Mackrodt, K. (2001) The role of an acute pain service. *British Journal of Perioperative Nursing* **11** (11), 492–7.

McNeil, M. (2004) Management of a CJD case Part 1 Preoperative organisation of the case. *British Journal of Perioperative Nursing* **14** (4), 164–70.

Neacsu, A. (2002) Predication of difficult intubation: A pre-assessment nurses' guide. *British Journal of Perioperative Nursing* **12** (7), 249–53.

Nelson, S. (1995) Preadmission clinics for thoracic surgery. *Nursing Times* **91** (15), 29–31.

Norton, D., McLaren, R. & Exton-Smith, A.N. (1962) *An Investigation of Geriatric Nursing Problems in Hospital*. National Corporation for the Care of Old People, London.

Quantrill, S. (2001) Deep vein thrombosis: Incidence and physiology. *British Journal of Perioperative Nursing* **11** (10), 442–51.

Roy, C. (1976) *Introduction to Nursing: An Adaptation Model*. Prentice Hall, Englewood Cliffs.

Roy, C. & McLeod, D. (1981) Theory of the person as an adaptive system. In: Roy, C. and Roberts, S.L. (eds) *Theory Construction in Nursing: An Adaptive Model*. Prentice Hall, Englewood Cliffs.

Schrecengost, A. (2001) Do humorous preoperative teaching strategies work? *AORN Journal* **74** (5), 683.

Scott, E.M. (2000) The prevention of pressure ulcers in the operating department. *Journal of Wound Care* **8** (1), 18–21.

Starritt, T. & Ewing, E. (1999) Implementing good practice in the prevention and management of pressure sores. *British Journal of Theatre Nursing* **9** (2), 60–3.

Tappen, R.M., Muzic, J. & Kennedy, P. (2001) Preoperative assessment and discharge planning for older adults undergoing ambulatory surgery. *AORN Journal* **73** (2), 464, 467, 469.

Thomas, S. (1999) Graduated compression stockings and the prevention of deep vein thrombosis (Part 2). *Journal of Wound Care* **8** (2), 93–5.

Waterlow, J. (1985) A risk assessment card. *Nursing Times* **81** (48), 49–55.

Waterlow, J. (1996) Operating table: The root of many pressure sores? *British Journal of Theatre Nursing* **6** (7), 19–21.

Wolfer, J.A. & Davis, C.E. (1970) Cited in: Copp, G. 1988 *Intraoperative Information and Preoperative Visiting*. Medical Group (UK), London.

Patient Care during Anaesthesia

8

LEARNING OUTCOMES

❏ Understand *roles and responsibilities of the anaesthetic practitioner*.
❏ Identify *principles and techniques of* general *anaesthesia*, regional, local anaesthesia and sedation.
❏ Understand and recognise *safe use of anaesthetic equipment*.

INTRODUCTION

Anaesthesia can be administered via different methods. Each method should be considered, taking into account the patient's medical condition and age, ideal operating condition, patient comfort and choice. The different techniques are: general anaesthesia, regional anaesthesia, local anaesthesia and sedation. These methods, use of anaesthetic equipment and the roles and responsibilities of anaesthetic practitioners will be discussed in this chapter.

Anaesthetic practitioners, who may be nurses or operating department practitioners (ODPs), are integral to operating practice and safe, effective patient care. They have responsibilities to the patients and their colleagues to maintain safe practice in the operating room environment, and for their own professional development. Patients are at their most vulnerable during their perioperative journey.

It is important that the practitioner displays a professional, confident and caring attitude to patients during their perioperative journey. They should provide a safe environment for the patient undergoing a general, regional or local anaesthesia, or sedation. The aim of the practitioner is to care for the patient during their perioperative journey, which includes: ·

- Reception area where the anaesthetic practitioner greets the patient and checks the preoperative document.
- Anaesthetic room where the anaesthetist establishes general anaesthesia, regional anaesthesia, local anaesthesia or sedation.
- Operating room where the anaesthetist and anaesthetic practitioner maintain anaesthesia.
- Recovery room where the recovery practitioner extubates and monitors patients until their condition is stable enough for the porter and ward nurse to escort them back to the ward.

This list does not include all the roles and responsibilities of the individual perioperative practitioners. These will be described in the different chapters of the book.

Anaesthetic practitioners have a duty to maintain their professional competence and development in operating room practice. They undertake an in-house training programme or a recognised university anaesthetic course before embarking on anaesthetic practice. They should be aware of the specialised anaesthetic equipment, relevant drugs and safe positioning of the patient within the operating room environment to ensure a safe perioperative journey. Other responsibilities include maintaining the correct temperature and humidity in the individual operating room for the particular surgical procedures.

Aitkenhead & Smith (1996) provide a summary of important factors which should minimise the risk of accidents during anaesthesia and the risk of litigation against the anaesthetist:

- Careful preoperative assessment should be undertaken to identify risk factors such as concurrent disease, chronic medication, history of allergy or other untoward reactions to anaesthesia and potential difficulties in tracheal intubation.
- Anaesthetic equipment must be maintained according to the manufacturer's recommendations and checked thoroughly before every operating room session, or when the equipment is changed during an operative session.
- The anaesthetic technique should be recognised as relevant for the individual patient and for the proposed type of surgery.

- The anaesthetist must always be present during anaesthesia.
- Appropriate monitoring, in accordance with national recommendations, should always be employed during anaesthesia and in the immediate recovery period. Alarms should be set at suitable levels and must not be disabled.
- All anaesthetists should be taught to manage common emergencies, such as failed intubation, anaphylaxis or malignant hyperthermia. It is advisable to have protocols available in every anaesthetising location to act as an aide-memoire for uncommon emergencies, and anaesthetists and operating room staff should rehearse emergency management regularly.
- The anaesthetist should keep careful records.

These issues are also applicable to anaesthetic practitioners in their practice within the operating room environment.

The roles and responsibilities of anaesthetic practitioners for the patient's perioperative journey are to:

- Prepare and check relevant equipment and drugs.
- Relieve the patient's anxiety by effective reassurance and communication throughout their perioperative journey (see Mitchell 2005).
- Undertake the preoperative checklist (see Figure 8.1).
- Locate any missing information or documentation before the start of the surgical procedure.
- Assist the anaesthetist in the chosen anaesthesia.
- Assist in the safe positioning of the patient, to prevent pressure damage. + NERVE DAMAGE
- Monitor the patient throughout anaesthesia.
- Complete effective documentation of patient's care.
- Communicate effectively with the multidisciplinary operating room team.

The role of the operating room support worker is to assist anaesthetists and anaesthetic practitioners in the anaesthetic and operating rooms with patient positioning and during anaesthesia. They are known by different names in different hospitals but undertake the same responsibilities.

Checklist	Comments of ward nurse	Comments of anaesthetic practitioner
Consent form completed correctly		
Identification bracelet		
Notes, investigations, preoperative assessment		
Operation site if applicable		
Site: left, right, both		
Allergies (please note)		
Jewellery removed or taped		
Dentures removed		
Loose teeth, dental work		
Hearing aid or prosthesis removed		
Baseline observations (blood pressure, pulse, temperature, respirations, oxygen saturation)		
Ward urinalysis		
Blood sugar		
Weight		
Waterlow score		
Deep vein thrombosis (DVT) risk (high, medium, low)		
Anti-embolitic stockings/deep vein thrombosis (DVT) prophylaxis aid used		
Last menstrual period (LMP)		
Is there any chance of the patient being pregnant? Yes or no If yes, pregnostician performed? Yes or no		
Medication Drugs accompanying patient: Premedicatiion: Time given: Prescribed drugs are:		
Nil by mouth from		
Interpreter required? If yes, booked for:		
Patient requests		
Patient accompanied by: Qualified nurse Student Health care worker Relative Other		

Fig. 8.1 Example of a preoperative checklist. (Continued on next page.)

Checklist	Comments of ward nurse	Comments of anaesthetic practitioner
Additional information (e.g. identify if patient is nervous and reassure patient in the anaesthetic room)		
Signature by ward nurse	Date	Time
Signature by theatre practitioner	Date	Time

Fig. 8.1 *Continued.*

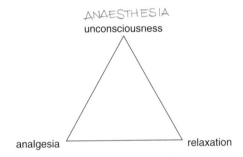

Fig. 8.2 Triad of anaesthesia.

GENERAL ANAESTHESIA

General anaesthesia can be divided into three components: unconsciousness (hypnosis), pain relief (analgesia) and muscle relaxation. All anaesthetic drugs produce anaesthesia by their effect on the brain. Anaesthetic gases are inhaled and then must be transferred from the lungs to the circulation and finally to the brain to be effective (Morton 1997).

Anaesthetists identify the 'Triad of anaesthesia' or 'Balanced anaesthesia'. This incorporates unconsciousness, analgesia and relaxation (Figure 8.2).

Airway management

The principal requirements of airway management in general anaesthesia are to:

- Ensure a patent airway.
- Deliver satisfactory ventilation:
  — spontaneous – patients breathe themselves;
  — mechanical or controlled – use of a ventilator and muscle relaxant and reversal drugs.
- Monitor and record patients' physiological observations.

The aim of airway management is to secure and maintain a patient's airway. Induction of anaesthesia may cause the patient's soft palate and epiglottis to move towards the back wall of the pharynx. During inspiration the walls of the pharynx can then collapse and obstruct the patient's airway.

Techniques that the anaesthetist or anaesthetic practitioner can use to secure a patent airway for patients with spontaneous breathing or ventilation are:

- *Head tilt and chin lift.* The head tilt and chin lift technique is administered by placing one hand on the forehead and tilting the head backwards while using the fingers of the other hand to draw the chin upwards and open (Griffiths 1999).
- *Jaw thrust.* A jaw thrust manoeuvre may be achieved by applying pressure on the mandible of the jaw, causing an anterior and upwards movement while using the thumbs to slightly open the mouth (Griffiths 1999). This is the technique of choice in the case of suspected cervical spine injury.

Anaesthetists can insert an oropharyngeal airway to maintain a patient's airway and to hold the tongue away from the posterior pharyngeal wall. It is inserted upside down and rotated 180° as it passes backwards into the mouth.

If a nasopharyngeal airway (lubricated well) is inserted into the nostril it is rotated gently into position – but they are not used for patients with suspected basal skull fractures.

The anaesthetic practitioner can help the anaesthetist during these techniques by repositioning the patient's head on the pillow, by flattening or plumping up the pillow or by removing hair accessories to ensure the correct position of the patient's head on the pillow. These techniques may be utilised within recovery care and this will be discussed in Chapter 10.

Spontaneous breathing
This may be observed in:

- patients with a face mask (with or without an airway) and a breathing circuit;
- patients with a laryngeal mask airway (LMA) and a breathing circuit;
- patients with an endotracheal tube (ET tube) and a breathing circuit.

Insertion of a laryngeal mask airway
The anaesthetist may insert an LMA and attach it to a breathing circuit to ensure that the patient breathes spontaneously throughout the surgical procedure. The role of the anaesthetic practitioner is outlined in Box 8.1.

Mechanical ventilation and tracheal intubation
Tracheal intubation is used to provide a secure and clear airway through which positive pressure ventilation can be applied. It also protects the airway from blood, vomit and regurgitation. An ET tube is inserted through the mouth and into the trachea through the vocal cords with the aid of a laryngoscope.

Preparation for induction and intubation procedure
The anaesthetic practitioner should check all relevant equipment for these procedures:

- the patient's trolley must have the facility of 'head down';
- monitoring equipment: heart rate, pulse, blood pressure, oxygen saturation, expiry carbon dioxide, measurement of vaporising agent;
- relevant induction drugs;
- face mask, angled piece and filter;
- oral and nasal airway;
- laryngoscope with appropriate sized blades;
- ET tube, lubricating jelly and relevant size of breathing circuit (adult or paediatric);
- introducer or bougie for ET tube;

- catheter mount;
- syringe to inflate the ET tube cuff;
- suction equipment;
- stethoscope for the anaesthetist to check the correct position of the ET tube;
- bandage or tape to secure the ET tube;

The correct size of ET tube is selected and checked for the adult patient and a size smaller size is made available in case of emergency.

- for the female adult: a size 8.0, 7.5, 7.0 or 6.5;
- for the male adult: a size 9.0, 8.5, 8.0 or 7.5;
- for the paediatric patient the size of the tube is determined by the age and weight of the patient and this is discussed later in this chapter.

The role of the anaesthetic practitioner is outlined in Box 8.2.

Rapid sequence induction (RSI)

This procedure is applied in emergency surgical procedures when the patient has a full stomach, in patients who have a hiatus hernia or with patients prone to reflux and therefore at risk of aspiration of the gastric contents into the lungs. It is the same procedure as tracheal intubation with cricoid pressure. The patient is preoxygenated for 3–5 minutes to maximise oxygen reserves. This prevents hypoxia and ensures oxygenation of the lungs in difficult intubation or airway obstruction. The ET tube is inserted by the anaesthetist. If any problems arise, he reapplies the face mask to ensure reoxygenation of the lungs and will attempt intubation again. The intubation procedure is as previously described in Box 8.2.

Cricoid pressure (Sellick's manoeuvre)

The unconscious patient, during tracheal intubation, is at risk from regurgitation or aspiration of stomach contents. Cricoid pressure can relieve these problems by occluding the oesophagus between the cricoid cartilage (ring) and the vertebral column (Figure 8.3). The anaesthetist discusses this procedure with the patient at their preoperative visit.

Box 8.1   Role of the anaesthetic practitioner prior to and during the insertion of an LMA

Before the procedure, check:

- All piped and cylinder gases are flowing efficiently. Replace any cylinders, if necessary.
- The breathing circuit, with valve closed and open. Ensure the valve is open before use.
- Vaporisers are full and replenish if necessary.
- Suction is working and appropriate accessories are available.
- LMA.
- Induction equipment.
- Relevant drugs.
- An intravenous infusion is available (with or without a fluid warmer and extension with a three-way tap for administration of intravenous drugs).
- All equipment and anaesthetic machines in the anaesthetic room and operating room environment.
- All stock is available.

When the patient is in the anaesthetic room:

- Reassure and communicate with the patient throughout procedure.
- Act as the patient's advocate.
- Attach all monitoring equipment and record observations before commencement of anaesthesia (a base reading).
- Maintain the patient's dignity at all times.
- Assist the anaesthetist in the venous cannulation of the patient.
- Attach a dressing to the venous cannula.
- Inform the anaesthetist of any allergies or medical conditions (arthritis, diabetes etc.) that the patient may have.

When the anaesthetist has administered the induction drugs the anaesthetic practitioner will:

- Pass the face mask and filter to the anaesthetist to preoxygenate the patient.
- Pass the lubricated LMA to the anaesthetist (and hold the patient's lower lip down for easy access).
- Pass the breathing circuit to the anaesthetist to attach to the filter.
- Inflate the cuff on the LMA until there is no obvious leak.
- Pass a catheter mount if necessary.
- Pass the tape or bandage to secure the LMA.
- Pass the tape for the eyes or eyegel to protect the eyes during the surgical procedure.

Have available:

- Muscle relaxants in case tracheal intubation is necessary.
- Intubation equipment as described below.

Be aware of the locality of all emergency equipment.

Box 8.2   Role of the anaesthetic practitioner prior to and during intubation

Before the procedure check:

- All piped and cylinder gases are flowing efficiently. Replace any cylinders, if necessary.
- The breathing circuit, with valve closed and open before the procedure. Ensure the valve is open before use.
- Vaporisers are full and replenish if necessary.
- Suction is working and appropriate accessories are available.
- Induction equipment.
- Relevant drugs.
- An intravenous infusion available (with or without a fluid warmer and extension with a three-way tap for administration of intravenous drugs).
- All equipment and anaesthetic machines in the anaesthetic room and theatre.
- All stock is available.

When the patient is in the anaesthetic room:

- Reassure and communicate with the patient throughout procedure.
- Attach all monitoring equipment and record observations before commencement of anaesthesia (a base reading).
- Maintain the patient's dignity at all times.
- Assist the anaesthetist in the venous cannulation of the patient.
- Attach a dressing to the venous cannula.
- Inform the anaesthetist of any allergies or medical conditions (arthritis, diabetes etc.) that the patient may have.

When the anaesthetist has administered the induction drugs:

- Pass the face mask and filter to the anaesthetist to preoxygenate the patient.
- Pass the laryngoscope – hold the patient's lower lip down for easy access of the laryngoscope. Have other laryngoscopes available as backup.
- Pass the ET tube and after insertion inflate the cuff on the ET tube until there is no obvious leak.
- Pass the breathing circuit to the anaesthetist to attach to the filter.
- Pass a catheter mount if necessary.
- Pass the tape or bandage to secure the ET tube.
- Pass the tape for the eyes or eye gel to protect the eyes during the surgical procedure.

Have available:

- Suction equipment and suction catheters (ready under the patient's pillow for easy access).
- Relevant size of oropharygeal airway.
- A bougie. The anaesthetist may have difficulty when inserting the ET tube.
- A stethoscope for the anaesthetist to check the correct position of the ET tube.

Box 8.2 *Continued.*

Be aware:

- Cricoid pressure may be necessary to ensure tracheal intubation is successful
- Where to find all emergency equipment.

The anaesthetist may connect the patient to the ventilator in the anaesthetic room or after transfer on to the operating table.

The person carrying out cricoid pressure must first identify the cricoid cartilage as the first prominence beneath the thyroid cartilage (Adam's apple). They centre it between the thumb and middle fingers of the (dominant) hand while pressing down firmly with the index finger. Good (firm) cricoid pressure sometimes pushes the neck down with the (dominant) hand while supporting the back of the neck with the (non-dominant) hand (bimanual cricoid pressure) (Morton 1997). If the operating room support worker performs single-hand cricoid pressure he or she will use the dominant hand only and not use the other hand to support the neck.

When anaesthetic practitioners or operating room support workers perform cricoid pressure, they:

- Inform the patient that they are going to apply pressure as the anaesthetist administers the induction drugs and commences intubation. They support the patient's neck with one hand and with the other hand apply the cricoid pressure.
- Maintain the correct pressure throughout the procedure (10 newtons until the patient is unconscious and 30 newtons thereafter).
- Do not remove this pressure until the anaesthetist is satisfied the ET tube is in the correct position and anaesthesia is established.
- Remove the cricoid pressure on instructions from the anaesthetist if the patient actively vomits. Vomiting may rupture the oesophagus if the cricoid pressure is not released.

During this procedure preparation is the key and all anaesthetic personnel need to be aware of their responsibilities and the

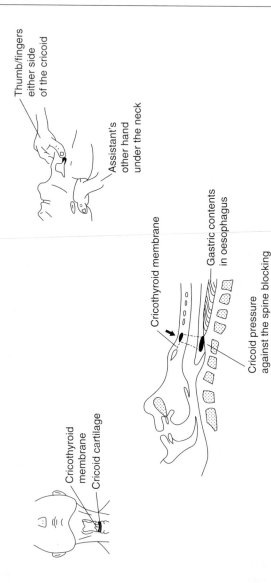

Thumb/fingers
either side
of the cricoid

Assistant's
other hand
under the neck

Cricothyroid membrane

Gastric contents
in oesophagus

Cricoid pressure
against the spine blocking
the oesophagus

Cricothyroid
membrane

Cricoid cartilage

Fig. 8.3 Position for cricoid pressure.

safety of the patient. Anaesthetists do not ask for cricoid pressure during the tracheal intubation procedure if the patient is actively vomiting.

Awake intubation

This technique is used principally if the anaesthetist suspects a difficult airway management problem such as difficult intubation. The patient is awake during the intubation and is breathing spontaneously and therefore is able to manage his or her own airway until the ET tube is securely in position. The anaesthetist can then administer induction drugs to maintain anaesthesia and ventilation of the patient.

A fibre-optic laryngoscope can be used during an awake intubation procedure. Before the procedure the anaesthetic practitioner or anaesthetist can thread the ET tube onto the scope ready for intubation.

Awake intubation is used to check the patient's airway anatomy (nose, larynx and trachea), for confirmation of the correct insertion of the ET tube, to evaluate trauma or the signs of infection. The patient's posterior pharynx is sprayed with local anaesthetic to minimise the gag reflex and other airway reflexes when the fibre-optic laryngoscope is inserted.

After use the anaesthetic practitioner cleans and sterilises the laryngoscope following local policy guidelines. The role of the anaesthetic practitioner in this procedure is outlined in Box 8.3.

Complications of tracheal intubation

Difficult intubation

Occasionally the anaesthetist may have difficulty in the tracheal intubation procedure because of the patient's anatomy or pathology. Cormack & Lehane (1984) classified difficult airways based on the view obtained at laryngoscopy:

- Grade 1: most of the glottis is visible and there should be no difficulty.
- Grade 2: if only the posterior aspect of the glottis is visible then there may be slight difficulty. Light pressure on the larynx will nearly always bring at least the arytenoids into view if not the vocal cords.

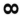

3: if no part of the glottis can be seen, only the epiglot-
n there may be fairly severe difficulty.
- Grade 4: if not even the epiglottis can be exposed then intubation may be impossible except by alternative methods.

Other anatomical issues may be observed, such as patient
limited head extension and difficulty in opening of the mouth,
restricted neck movements, tracheal stenosis or deviation that
might produce a difficult intubation procedure.

Anaesthetic practitioners will prepare the equipment for
tracheal intubation but have all laryngoscopes including the

Box 8.3   Role of the anaesthetic practitioner prior to and during the awake intubation procedure

Prepare:

- Fibre-optic laryngoscope, bite guard and light source (battery or mains).
- Reinforced or oral ET tube (6.0 / 7.0).
- Difficult intubation tray.
- Local anaesthetic throat spray.
- Nasal spray.
- Syringe, needles, kwill and normal saline.
- Suction tubing.
- Nasal oxygen.
- Vomit bowl.
- Tape to secure the ET tube.
- A stethoscope available for the anaesthetist to check the position of the ET tube.

During procedure:

- Reassure and communicate with the patient.
- Attach all monitoring equipment and record observations before the start of the anaesthetic to have a base reading.
- Assist the anaesthetist in the venous cannulation of the patient.
- Attach a dressing to the intravenous cannula.
- Have available an intravenous infusion (with or without a fluid warmer and extension with a three-way tap for administration of intravenous drugs) for the anaesthetist.

Have:

- Relevant induction drugs.
- A breathing circuit.
- Suction ready for use.
- Emergency equipment to hand.

McCoy and short-handle laryngoscopes, the fibre-optic laryngoscope and cricothyroid needle set available during the procedure.

The anaesthetists can use either a bougie or an introducer:

- A bougie aids the insertion of the ET tube. They insert the bougie through the larynx and vocal cords under direct vision or blind. The anaesthetic practitioner passes the ET tube over the bougie and the anaesthetist feeds the tube through the vocal cords. The anaesthetic practitioner removes the bougie on the instructions of the anaesthetist.
- An introducer alters the shape of the ET tube. The anaesthetic practitioner inserts it into the selected ET tube and ensures it does not protrude beyond the distal end of the tube as this might cause damage to the larynx. The anaesthetic practitioner removes the introducer on the instructions of the anaesthetist after correct insertion of the ET tube.

Failed intubation

The anaesthetist will attempt to oxygenate the patient by any means necessary. He or she will try to insert an oropharyngeal airway and oxygenate the patient with 100% oxygen. He or she will:

- Request help from other anaesthetists.
- Ask for cricoid pressure and try to intubate the patient with a size 6 ET tube
- Insert an LMA.
- Wake the patient and undertake a regional anaesthetic technique.
- Undertake an awake intubation.
- Attempt an needle cricothyroidotomy. Complications from this procedure are pneumothorax, surgical emphysema and problems with exhalation. The role of the anaesthetic practitioner in this procedure is outlined in Box 8.4. Figure 8.4 shows the equipment used.
- Postpone the surgery.

Laryngospasm

Laryngospasm is a reflex, prolonged closure of the vocal cords in a response to a trigger, usually airway stimulation during

---

Box 8.4

(a) Role of the anaesthetic practitioner during a cricothyroidotomy procedure using a needle

- Assist the anaesthetist in the procedure.
- Prepare a cricothyroidotomy needle.
- Have the venturi injector device to provide a high pressure oxygen source through the cricothyroidotomy needle (50 psi pressure).
- Have available an intravenous infusion (with or without a fluid warmer and extension with a three-way tap for administration of intravenous drugs) for the anaesthetist.
- Pass tape to secure the needle.

Have:

- Suction ready for use.
- Emergency equipment to hand.

(b) Role of the anaesthetic practitioner during a surgical cricothyroidotomy procedure using an ET tube

- Assist the anaesthetist in the procedure.
- Prepare the ET tube or tracheostomy tube.
- Have a syringe for inflation of tube.
- Have a breathing circuit to attach to the ET tube or tracheostomy tube.
- Have available an intravenous infusion (with or without a fluid warmer and extension with a three-way tap for administration of intravenous drugs) for the anaesthetist.
- Pass tape or bandage available to secure the tube.

Have:

- Suction ready for use.
- Emergency equipment to hand.

---

light anaesthesia. It is most common during induction, premature insertion of an oropharyngeal airway, presence of pharyngeal secretions or blood or airway irritation from volatile agents (Aitkenhead *et al.* 2001).

The laryngeal muscles contract and occlude the glottis. The anaesthetist will use appropriate suction, administer 100% oxygen and deepen the anaesthesia to relieve it or administer muscle relaxants and ventilate the patient.

Aspiration of gastric contents

Patients with a history of hiatus hernia, acid reflux or other intra-abdominal pathology that may cause the possibility of

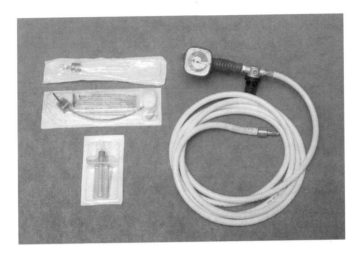

Fig. 8.4 Cricothyroid equipment.

aspiration of gastric contents at intubation are identified. In this case the anaesthetist will carry out an RSI procedure. He will advise the anaesthetic practitioner or operating room support worker of the need to undertake cricoid pressure during the RSI procedure. Complications of aspiration are bronchospasm, acute (adult) respiratory distress syndrome (ARDS), sepsis and eventually death.

Bronchospasm

Bronchospasm is temporary narrowing of the bronchi and any irritants present can cause this. The anaesthetist will administer 100% oxygen to the patient and, if necessary, administer bronchodilator drugs.

General anaesthesia can alter airway resistance by influencing bronchomotor tone, lung volumes and bronchial secretions (Aitkenhead *et al.* 2001). The anaesthetist will use appropriate suction, administer 100% oxygen, maintain the airway and reposition the ET tube if necessary.

Box 8.5   Role of the anaesthetic practitioner during an anaphylactic attack

Assist the anaesthetist:

- Provide appropriate emergency drugs (oxygen and adrenaline).
- Prepare an intravenous infusion.
- Record all physiological readings.
- Record all relevant care.

Have available:

- Resuscitation equipment.

Undertake cardiopulmonary resuscitation if necessary.

Acute (adult) respiratory distress syndrome

Acute (adult) respiratory distress syndrome (ARDS) is a syndrome when the alveoli become inflamed, causing them to fill up with liquid and then they collapse. Gas exchange ceases and the body becomes starved of oxygen. Mechanical ventilation is necessary.

Other induction complications

Anaphylaxis

Anaphylaxis is an exaggerated response to a drug or foreign substance (Morton 1997). The response may occur during or after the induction procedure. The patient may develop a rash or swelling and bronchospasm. It may be difficult to ventilate the patient. Hypotension and tachycardia are identified by observation of the patient's physiological readings. The anaesthetist will stop all administration of anaesthetic drugs, will administer 100% oxygen and maintain the airway and give emergency drugs as necessary. The role of the anaesthetic practitioner in this instance is outlined in Box 8.5.

Malignant hyperpyrexia

In malignant hyperpyrexia the patient's muscles unexpectedly increase their rate of metabolism. They use oxygen at a huge rate and produce carbon dioxide, acids, potassium and heat. In susceptible individuals it is triggered by suxamethonium and by any volatile agents (Morton 1997).

> **Box 8.6 Role of the anaesthetic practitioner during malignant hyperpyrexia**
>
> Assist the anaesthetist:
>
> - Provide dantrolene and intravenous infusions including sodium bicarbonate.
> - Provide ice packs to reduce the patient's temperature.
> - Record all physiological readings.
> - Prepare any relevant equipment for further treatment: e. g. arterial and central venous pressure.
>
> Have available:
>
> - Resuscitation equipment.

Increased expiry carbon dioxide and tachycardia are observed from the physiological recordings. The anaesthetist will stop all administration of anaesthetic drugs and volatile agents, will administer 100% oxygen and maintain the airway and administer dantrolene and sodium bicarbonate intravenously. The role of the anaesthetic practitioner in this instance is outlined in Box 8.6.

ANAESTHETIC EQUIPMENT

Face masks
These are available in black rubber or transparent plastic and in different sizes (Figure 8.5). Their design aims to fit the patient's face without any leaks (the anaesthetic team can observe any secretions through a transparent mask). The air-filled cuff of the mask helps to minimise the mask's pressure on the patient's face. Suitable sizes should be available for the patient. An angle piece and an airway filter fits onto the face mask and a catheter mount and the breathing system fits onto the airway filter.

Airway filter
Airway filters are single use and prevent the spread of infection from the patient into the breathing circuit or ventilator.

Catheter mount
The catheter mount is a corrugated disposable tubing (single use) which may have a concertina design. It lessens the trans-

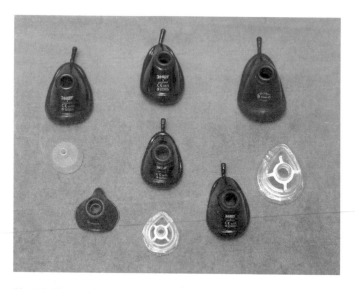

Fig. 8.5 Face masks.

mission of accidental movements and allows adjustment of the breathing system to the ET tube. Its length contributes to the apparatus dead space.

Laryngeal mask airway (LMA)

The LMA, invented by Brain in 1981, is a general-purpose airway that fills a niche between the face mask and ET tube, both in anatomical location and degree of invasiveness. It sits with its tip in the hypopharynx at the interface between the gastrointestinal and respiratory tracts and here it forms a circumferential low-pressure seal around the glottis. This has the advantages in maintaining the gas flow through the upper airway and in providing direct access to the glottis without loss of airway control. The LMA allows the administration of gases through a minimally stimulating airway (Intavent 1999).

The advantages over the ET tube include avoidance of laryngoscopy, less invasion of the respiratory tract, avoidance of the risks of endobronchial or oesophageal intubation and less trauma to local tissues. The main disadvantage of the LMA compared with the ET tube is that air leakage and gastric insufflation are more likely. It also does not secure the airway as effectively as an ET tube and airway obstruction at the glottic and subglottic level cannot be prevented (Intavent 1999).

Anaesthetists insert LMAs for general anaesthesia when the patient breathes spontaneously throughout the surgical procedure. The LMA is lubricated by the anaesthetic practitioner just before insertion so that the lubricant does not dry out. It is only necessary to lubricate the back of the mask. If the front of the LMA is lubricated, globules of lubricant may block the tube, especially in children, or the patient may inhale the lubricant after insertion, causing laryngeal spasm or coughing.

The LMA has an inflatable silicone ring and cuff. When the cuff is inflated by the anaesthetic practitioner the mask fills the space around and behind the larynx. This ensures a tight seal and no detection of any leak. The LMA is secured by using either bandage or tape. Different sizes of the various LMAs are available for patients of all ages. It is essential to check the laryngeal mask before use.

Consultant anaesthetists may use an LMA in the tracheal intubation procedure in the place of an ET tube. The anaesthetic practitioner should always have an ET tube available in case of inadequate ventilation.

Standard LMA

The LMA is of medical grade silicone rubber, it is latex free and is reusable and sterilised by steam autoclaving. It consists of a flexible curved opening into the lumen at the distal end of a small elliptical mask that has an inflatable outer rim (Figure 8.6).

Reinforced LMA

This LMA design is ideal for use in surgery to the head, neck and upper torso where the standard LMA would either interfere with the surgical field or occlude or be displaced by the surgeon. It is crushproof and kink-free but not bite proof.

Disposable LMA

This has similar properties to the standard LMA but is more rigid and has a thicker cuff than the reusable LMA.

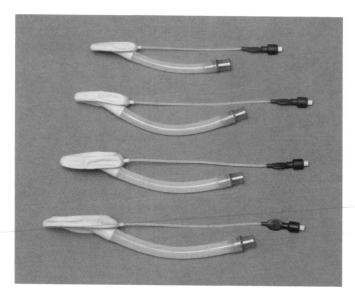

Fig. 8.6 Standard laryngeal masks.

Intubating LMA

This has better intubation characteristics than the standard LMA. It consists of an anatomically curved, short, wide-bore, stainless steel tube sheathed in silicone, which bonds to an LMA and a guiding handle. It has a single moveable epiglottic elevator bar, a guiding V-shaped ramp and can allow up to an 8 mm tracheal tube. The LMA has a dedicated straight-cuffed silicone tracheal tube with a soft bevelled tip.

Proseal LMA

The proseal LMA is designed to conform to the contours of the hypopharynx, with its lumen facing the laryngeal opening. The mask has a main cuff that seals around the laryngeal opening and a rear cuff helps increase the seal. Attached to the mask is an inflation line terminating in a pilot balloon and valve for mask inflation and deflation. A removable introducer tool is available to aid insertion of the LMA to avoid placing a finger in the mouth on insertion.

Cleaning and sterilisation

The LMA is a reusable and it is autoclaved by the Hospital Sterilisation and Decontaminations Unit (HSDU) before its first use and before each following use (following local policy). If it is placed in water after removal, secretions will not become dried on to it. Standard precautions should be followed during cleaning of the LMA and it is washed in warm water. The cuff is deflated before sterilisation. The temperature should be 134°C for steam autoclaving following the standard procedure for porous loads.

Pre-use tests

- Test 1: Examine the interior of the tube to ensure free from blockage or loose particles. Then flex the tube to increase its curvature. Kinking of the tube should not occur when it bends around 180°. Do not bend beyond 180° to avoid permanent damage to the tube.
- Test 2: The tube should be transparent so any fluids or contaminants within it are readily obvious. Discoloration of the tube usually indicates considerable use beyond the warranty use (40 uses), and hinders the ability to detect potential airway problems. Ensure the connector has a secure fit.
- Test 3: Examine the opening in the mask to ensure integrity of the mask open bars. The spaces between the bars must be free from any particulate matter.
- Test 4: Deflate the mask cuff to a high vacuum so the cuff walls are flat tightly against each other. Remove the syringe from the syringe port with a rapid twisting action. Now examine the cuff walls to ensure they remain tightly flattened against each other. Gradual inflation suggests there is a faulty valve or a leaking cuff.
- Test 5: Inflate the cuff from complete vacuum as follows: size 1 – 7 ml, size 2 – 10 ml, size 2.5 – 14 ml, size 3 – 20 ml, size 4 – 30 ml, size 5 – 40 ml. If no leak is apparent inflate 50% more air into the cuff and again check for leaks. There should not be uneven bulging of the cuff or either end or on one or other of the sides (Intavent 1999).

Equipment for tracheal intubation

Other equipment for tracheal intubation includes face masks, airway filter and catheter mount which have been described earlier for spontaneous breathing.

Laryngoscope

The anaesthetist uses the laryngoscope to examine the larynx and to aid insertion of the ET tube. It consists of a handle and a blade. The handle contains the power source, batteries and the blade has a light carrier with a bulb. The electrical current flows from the battery to the bulb through an insulated contact at the top of the handle. When the laryngoscope blade is opened, the light comes on and it is ready for use. When the blade is closed the light switches off. The bulb illuminates the larynx. The relevant size of blade is used for the particular type of laryngoscope. Blades are also of different sizes to accommodate all ages and sizes of patients.

All types of laryngoscope are checked by the anaesthetic practitioner before use. Failure of the batteries or light bulb can cause a delay in intubation, a worry for the anaesthetist and anaesthetic practitioner and danger to the patient's care. Usually two laryngoscopes are available with different size blades (4 and 3), for intubation of female and male adults. The other one is available as backup if the light or batteries fail. The most commonly used adult laryngoscope blade is the MacIntosh curved blade which is manufactured in several sizes and the Magill laryngoscope (Figure 8.7) and blades for children (Shields & Werder 2002).

The McCoy laryngoscope is based on the standard MacIntosh blade but has a hinged tip (Figure 8.8). When the lever on the handle is pressed the tip of the blade bends forward and this improves the view of the larynx. This laryngoscope is used in the difficult intubation procedure.

Anaesthetic practitioners should be familiar with the identified laryngoscope and blades and the other different types available in their operating departments.

After use the laryngoscope blade is cleaned following local policy, for example:

- The blade is detached and the light carrier is removed.
- The blade is cleaned and sent to the HSDU.
- A new blade is attached to the handle and the light is checked ready for the next patient.

The light carrier or batteries are changed if the light does not work. Standard precautions are followed during the cleaning procedure. If the policy is to use disposable laryngoscope blade covers the anaesthetic practitioner will dispose of the laryngoscope blade cover and attach a new one.

Fibre optic laryngoscope

The laryngoscope consists of an eye piece and insertion tube (Figure 8.9). A light source and suction is necessary for these procedures. Anaesthetic practitioners and anaesthetists should take care with the preparation and use of the instrument because the optic fibres are delicate and easily damaged.

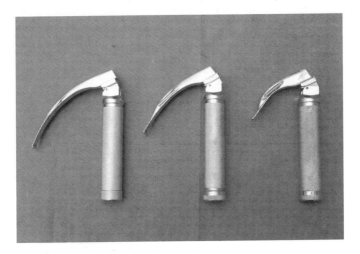

Fig. 8.7 Magill laryngoscope.

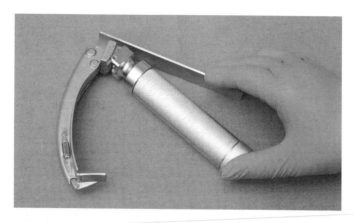

Fig. 8.8 McCoy laryngoscope.

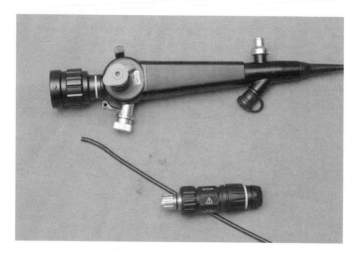

Fig. 8.9 Fibre-optic laryngoscope.

ET tube

ET tubes provide a safe way of securing the patient's airway. They are plastic and transparent for reduction of trauma and

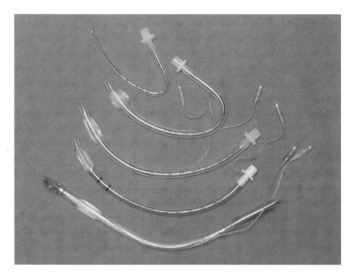

Fig. 8.10 Endotracheal tubes. From top to bottom: RAE tube, RAE tube (cuffed), Lo-pro tube, MLT tube, endobronchial tube.

easy view of secretions (Figure 8.10). They are for single use, and they have a radio-opaque line running along their length to enable easy identification of anatomical position on chest X-rays.

The usual size for a female adult patient is 7–8 mm and for a male adult is 8–9 mm. The anaesthetist decides on the choice of size for paediatric patients depending on the weight and size of the patient. Some anaesthetists prefer their ET tubes cut and some prefer to insert them uncut. Anaesthetists observe the desired length of the ET tube on the outside of the patient's mouth. Anaesthetic practitioners should ensure the connection (cut or uncut) at the end of the ET tube is secure. There are marks on the ET tubes which signify the internal diameter (mm) and the length of the tube (cm).

There is a risk of advancing the tube into one of the main bronchi, usually the right side, if the anaesthetist inserts the tube too far. Correct choice of the ET tube size is essential to minimise the risk of trauma of the larynx.

The ET tube may have a cuff which the anaesthetic practitioner inflates and this provides an airtight seal between the ET tube and trachea. This protects the patient's airway from aspiration of gastric fluid and allows the efficient ventilation during intermittent positive pressure ventilation (IPPV). Non-cuffed ET tubes are used for paediatric anaesthesia under the age of eleven as cuffed tubes may damage the patient's larynx and trachea.

There are different types of tubes and sizes (adult and paediatric) used in anaesthesia:

- Oral. They are made of plastic and have a gentle curve to ease insertion. Adult tubes have a cuff to provide an air-tight fit.
- Ring–Adair–Elwyn (RAE). RAE tubes have a preformed shape to fit the mouth or nose without kinking. They have a bend located just as the tube emerges so the tube connections to the breathing system are at the level of the chin or forehead and they do not interfere with surgical access.
- Reinforced (armoured). Reinforced tubes are plastic or silicone. They are thicker and contain a spiral of metal wire or tough nylon. This prevents kinking and occlusion of the tube when the head or neck rotates or flexes during surgery. Anaesthetic practitioners cannot cut this tube so there can be a risk of bronchial intubation. There are markers just above the cuff to advise the anaesthetist of the correct position of the tube.
- Laser. These tubes are used for laser surgery on the larynx or trachea. Laser tubes can withstand the laser beam. The tube has two cuffs to inflate and the anaesthetic practitioner fills these with normal saline instead of air to prevent the hazard of fire from the laser beam. The anaesthetic practitioner covers the patient's eyes with damp gauze swabs and padding during the surgical procedure.
- Endobronchial or double lumen tubes. During thoracic surgery there is a need to deflate one lung. This offers the surgeon easier and better surgical access. Either a right-hand or left hand tube is selected to allow deflation of one lung while the patient is ventilated using the other lung.
- Montandom. The tube allows the anaesthetist to ventilate a

patient through laryngectomy access. It has a curve at one end to ensure easy access.

- Tracheostomy. These are plastic or metal tubes (curved) that the anaesthetist usually inserts through the second, third or fourth tracheal cartilage rings. They are used for:
  — long-term intermittent positive pressure ventilation;
  — avoidance of an upper airway obstruction that cannot be bypassed with an oral or nasal tracheal tube;
  — maintenance of the airway after the laryngectomy surgical procedure;
  — control of excessive bronchial secretions especially in patients with a reduced consciousness over a long period.

Introducer

Anaesthetists may use this to alter the shape of the ET tube and to aid them in a difficult intubation procedure. Figure 8.11 shows an introducer and bougie.

Bougie

A bougie can be used in a difficult intubation procedure. This can be a single-use item or be sterilised following local policy.

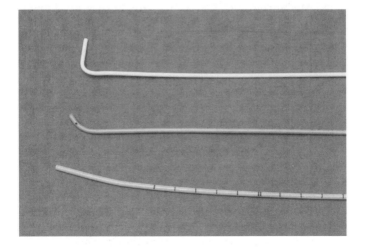

Fig. 8.11 Introducer with bougie.

There are a range of different sizes available for adult and paediatric patients.

If it is not possible to see the larynx in the tracheal intubation procedure the anaesthetist will pass and insert the bougie blind through the vocal cords. The anaesthetic practitioner threads the ET tube on to the bougie and the anaesthetist pushes it down into position. The anaesthetist holds the ET tube and the anaesthetic practitioner removes the bougie once the ET tube is in position. Figure 8.12 shows a bougie within an ET tube.

Oropharyngeal airway

Airways are available in different sizes for adult and paediatric patients. They are inserted through the mouth into the oropharynx above the tongue to protect the airway. There are different sizes for adult and paediatric patients (Figure 8.13).

An airway should never be inserted if the patient has epiglottitis. Total airway obstruction may be precipitated (Illingworth & Simpson 1994).

Nasopharyngeal airway

These airways are inserted through the nose into the nasopharynx. Care must be taken with insertion. They are not used with patients who have bleeding disorders, nasal deformities, head or neck trauma or sepsis. Their role is to provide a patent airway between the nostril and laryngeal opening. These

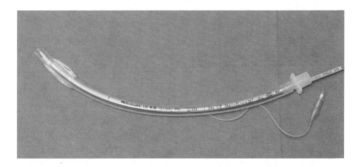

Fig. 8.12 Bougie within an endotracheal tube.

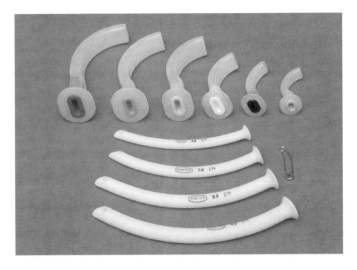

Fig. 8.13   Oropharyngeal and nasopharyngeal airways.

airways are available in different sizes for adult and paediatric patients.

Ryles tube (nasogastric tube)
A Ryles tube can be inserted through the nasopharnyx, down the oesophagus into the stomach to allow emptying of the liquid contents of the stomach before or during the surgical procedure. The ET tube is inserted before the Ryles tube or afterwards depending on the preference of the anaesthetist. The anaesthetist will need Magill forceps and a laryngoscope available for insertion. The role of the anaesthetic practitioner is illustrated in Box 8.7.

Magill forceps
Magill forceps are used when the anaesthetist inserts a Ryles tube or a throat pack or in the removal of foreign body or bodies from the oropharynx and larynx. There are suitable sizes for the adult and paediatric patient.

Box 8.7   Role of the anaesthetic practitioner during the insertion of a Ryles tube

Assist the anaesthetist:

- Select the correct size of tube. Have a smaller and larger size available.
- Pass the lubricated Ryles tube to the anaesthetist.
- Pass the laryngoscope to the anaesthetist.
- Pass the Magill forceps to the anaesthetist to help position the Ryles tube.
- Have suction ready for use.

After insertion:

- Attach a bag to the end of the Ryles tube. Do not forget to close the valve on the end of the bag to prevent leakage. The bag has markings on to identify the quantity of the contents of the bag.
- Secure the Ryles tube to the nose with a nasal dressing.
- Clean the Magill forceps following local policy and then send them to HSDU for sterilisation.

The anaesthetist will not insert a Ryles tube for patients with:

- Head injuries.
- Fracture of the base of the skull.

Oxygen mask

Patients can receive oxygen from a mask which attaches via tubing to the cylinder or piped gas fitting (Figure 8.14). A venturi mask delivers different concentrations of oxygen and anaesthetic; recovery practitioners use this mask when they need to deliver a specific concentration of oxygen to the patient. Different colour attachments represent different concentrations of oxygen.

Oxygen is passed through a narrow orifice within the mask and the sub-atmospheric pressure created by the accelerating oxygen stream entrains room air through openings (side ports) at right angles to the jet stream. The performance of these masks is not appreciably affected by the patient's ventilatory pattern. Masks are available for delivering 24%, 28%, 31%, 40% or 50% oxygen (Morgan & Mikhail 1996).

Nasal cannula

The nasal cannula delivers 2–4 litres of oxygen per minute to the patient. There are two prongs that fit inside the nose and the

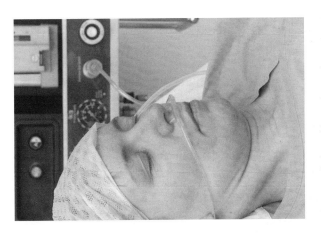

Fig. 8.15 Patient with nasal cannula.

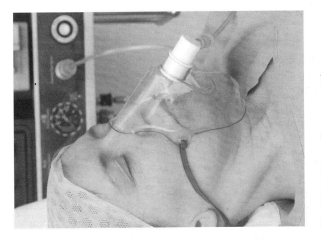

Fig. 8.14 Patient with oxygen mask.

tubing attaches to the oxygen cylinder or piped oxygen (Figure 8.15). There is the potential for trauma to the nasal cavity by the dry airflow but humidified oxygen can reduce this.

MAINTENANCE AND EMERGENCE FROM ANAESTHESIA

Anaesthesia is maintained by the anaesthetist by two methods:

- anaesthesia with inhalational agents and oxygen;
- anaesthesia with total intravenous anaesthesia (TIVA).

Other drugs that may be administered throughout the anaesthesia are:

- analgesics;
- muscle relaxants;
- anti-emetics;
- antibiotics;
- anticholinergics;
- antipressors;
- antidisarrythmias;
- emergency drugs.

These drugs are discussed in further detail in Chapter 3.

The anaesthetic practitioner will also ensure that the following effective care is given to the patient:

- patient monitoring;
- fluid management;
- temperature management: operating room temperature and humidity control, intravenous fluids and warming blankets;
- deep vein thrombosis (DVT) prophylaxis;
- pressure area care;
- documentation.

The role of the anaesthetic practitioner is summarised in Box 8.8 and the documentation completed in the operating room during the maintenance of anaesthesia is summarised in Figure 8.16.

REGIONAL ANAESTHESIA

Regional anaesthesia is the reversible blocking of nerve conduction leading to the abolition of the transmission of impulses

Box 8.8   Role of the anaesthetic practitioner during the maintenance and emergence of anaesthesia in the operating room

- A safe transfer of the patient onto the operating table.
- All attachments (intravenous infusion, catheter etc.) are safe during transfer.
- The patient is comfortable and the use of relevant accessories to prevent any nerve or tissue injuries.
- Attachment of all patient monitoring devices to the monitoring machine.
- All patient physiological recordings are within normal limits.
- The use of warming blankets and temperature probes (following local policies) to prevent the occurrence of hypothermia.
- Availability of relevant intravenous infusions or blood throughout the surgical procedure.
- Availability of any further equipment or anaesthetic requirements for the anaesthetist.
- Availability of the relevant trolley, using an aseptic technique, for any further required procedures.
- Availability of relevant pain management equipment and documentation.
- Completion of documentation for the establishment of anaesthesia and patient care throughout the surgical procedure.
- Locality of emergency equipment and daily checks for immediate use.

Have:

- Reversal drugs available for the anaesthetist.
- Suction equipment available.
- Syringe available to deflate the ET tube cuff if appropriate.
- Patient's facemask, oxygen cylinder and breathing circuit available to transfer the patient from the operating room to the recovery area.
- Scissors to cut the bandage securing the ET tube.

Give:

- An effective handover to the recovery practitioner of the patient's care in the operating room (anaesthesia, intravenous drugs, surgical procedure, method of pain management, drains, catheters, etc. and any issues from the preoperative checklist (allergies, loose teeth, hearing aid etc.).

Ensure:

- Recovery practitioner is satisfied with handover and patient's condition.
- Transfer of any postoperative management equipment into the recovery area. The anaesthetist may start pain management in the anaesthetic room or operating room.
- Attach the patient's monitoring equipment to the recovery monitor.

Relevant equipment checked and available (Sign)	
Ensure check list corresponds to theatre list (Sign)	

Monitor and assess patient throughout induction and surgical procedure:

Induction	**Perioperative**
Oxygen saturation	Oxygen saturation
ECG, Heart rate	ECG, Heart rate
Non-invasive blood pressure	Non-invasive blood pressure
Arterial blood pressure	Arterial blood pressure
Central venous pressure	Central venous pressure
Respirations	Respirations
Temperature	Temperature
Other	Other

Transfer patient to operating table as per local policy

Patient's position:

Aids used to minimise potential risk of pressure or nerve damage:

Temperature maintained by:

Ensure diathermy or tourniquet is applied and used as per local policy

Diathermy site:
Site checked postoperatively:

Tourniquet site:
Tourniquet on:
Tourniquet off:

Assess viability of existing intravenous access
Assist in and perform in intravenous cannulation
Cannula site:
Cannula size:

Record intravenous fluids given and expiry date:

Record urological fluid regime
Record initial urine output if catheterised
Preoperatively: Postoperatively:

Additional information (for example note of allergies, loose teeth, etc.)
Any inhalers with patient:
Application of flowtron boots:
Waterlow score:
Blood sugar result and time if appropriate:

Anaesthetic practitioner signature:
Print name:

Fig. 8.16 Outline of a patient care plan.

in sensory, motor and autonomic nerves and ultimately their sensation. It may be applied to the peripheral nerves or to the spinal cord. Consciousness is maintained. Local anaesthetic agents are used that block the sodium channels of the nerve fibres, thereby blocking the impulses passing along them (Shields & Werder 2002).

Regional anaesthetic techniques

These techniques produce analgesia in a specific part of the body. A local anaesthetic is injected near suitable nerves to achieve regional anaesthesia of the chosen area. The chosen local anaesthetic is injected at or near the nerves of the surgical site and it temporarily interrupts sensory nerve impulses during manipulation of sensitive tissues.

Regional anaesthetic techniques decrease intraoperative stimuli and diminish the stress response to surgical trauma. Regional anaesthesia reduces the stress response and increases the blood flow, which can have benefits for wound healing and diseases such as thrombophlebitis. It can reduce pain intraoperatively and postoperatively.

The patient can solely have a regional anaesthetic for the surgical procedure and will be awake or lightly sedated. In addition the patient may receive oxygen via a nasal cannula or mask. The regional anaesthetic may also be supplemented (for pain management postoperatively) with a general anaesthetic.

The anaesthetic practitioner communicates with, supports and reassures the patient during the following procedures. The patient's correct position is maintained by the anaesthetic practitioner as this is essential for anaesthetist to achieve the procedure successfully.

There are different types of regional anaesthesia and the most common are spinal and epidural.

Spinal

Spinal anaesthesia, also referred to as an intrathecal block, causes desensitisation of spinal ganglia and motor roots. A local anaesthetic is injected into the lumbar intrathecal space. The local anaesthetic blocks conduction in the spinal nerve roots and dorsal ganglia. Paralysis and analgesia occur below the level of the injection.

During a spinal anaesthesia the anaesthetist selects and injects the local anaesthetic drug into the cerebrospinal fluid in the subarachnoid space to produce motor, sensory and autonomic blockade by bathing the nerve roots as they leave the spinal cords. This injection will anaesthetise the spinal nerves resulting in analgesic properties, muscular relaxation and sympathetic blockade. The drug diffuses into the cerebrospinal fluid around ganglia and the nerves before they absorb it into the bloodstream. This technique is used in lower abdominal, inguinal, perineal and obstetric surgical procedures.

This procedure is applied with the patient either in the sitting position (patient is awake), or in the lateral position (patient awake or anaesthetised; Figure 8.17). The patient flexes his or her spine for easier access for the anaesthetist to undertake this procedure. The circulating practitioner supports the patient throughout the procedure and gives reassurance throughout. Figure 8.18 illustrates the position of the injection site within the spine.

Box 8.9 details a checklist for the preparation of the spinal anaesthesia equipment before the procedure.

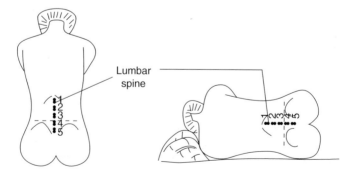

Lumbar spine

Fig. 8.17 Positioning for spinal anaesthesia.

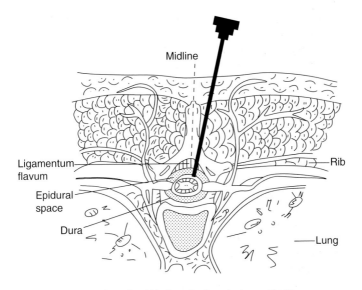

Fig. 8.18 Position of needle within the spine for spinal anaesthesia.

Epidural

The local anaesthetic is injected into the extradural space (epidural space; Figure 8.19). The results are similar to a spinal anaesthetic. During an epidural, the local anaesthetic is injected into the potential space immediately outside the dura mater and this permeates the fatty areolar tissue, contacting the nerves as they transverse into the epidural space. The epidural space lies between the vertebral ligaments and the dura mater of the spinal cord. An injection into the epidural space affects the spinal nerves and causes anaesthesia along these nerves (dermatomes; Figure 8.20).

Anaesthetists use an epidural as an anaesthetic, as an adjuvant to general anaesthesia and for postoperative analgesia in procedures involving the lower limbs, perineum, pelvis, abdomen and thorax (Visser 2001). The amount of local anaesthetic affects the efficiency and amount of nerves affected. The

---

Box 8.9   Role of the anaesthetic practitioner before spinal anaesthesia

- An aseptic technique to prepare the relevant trolley and equipment.
- Relevant size of sterile gown and gloves for the anaesthetist.
- The relevant skin cleansing solution.
- The relevant drape.
- Relevant syringes for local anaesthetic (skin and spinal).
- Relevant needles and filter needle.
- Normal saline.
- Relevant dressing.
- Documentation labels.

Before the procedure:

- Attaches all monitoring equipment.
- Reassures the patient.
- Helps to position the patient correctly before the procedure.
- Maintains the dignity of the patient throughout the procedure.
- Communicates and reassures the patient throughout the procedure.
- Documents physiological recordings throughout the procedure.
- Relevant intravenous infusion with warming coil.

Have:

- All relevant monitoring available. Record all physiological readings.
- Nasal cannula or oxygen mask available.
- Tracheal intubation equipment available.
- Relevant drugs available.
- Emergency equipment available.

---

surgical procedure determines the different levels of the spinal cord (cervical, thoracic, lumbar and caudal spine).

A continuous infusion is commenced in the operating room for postoperative analgesia. A test dose of local anaesthetic is injected to ensure the infusion catheter is correctly in place before the catheter is secured with a dressing. Normal saline is injected into the epidural space through the epidural needle and the epidural tubing is flushed for the epidural infusion. Normal saline can be differentiated from cerebrospinal fluid as the cerebrospinal fluid will be at body temperature and not as cold as the normal saline.

Preparation of equipment for an epidural important for the anaesthetist is outlined in Box 8.10.

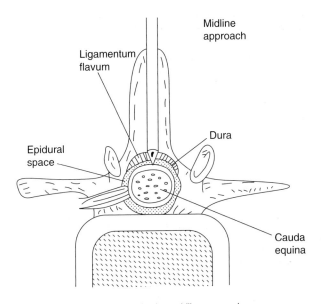

Fig. 8.19 Lumbar epidural anaesthesia – midline approach.

Complications and side effects of a spinal anaesthetic

Spinal anaesthesia is a common procedure but the anaesthetic practitioner must be aware of the risks associated with it:

- toxicity;
- higher volume;
- less predictable block;
- less dense block.

High or total spinal

This can occur if the anaesthetist injects an excessive quantity of local anaesthetic into the subarachnoid space. The block can increase upwards causing a high block and will cause the side effect of hypotension. The recovery team may observe the patient having difficulty in breathing. To assist the patient's breathing both preoperatively and postoperatively the

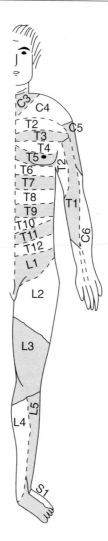

Fig. 8.20 Dermatomes.

Box 8.10   Role of the anaesthetic practitioner before an epidural procedure

- An aseptic technique to prepare the relevant trolley and equipment.
- Relevant size of sterile gown and gloves for the anaesthetist.
- Skin cleansing solution.
- Relevant drape.
- Epidural pack (Tuohy needle, catheter, filter). The catheter allows the topping up of the epidural local anaesthetic.
- Relevant syringes and needles for local anaesthetic (skin).
- Normal saline for flush of epidural tubing and filter.
- Relevant dressings.
- Documentation labels.
- Equipment for the epidural infusion:
  — infusion bag – relevant infusion local anaesthetic and opiate (e.g. bupivacaine and fentanyl);
  — infusion pump with batteries;
  — infusion set;
  — documentation labels.

Before the procedure:

- Communicates and reassures the patient throughout the procedure.
- Helps to position the patient in the relevant position.
- Maintains the dignity of the patient throughout the procedure.

Have:

- All relevant monitoring available. Record all physiological readings.
- Intravenous infusion with warming coil.
- Nasal cannula or oxygen mask available.
- Tracheal intubation equipment available.
- Relevant drugs available.
- Emergency equipment available.

---

anaesthetist may intubate the patient. They may also treat the hypotension with the appropriate drug.

Headache

There is a possibility of a headache after a spinal procedure. Leakage of the cerebrospinal fluid may cause this. The anaesthetic team position the patient flat and administer relevant analgesia. If the headache persists anaesthetists apply an 'epidural patch' to the leakage area to seal the leak. This may occur postoperatively on the ward.

A blood patch may be performed by removing 20 ml of the patient's blood, under aseptic conditions, and injecting it extradurally at the same interspace as the spinal was performed. This procedure should be stopped if discomfort is experienced. This is an effective cure for lumbar puncture headache and appears to be remarkably free from adverse effects (Aitkenhead & Simpson 1996).

Side effects of an epidural

Dural puncture
If the epidural needle punctures the dura the anaesthetist may give a spinal by accident. Leakage of cerebrospinal fluid will occur from the epidural needle.

Side effects of a spinal and epidural anaesthetic

Hypotension
It is essential to monitor the patient during this procedure. Hypotension can arise because of the use of the local anaesthetic. The appropriate drug should be available to reverse the hypotension.

Infection
To prevent an infection the anaesthetic practitioner will set up the relevant trolley using an aseptic technique. Anaesthetists do not undertake these procedures if there are any problems with an underlying infection or clotting problems.

High block
When a high block occurs anaesthetists will sit the patient up and monitor the patient's physiological recordings. To relieve the patient's breathing both preoperatively and postoperatively the anaesthetist may intubate the patient. Hypotension may also be treated with appropriate drugs.

Urinary retention
The patient may have problems urinating after these procedures. The surgeon may catheterise the patient to alleviate this preoperatively or postoperatively.

Other problems of regional anaesthesia are failure of the blocks, nausea and vomiting, respiratory depression, toxic reactions, pneumothorax or neurological damage.

Use of regional techniques

For all regional techniques the anaesthetist will secure venous access before the start of the regional anaesthetic procedure. The anaesthetic team monitor the patient throughout the regional anaesthetic within the anaesthetic room and operating room environments. If the patient is awake, throughout the surgical procedure, anaesthetic practitioners will fit a nasal cannula or oxygen mask on to the patient and they will support and observe the patient during the surgical procedure.

If the regional anaesthetic is not effective or if any complications occur the anaesthetist may consider a general anaesthetic. The anaesthetic practitioner will have tracheal intubation and resuscitation equipment ready for this event.

Resuscitation equipment including oxygen, a means of ventilating the patient, suction and drugs must be available. The anaesthetic practitioner must be aware of potential side effects and must monitor the patient for these both during the procedure and following its completion (Shields & Werder 2002). Factors to consider with regional anaesthesia are listed in Box 8.11.

LOCAL ANAESTHESIA, LOCAL INFILTRATION AND NERVE BLOCKS

Local infiltration is a technique that surgeons or anaesthetists use to block a nerve to produce local anaesthesia. The local anaesthetic diffuses into the cell membrane to produce this effect. Efficacy depends on the degree of myelination, size of nerve and the position of the fibre within the nerve. Infiltration of the local anaesthetic will act on the sensory nerve ending.

Anaesthetists and surgeons use a local anaesthetic for many reasons:

- an anaesthetic for minor surgery;
- the patient has a medical condition which prevents the anaesthetist administering a general anaesthetic;

- preference by the patient, anaesthetist or surgeon;
- local infiltration for pain management after an invasive procedure.

Local field block

Anaesthetists or surgeons can inject a local anaesthetic subcutaneously to produce a local field block. This allows the surgeon to remove lumps and bumps after injecting a local anaesthetic into the relevant site to freeze the surgical procedure area. A local anaesthetic can also be injected with a vasoconstrictor (adrenaline), which can increase the speed of action of the local anaesthetic by local vasoconstriction. The latter can never be used in nasal, digit or penile surgery.

Local infiltration

Surgeons use a local anaesthetic to infiltrate a surgical wound subcutaneously (before or after suturing the skin) for postoperative management of a surgical procedure in coordination with other methods.

Local nerve block

A local anaesthetic can be injected into nerve plexuses (brachial, lumbar, cervical), a major or a minor nerve to produce local anaesthesia for intraoperative and postoperative pain management for a surgical procedure. Major nerves (e.g. femoral or sciatic) and minor nerves (e.g. ulnar or digital) are examples of nerve blocks that the anaesthetist might perform.

The anaesthetic practitioner will prepare and check all relevant equipment before the procedure, illustrated in Box 8.12.

Topical anaesthesia

Anaesthetists may request a topical cream (e.g. Emla) for paediatric patients before they perform venous cannulation. This cream desensitises the skin and aids pain management in this procedure. This cream can also be used for adult patients who have a needle phobia. It is preferable that the

Box 8.11   Factors to consider with regional anaesthesia

Level of insertion

- Cervical
- Thoracic
- Lumbar
- Caudal

Choice of drug/dosage
Local anaesthetic

- Bupivacaine or lidocaine

Opioid

- Fentanyl
- Diamorphine

Considerations before procedure

- Patient choice/cooperation
- Abnormalities of spinal cord
- Coagulopathy
- Vascular disorders
- Skin infection
- Raised intracranial pressure
- Hypvolaemia

Infusion/rate of infusion

- Continuous infusion
- Intermittent boluses

Monitoring

- ECG
- Pulse oximeter
- Blood pressure
- Respiration
- Level of block
- Temperature
- Oxygen administration if applicable

Treatment

- Drugs (e.g. vasopressors, anti-emetics, emergency IV infusion)
- Resuscitation equipment

Box 8.12 Role of the anaesthetic practitioner for a local nerve block procedure

- An aseptic technique to prepare the relevant trolley and equipment.
- Relevant size of sterile gown and gloves for the anaesthetist.
- Skin cleansing solution.
- Relevant drape.
- Relevant size of nerve block needle.
- Relevant syringes and needles for local anaesthetic (skin and nerve block).
- Normal saline.
- Relevant dressings.
- Intravenous infusion with warming coil.

Before the procedure:

- Communicates and reassures the patient throughout the procedure.
- Helps to position the patient in the relevant position.
- Maintains the dignity of patient throughout the procedure.

Have:

- All relevant monitoring available. Records all physiological readings.
- Nasal cannula or oxygen mask available.
- Tracheal intubation equipment available.
- Relevant drugs available.
- Emergency equipment available.

---

ward staff apply this an hour before the anaesthetic for it to be effective.

SEDATION

Sedative drugs may be administered during a regional or local anaesthetic. Surgeons may use them during an endoscopy procedure. Sedative drugs can reduce the patient's anxiety and produce sleep. They can produce airway problems and hypotension so the appropriate oxygen and reversal drug should be available.

The anaesthetic practitioner will prepare and check all relevant equipment before the procedure, illustrated in Box 8.13.

THE PAEDIATRIC PATIENT

It is important to reassure, support and involve the paediatric patient and parent or carer in the reception area and anaesthetic

---

Box 8.13   Role of the anaesthetic practitioner during sedation

- Reassure and communicate with the patient throughout procedure.
- Attach all monitoring equipment and record observations.
- Assist the anaesthetist or surgeon in the venous cannulation of the patient.
- Attach a dressing to the venous cannula.
- Ensure an intravenous infusion is available if required.
- Have a nasal cannula available.
- Measure the level of consciousness of the patient.

Have available:

- Reversal of the sedative drug.
- A face mask and filter.
- Tracheal intubation equipment.
- Suction equipment and suction catheters.
- Relevant size of oropharyngeal airway.
- A gum elastic bougie. Anaesthetists may have difficulty when they insert the ET tube.
- A stethoscope for anaesthetists to check the correct position of the ET tube.
- Emergency equipment.

---

room. Mallet & Dougherty (2001) state that paediatric patients have special communication needs within the operating room environment. They have the same anxieties as adult patients, it is simply that they are unable to articulate them as well. The anaesthetic practitioner needs to involve the parents of the patient in the preoperative care and promote security and comfort in the anaesthetic room for the patient and the parent(s) or carer(s). Anaesthetic practitioners may use distraction techniques during the care of the patient especially during the intravenous cannulation and induction of the patient.

Occasionally the patient will need to have a gas induction as it is too distressing for the patient to undergo venous cannulation. The anaesthetic practitioner can help to relax the patient and parent and can ensure that the induction procedure is as comfortable as possible. Keeping calm and confident can help the patient, the anaesthetist and the parent.

Monitoring of the patient is essential before and during induction as the paediatric patient's condition can deteriorate more quickly than an adult's. Because of the possibility of rapid deterioration during anaesthesia it is especially important to check that all drugs and apparatus are ready before induction (Rusy & Usaleva 1998). Therefore before commencing induction of the paediatric patient the anaesthetic practitioner must prepare two laryngoscopes, suction apparatus, a range of ET tubes, LMAs and masks. Clear facemasks are the choice of most anaesthetists as the patient's colour and secretions can be checked during the intubation procedure.

The intubation technique is the same as for adults but the paediatric patient has some anatomical differences from the adult patient (Avidan *et al.* 2002). Important implications with regard to airway management as indicated by the Association of Anaesthetists of Great Britain and Ireland (AAGBI 1998a) suggest that that there are some special features peculiar to the paediatric airway. The head is relatively large with a prominent occiput, the neck is short and the tongue is large and furthermore, infants breathe mainly through their nasal airway, although their nostrils are small and easily obstructed. As a consequence the airway is prone to obstruction because of these differences (Rusy & Usaleva 1998).

The infant's larynx is higher in the neck than the adult and may be more difficult to visualise. The epiglottis is relatively large and floppy. It is therefore best to use a straight-bladed laryngoscope for infants up to the age of 6 months. The narrowest part of the glottis in an adult is between the vocal cords but in a child it is at the cricoid ring (Illingworth & Simpson 1994).

With regards to the preparation of airway management the anaesthetic practitioner must consider the size and weight of the paediatric patient. The size of the ET tube is critical, as one that is too large will exert pressure on the internal surface of the cricoid cartilage resulting in oedema. This could lead to airway obstruction when positive pressure is applied to it. Box 8.14 provides details of the recommended size of ET tube to use, depending on the patient's age.

The anaesthetic practitioner selects the size of the ET tube according to the width and length of the trachea. The anaesthetist uses an uncuffed ET tube in the paediatric patient under 11 years of age. This allows for a slight space around the exte-

---

Box 8.14 Recommended endotracheal tube sizes (Rusy & Usleva 1998)

Internal diameter

Age	*Size of tube*
Premature	2.5–3.00 mm
Neonate – 6 months	3.0–3.5 mm
6 months – 1 year	3.5–4.00 mm
1–2 years	4.0–5.0 mm
>2 years	Use the formula 4 + (age ÷ 4)

Length in cm
(Age in years ÷ 2) + 12

---

rior circumference. Soft tissue at the narrowest level of the cricoid cartilage located just below the vocal cords forms a loose seal around the tube.

Preparation for intubation

Anaesthetic practitioners should check all relevant equipment for this procedure as for the adult procedure.

The anaesthetic practitioner must take meticulous care to preserve body heat to prevent the development of hypothermia. The paediatric patient is vulnerable to hypothermia because of the high surface area to body weight ratio and the small amount of subcutaneous fat; 70% of an infant's heat loss is through conduction (Booker 1999). Therefore perioperative thermal management is clearly important for decreasing morbidity and accurate measurement of body temperature is necessary for timely detection of temperature disturbances and appropriate thermal management. Rusy & Usaleva (1998) advocate that measures should taken by the anaesthetic practitioner to reduce hypothermia, including: warming the environment, using warming devices and blankets, warming inspired gases and intravenous fluids.

THE PREGNANT PATIENT: CAESAREAN SECTION

Anatomical and physiological changes during pregnancy result in the pregnant patient being at greater risk from airway problems and difficult and failed intubation than a non-pregnant patient (Kuczkowski 2003). These difficulties can be due to capillary engorgement of the respiratory mucosa, predisposing upper airways to trauma, bleeding and obstruction. The anaesthetic practitioner therefore must have all airway and resuscitation equipment available before induction of a general or spinal anaesthetic.

Gastro-oesophageal reflux and delayed gastric emptying are features of pregnancy and therefore the risk of aspiration is taken into consideration at intubation. Anaesthetists administer sodium citrate before induction. If anaesthetists undertake induction the anaesthetic practitioner applies cricoid pressure to prevent the regurgitation of gastric contents into the pharynx.

The anaesthetic practitioner attaches routine monitoring equipment as hypertension is one of the frequent complications of pregnancy. It is important that the patient's physiological readings are checked and recorded frequently. The AAGBI (1998b) advises that all anaesthetic practitioners and obstetric staff should have agreed and regularly updated guidelines on failed intubation drill. Airway management is compromised with the physiological changes to the gastrointestinal system.

Cardiovascular stability is further compromised during preoperative positioning. In the supine position the enlarged uterus compresses major abdominal vessels causing a decrease in cardiac output and venous return. Morgan & Mikhail (1996) convey the view that the gravid uterus compresses the aorta of the parturient when she is in the supine position, diminishing the blood flow to the uteroplacental circulation. Uteroplacental circulation is vital in the development and growth of the healthy fetus. The fetus depends on the placenta for nutrients, gas exchange and eliminating waste. Also the compression of the vena cava decreases venous return. Tilting of the operating table 30° to the left will shift the uterus away from the major vessels to help avoid maternal hypotension. The anaesthetic practitioner can help to position the patient correctly when induction and surgery is necessary.

THE ELDERLY PATIENT
Surgical risk increases with age, and complications are poorly tolerated by the elderly patient. Although surgical risk is

significant, careful preoperative assessment, risk assessment and intraoperative management offers the patient the best possible outcome.

Obtaining vascular access may be more difficult in the elderly patient because their veins may be fragile making it difficult to place monitoring devices and for the administration of intravenous drugs, fluids and blood products. Arthritic changes could make patient intubation and operative positioning difficult and these aspects need particular consideration by the anaesthetic practitioner.

Age-related changes in temperature regulation mean that the elderly are at more risk during surgery and the use of warming devices is necessary to maintain satisfactory temperature levels. Atkinson *et al.* (1997) state that it has been shown that maintaining an effective body temperature during the surgical procedure can have significant beneficial effects on wound healing for perioperative patients.

Careful monitoring is essential in the elderly as tolerance to intravenous drugs and anaesthesia may be poor and detoxification can be slow in the elderly patient. Patients must be monitored for hypoxia because oxygenation to the heart, kidneys and brain will be less efficient (Fortunato 2000).

Anaesthetic practitioners need to be vigilant in the positioning of elderly patients as they may have frail skin and correct positioning is important to prevent damage on pressure areas such as heels, sacrum, elbows and all areas where monitoring equipment comes in contact with the skin. Care must be taken when moving the patient's limbs as the patient may suffer from degenerative conditions such as arthritis or osteoporosis.

CONCLUSION

To deliver and maintain effective patient care in their anaesthetic practice practitioners must be aware of their roles and responsibilities and provide efficient collaboration within the multiprofessional team of the operating department.

REFERENCES

Aitkenhead, A.R. & Smith, G. (1996) *Textbook of Anaesthesia*, 3rd edn. Churchill Livingston, Edinburgh.

Association of Anaesthetists of Great Britain and Ireland (1998a) *Paediatric Surgery Standards of Care.* AAGBI, London.

Association of Anaesthetists of Great Britain and Ireland (1998b) *Guidelines for Obstetric Services.* AAGBI, London.

Aitkenhead, A.R., Rowbotham, D.J. & Smith, G. (2001) *Textbook of Anaesthesia.* Churchill Livingstone, Edinburgh.

Atkinson, R., Smith, E., Bern, D. & Hilgard, E. (1997) *Introduction to Psychology*, 10th edn. Washington Health, Washington.

Avidan, M., Ponte, J. Wendon, J. & Jinsburg, P. (2002) *Perioperative Care, Anaesthesia, Pain Management and Intensive Care.* Churchill Livingstone, Edinburgh.

Booker, P. (1999) Equipment and monitoring in paediatric anaesthesia. *British Journal of Anaesthesia* **83**, 78–90.

Cormack, R.S. & Lehane, J. (1984) Difficult tracheal intubation in obstetrics. *Anaesthesia* **39**, 1105.

Fortunato, R. (2000) *Operating Room Technique.* Mosby, St Louis.

Griffiths, R.V. (1999) Anaesthesia: airway management. *British Journal of Nursing* **9** (10), 480–4.

Illingworth, K.A. & Simpson, K.H. (1994) *Anaesthesia and Analgesia in Emergency Medicine.* Oxford University Press, New York.

Intavent (1999) *Anaesthesia: LMA. Instructions for Use*, 4th edn. Intavent Research Ltd., Coalville, Leicestershire.

Kuczkowski, K.M. (2003) Airway problems and new solutions for the obstetric patient. *Journal of Clinical Anaesthesia* **15**, 552–63.

Mallet, J. & Dougherty, L. (2001) *The Royal Marsden Hospital: Manual of Nursing Procedures*, 5th edn. Blackwell Science, London.

Mitchell, M.J. (2005) *Anxiety Management in Adult Day Surgery. A Nursing Perspective.* Whurr, London.

Morgan, G.E. & Mikhail, M.S. (1996) *Clinical Anaesthesiology.* McGraw-Hill, New York.

Morton, N.S. (1997) *Assisting the Anaesthetist.* Oxford University Press, Oxford.

Rusy, L. & Usaleva, E. (1998) *Paediatric Anaesthesia Review.* www.nda.ox.ac.uk/wfsa/html/u08/u08_003.htm

Shields, L. & Werder, H. (2002) *Perioperative Nursing.* Greenwich Medical Media, London.

Visser, L. (2001) *Epidural Anaesthesia.* www.nda.ox.ac.uk/wfsa/html/u13/u/311-01.ht#epid

9

LEARNING OUTCOMES

❏ Discuss the *role of the scrub and circulating practitioner* in the surgical team.

❏ Discuss the *key clinical skills and knowledge* required in the following areas of care:

- *infection control* in the operating room;
- *positioning* the patient;
- *surgical skills* – managing recordable items, haemostasis and wound management.

INTRODUCTION

The perioperative team must provide a holistic approach to the evidence-based, safe and effective care of the patient. The team must achieve this in the short time available while the patient undergoes their anaesthesia and surgery.

The scrub practitioner works within the perioperative team to provide care and clinical expertise to help the surgical procedure to progress smoothly and efficiently. Because of this, the role of the scrub practitioner merits special considerations. As part of the more holistic perioperative role, the scrub practitioner is central to the patient's treatment. The work of the scrub practitioner can make the difference between a smooth, efficient procedure and a procedure fraught with delays, frustrations and errors (Taylor & Campbell 1999a). Specific roles include providing supplies to surgeons and assistants undertaking the surgery, managing instruments and medical devices and providing skilled help to the surgeon with the surgical procedure.

The circulating practitioner is responsible for supporting the surgical team and providing skilled care and support for the patient. This includes, for example, positioning of the patient, protecting the patient from pressure damage, keeping the patient safe from harm during long procedures and safe transfer to and from the reception and recovery areas.

Chapter 3 of this book shows how to improve care by preparing the patient and the perioperative team for this experience. Chapter 6 'A route to enhanced competence in perioperative care' describes in detail the competencies required of scrub and circulating practitioners. This chapter discusses the underpinning skills and knowledge in three particular areas of care:

- infection control in the operating room;
- positioning the patient;
- surgical skills – managing recordable items and haemostasis and wound management.

INFECTION CONTROL IN THE PERIOPERATIVE ENVIRONMENT

The control of infection in the perioperative environment is one of the most important roles for practitioners. Some 75% of nosocomial (hospital acquired) infections occur in surgical patients. Most postoperative infections arise from the patient's own flora and the commonest sites of infection include the urinary tract, respiratory tract and blood (septicaemia) (Surgical Tutor 2005a) (Table 9.1). Other common sites of infection include wounds and areas of the body involved in the surgery.

Practitioners must therefore be aware of potential sources of contamination and measures that they can take to prevent or reduce perioperative infection. Hand washing is the single most important measure for preventing nosocomial infections (Fell 2000; Pinney 2000).

Standard precautions

'Standard precautions' is the term used to describe an approach to infection control which offers protection for individuals against contamination from all sources, whether or not they carry a known infection risk (Wicker 1991; Pearson 2000; Gruendemann & Mangum 2001; Beesley & Pirie 2005). It involves assessing the risk of contamination by any blood and

Table 9.1 Common sites of perioperative infection.

Infection	Common causes	Prevention
Urinary tract (40%)	Urinary catheterisation, renal disease	Aseptic technique, hand washing
Respiratory tract (15%)	Bypassing respiratory defence systems, for example ET tubes, oral airways. Aspiration of stomach contents	Prophylactic antibiotics, aseptic technique, patient education on coughing and breathing exercises
Bacteraemia (5%)	Infection of the blood often caused by contaminated intravenous lines, catheters and other invasive devices	Aseptic technique, regular changing of catheters and lines, checking solutions before infusing
Other (40%)	Wound and surgical sites	Aseptic technique, careful instrument management, good draping techniques, good surgical techniques

body fluids (organic matter) and providing protection against it.

Practising standard precautions involves confining and controlling spillages of contamination, and providing a barrier between the contamination and the practitioner. Following standard precautions helps to ensure the safety of practitioners and patients. Confining and controlling spillages includes such measures as:

- wiping up blood spillages immediately rather than waiting to the end of the case;
- decontaminating spillages with suitable solutions;
- using suction with lavage to prevent spillages on the floor;
- soaking excess lavage with packs and disposing safely;
- using suitable drapes for containing spillages when anticipating large amounts of fluid;
- changing contaminated clothing immediately;
- providing protection from contamination for practitioners involves using protective clothing – this includes surgical masks, hats, gloves, shoes and gowns.

Each of these items can provide different levels of protection. For example, a simple paper mask may offer some protection against splashing to the face, whereas high filtration surgical masks can offer hours of protection against fluid splashes and inhalation of aerosols or surgical smoke. The quality of surgical gowns also differs widely from simple cotton gowns with almost no fluid repelling properties, to high-tech gowns which are impermeable to any fluid.

Similarly, some surgical procedures carry more risk of contamination than others. For example, removing a sebaceous cyst on the hand carries much less risk of contamination than a hemiarthroplasty of the hip joint, where the risk of contamination by blood and aerosols is much higher.

The ability to assess the risk of contamination is therefore a key skill for the perioperative practitioner. Risk assessment is a measure of the perceived likelihood of something happening and the impact if it does happen. The Association for Perioperative Practice's *Risk Assessment Guide* (NATN 2004) offers guidelines on the risk assessment of clinical situations, including standard precautions. This tool uses standards, assessment of criteria to meet the standard, and allocation of a score to help practitioners assess risk.

Practitioners do not always need such a detailed risk assessment if the practitioner understands the features of the clinical situation, the appropriate standards of practice and the criteria that must be met. For example, a scrub practitioner may identify a high risk of glove perforation and inhalation of aerosols from pulse lavage during a major orthopaedic case. The relevant standards include protection from contamination, so the practitioner should use a high filtration face mask and visor, waterproof barrier gown and double gloves. Similarly, a circulating practitioner who needs to clean potentially contaminated operating room furniture, following the removal of a sebaceous cyst, may decide that gloves are sufficient. The standard in both situations is identical – protection from contamination – but the risk assessment has shown the way to different practices which are equally safe. The ability to undertake such assessments is one which experienced practitioners develop through continual professional development and learning from experience.

Sources of perioperative contamination

The spread of contamination occurs when organisms move from one area to another. If the organisms infect a human being, then disease can occur. Continued vigilance and following the principles of standard precautions is essential to reduce the possibility of infection from contamination.

Operating departments normally provide a low infection risk environment for patient care. However, the biggest infection source is from people and often clinical requirements and operational demands increase infection risk. For example, the need to perform extended surgery increases infection risk because of exposed instruments, increased possibility of contamination and exposure of the wound site. However, the patient's well-being may be dependant on the successful completion of the surgery, regardless of the time taken. Similarly the constant opening of doors to and from the anaesthetic or disposal room may disturb ventilation systems, but may be essential to carry out clinical procedures safely and efficiently (Line 2003).

Potential problems in infection control in the operating department include:

- staff;
- patients;
- ventilation systems;
- equipment;
- surgical gowns and drapes.

Staff

The purpose of the surgical scrub is to reduce the transfer of organisms from the surgical team to the patient's open wound. The scrub procedure, disinfectant or skin cleaner used are important to reduce skin flora as far as possible (Beesley & Pirie 2005).

However, despite the surgical scrub, even thorough hand washing does not permanently reduce the number of micro-organisms on the skin – organisms from deep within skin pores reappear on the skin surface in 10–20 minutes. Therefore, practitioners must also wear sterile surgical gloves to help reduce the risk of contamination. Several makes of surgical glove are available but all aim to reduce organisms spreading to and from the patient (Fell 2000; Pinney 2000).

The use of masks in the operating room remains controversial (Lipp & Edwards 2002). Masks filter bacteria and can reduce the number of organisms inhaled or given off into operating room atmosphere. They also provide a physical barrier to contamination from the blood or body fluids of the patient. However, there are several issues associated with masks which make them less effective. For example:

- Removing the mask transfers organisms on to the hands.
- Masks become ineffective when wet.
- Contaminated air can easily escape from badly fitting masks.

Poor compliance with mask wearing can occur when practitioners do not understand the need for reducing infection or the features of the mask (Pearson 2000). For example, practitioners should be aware that standard masks do not always protect users against inhaling surgical smoke, especially if they are badly fitting.

The practitioner should use a mask for protection:

- when the operating room doesn't have plenum air ventilation;
- when the practitioner is close enough to the surgical site to be exposed to contamination from splashing by blood or body fluids;
- when frequently opening operating room doors (reducing the efficiency of the ventilation system).

Patients

Normal bacterial flora live in the nose, groin, armpit, gut, skin and hair of everybody, including patients (Table 9.2). Organisms may become pathogenic when they move out of their normal area on the body to an open wound. For example, healthy people's noses often contain *Staphylococcus aureus*, which can cause wound infection. Organisms normally resident in the gut can cause wound and other infections and good surgical technique is essential to prevent their transfer to other areas of the body. Prophylactic antibiotics can help to reduce the possibility

Table 9.2 Normal body flora.

Body area	Normal flora
Skin	*Staphylococcus aureus*, *Streptoccoccus pyogenes*, methycillin resistant *Staphylococcus aureus* (MRSA)
Oral cavity	Staphylococci, streptococci and anaerobes
Nasopharynx	Staphylococci, streptococci, *Haemophilus* and anaerobes
Large bowel	Gram-negative rods (for example *Escherichia coli*, *Enterobacter*), enterococci and anaerobes *Clostridium*
Urinary tract	Normally sterile

of infection when a surgical procedure has a known high infection risk (Line 2003).

Practitioners use a wide range of skin disinfectants to reduce the risk of skin organisms infecting wounds. Despite these precautions, normal surgical activities may still transfer organisms from exposed areas of the patient's skin to the wound area. Practitioners still require good aseptic technique to keep a barrier between the environment and the patient (Gruendemann & Magnum 2001).

Preoperative skin preparation sometimes takes place on the ward, although it is much more common nowadays to undertake skin preparation within the operating department. Figure 9.1 illustrates the typical surgical preparation of the patient's skin. Research is still ambiguous about the benefits of skin preparation (Doebbeling *et al.* 1992).

Skin shaving helps to keep hair away from the wound site and is most effective at reducing wound infection when performed immediately before surgery. Infection rate increases from 1% to 5% if performed more than 12 hours before surgery, because of organisms moving from deeper levels of the skin to the surface, and because of the damage to skin caused by shaving. Abrasions can cause colonisation, which can lead to wound infection, and clippers or depilatory creams may reduce infection rates to less than 1% (Surgical Tutor 2005a).

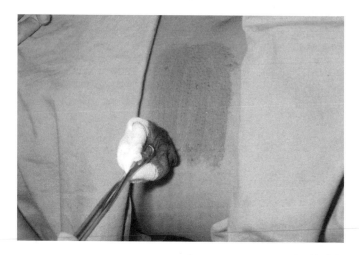

Fig. 9.1 Patient skin preparation.

Skin preparation solutions

There are several skin preparation solutions available with the commonest being alcoholic or aqueous iodine solutions and clear or coloured alcohol based chlorhexidine solution (Surgical Tutor 2005b) (Table 9.3). Surgical likes and dislikes, the presence of allergies or whether the procedure requires electrosurgery or laser often influences choice of solution. For example, alcohol-based solutions may ignite through heating by electrosurgery or laser beams, causing patient burns. Patient skin sensitivity to these lotions can sometimes cause a chemical burn or irritation which resembles an electrosurgery burn, especially when associated with pooling of solutions underneath the return electrode.

Ventilation systems

The cleanest areas in the operating room should be the surgical site and instrument table. Although aseptic technique and prophylactic antibiotics can reduce wound infection, suitable ventilation can reduce bacterial contamination of these areas.

Table 9.3 Skin preparation solutions.

Solution	Actions
70% Isopropyl alcohol	Acts by denaturing proteins. Bactericidal and short acting. Effective against Gram-positive and Gram-negative organisms, fungicidal and virucidal
0.5% Chlorhexidine	Quaternary ammonium compound which acts by disrupting the bacterial cell wall. Bactericidal but does not kill spore-forming organisms. It is persistent and has a long duration of action (up to 6 hours). More effective against Gram-positive organisms
70% Povidone-iodine	Acts by oxidation and substitution of free iodine. Bactericidal and active against spore-forming organisms. Effective against both Gram-positive and Gram-negative organisms. Rapidly inactivated by organic material such as blood and body tissues

Panels in the operating room ceiling provide large volumes of clean air filtered over the surgical site. Infectious particles shed by the operating team therefore move away from the operating table toward the margins of the room.

Laminar flow ventilation with filtration is common in orthopaedic cases to prevent the often catastrophic results of surgical site infection of bone or implants. A canopy, which drops from the ceiling, encloses the operating team. This provides a protective environment which is in positive pressure compared with the rest of the operating room and therefore encourages particles to move away from the wound, surgical team and equipment.

Ventilation systems provide airflow out of the operating room. Maintaining the pressure gradient is a problem when windows or doors are left open, resulting in air moving in and out of the operating room. Doors and windows should therefore be closed, apart from necessary use, while the surgical site is open (Beesley & Pirie 2005).

The surgical team is a potential reservoir of infection because people shed potentially infectious particles of sloughed skin.

However, with proper ventilation, such shedding should not pose an infectious risk to patients. For orthopaedic procedures involving insertion of an implant the surgical team may also wear evacuated gowns which reduce contamination by skin shedding.

Equipment

Practitioners should keep equipment outside the operating room as far as possible, given the requirements for the surgical procedure. Storage of equipment within the operating room is not advisable because it may provide a surface for dust, lint and other potential sources of contamination. However, it may be necessary if storage space is lacking externally. Equipment stored in the operating room should be kept away from clinical activities and if possible kept under cover or in a cupboard. Using plastic covers for delicate or sensitive equipment protects them from contamination and risk of damage to the equipment. However, these covers can also become contaminated and when removed transfer their contamination to practitioner's hands. Bacteria and viruses can live for significant lengths of time if surrounded by contamination from blood or body fluids and so may cause cross infection by contaminating practitioners working with the same equipment later (Line 2003).

Applying the principles of standard precautions to equipment ensures their protection from contamination, but if they do become contaminated then the practitioner should control it through immediate cleaning and removal of the contaminant. The most effective way of cleaning such equipment is normally using a damp cloth with a suitable hospital detergent. Disinfectants are at best useless, because they require prolonged contact times to be effective, and at worst could damage equipment (Gruendemann & Fernsebner 1995).

Equipment brought into the operating room is also a risk. There are many examples of equipment sharing between areas. For example, instruments trays from storage areas or X-ray machines and clinical monitors transferred from another operating room. Effective cleaning policies with good documentation may help to reduce incidents of cross contamination.

Equipment leaving the operating room also poses a potential problem for staff transferring and repairing the equipment. Documented evidence of cleaning verifies that cleaning has taken place before the equipment leaves the clinical area.

Local instrument reprocessing

During litigation, a Trust may have to prove that their instruments did not cause infection, rather than the patient having to prove that they did. A decontamination survey conducted by NHS Estates in September 2000 (NHS Estates 2000) identified major concerns with the local reprocessing of instruments. As a result, reprocessing within the operating room has reduced following the implementation of safer alternative methods. The survey also found that many of the smaller reprocessing units were inadequate; as a result they were closed and the work moved to larger purpose-built sterile supply departments (Line 2003).

There are several advantages to reprocessing surgical items locally. These include quicker turnaround especially where there are limited numbers of instruments; local control over expensive and fragile equipment and reduced chance of losing equipment in the system. However, there are also significant problems with local reprocessing. For example equipment must be clean to sterilise it effectively, however, it is difficult to clean equipment or instruments with lumens and, unlike larger sterilising units, few operating rooms have quality assurance systems associated with cleaning by practitioners. Therefore, if for example a patient acquired HIV following a surgical procedure, the hospital would find it difficult to prove the equipment was clean before sterilisation, and therefore that the sterilisation process had been effective.

Other problems with local reprocessing include hazards to operators and patients from hand washing of contaminated instruments, aerosols produced by rinsing instruments under a tap, contamination of the surrounding area and clothing, operator time required, no testing scheme and lack of documentation. Where local instrument reprocessing is essential, the controls and guidance in HTM2030 are essential to make these procedures safe (Beesley & Pirie 2005).

Surgical gowns and drapes
Surgical gowns and drapes are medical devices which are subject to legally binding minimum standards in areas such as microbial penetration, tensile strength, linting and permeability to fluids. Surgical gowns and drapes are either reusable or single use. Figure 9.2 shows the surgical draping of a patient.

Reusable gowns and drapes
Polycotton is one of the most widely used materials for reusable gowns because it is cheap and easy to produce, comfortable to wear, permeable to perspiration and durable in use. However, polycotton is also permeable to bacteria and fluids which can be a problem during major procedures.

Because of these limits, other reusable materials have developed which offer better protection from contamination, while being comfortable to the wearer. Rotecno, made by Lojigma UK, is an example of a modern material. While being more expensive, such materials offer excellent protection, especially during surgical procedures where there is a high risk of contamination.

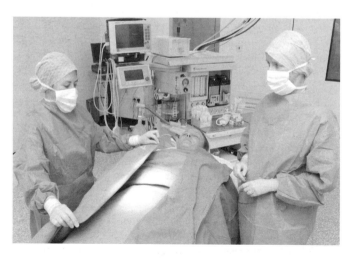

Fig. 9.2 Surgical draping of a patient.

However, there are several disadvantages with reusable gowns. For example, laundering may affect surface treatment of reusable materials and testing can be expensive. Many hospital-run laundry departments have closed, which affects fast processing and safe transport of large amounts of contaminated material. For these reasons, many Trusts use single-use materials as an economic and safe way of providing surgical drapes and gowns (Line 2003).

Single-use gowns and drapes

As a result of the increased focus on quality and risk assessment, single-use materials are now the materials of choice in most situations and are available from several manufacturers. They also take several different forms, including single layer and multi-layer materials and plastic materials. All try to provide properties similar to or better than reusable materials, for example resistance to bacterial penetration, wetting and tearing and increased comfort and durability in use. Manufacturers are usually responsible for sterility and fitness for purpose of single-use gowns. The Trust may see this as an advantage if litigation raises questions of sterility or wound infection.

The single-use against multi-use materials argument is complex and involves financial, environmental and risk-assessment factors. However, as standards of use rise it is likely that single-use drapes and gowns will continue to be popular (Gruendemann & Fernsebner 1995; Beesley & Pirie 2005).

POSITIONING THE PATIENT

The ability to position a patient safely and effectively for surgery can take many years to develop and is an essential skill for the safe care of patients. The practitioner must be able to display and apply safe principles of surgical positioning for anaesthetised patients. This involves consideration in such areas as positioning unconscious patients, understanding the physiological effects of surgical positioning, considering surgical, anaesthetic and patient-related factors when positioning the patient and managing potential problems of patient positioning.

Careful positioning of the surgical patient helps to provide surgical access to carry out the surgical procedure. Therefore, practitioners place patients in a large variety of positions, many of which are potentially dangerous, uncomfortable or painful.

At the same time, there are many other considerations apart from the need for surgical access. For example, the anaesthetist must be able to gain access to the patient's airway, even, for example, when undergoing surgery to the head, which would normally exclude non-sterile personnel from the area. The anaesthetist will also need access to other anaesthetic equipment such as intravenous lines, monitors and catheters.

Practitioners must also consider the patient's privacy and dignity. If the patient is awake, unnecessary exposure can cause embarrassment and increase anxiety. As well as being unpleasant for the patient, this can lead to anger, frustration, disempowerment and justifiably result in non-cooperation. If the patient is asleep, then the main effect of neglecting the patient's privacy is on the perioperative team itself. Treating the unconscious patient as less than human, also dehumanises the perioperative team. The team may develop a lack of respect for the patient which can make members of the team less concerned about the patient's well-being.

Preparation and planning are the key to effective and safe positioning techniques. The practitioner should position the operating table in the best position within the operating room. This will involve considering such issues as position of the anaesthetist and anaesthetic equipment, lighting, space for surgical instrument trays and access for X-ray machines. All table fittings should be available before the patient enters the operating room. This involves discussing requirements with the surgeon and anaesthetist and agreeing the best position to adopt for the patient.

It is essential to adopt a team approach to position the patient safely and effectively. A coordinated approach is necessary to avoid damage by sudden jerky movements of limbs, or abnormal twisting or torsion of parts of the patient's body. At the same time, practitioners should ensure that they adopt a slow, careful and ergonomical approach to moving the patient (Clarke & Jones 1998).

Various positioning aids help to maintain the patient's position. Foam wedges or bolsters help to support or position the patient's limbs or back when in a lateral position. Laminectomy frames support the patient in a modified prone position, which encourages the gap between vertebrae to open for lumbar laminectomies. Limbs can be flexed against posts fixed to the table – for example when undertaking an arthroscopy or for supporting the patient from the front in the lateral position. Placing kidney elevators beneath the patient's iliac crest while in the lateral position causes the operative area between the 12th rib and the iliac crest to lift. Gel pads have various uses for supporting and protecting bony prominences and limbs. Stabilising the head is especially important because of the potential risk to the airway and the neck. Various positioning aids are available for the head, including the 'doughnut' or ring, sandbags or gel pads (Gruendemann & Fernsebner 1995).

Physiological effects of positioning

One of the major implications of poor positioning is its effects on the respiratory and circulatory systems (Taylor & Campbell 1999b). Unnatural positioning leads to muscle fatigue and inefficiency of muscle pumps and vasomotor systems, or compression of the respiratory muscles and organs. The reduced ability of the body's homeostatic system to maintain a natural balance makes this worse and can affect the body systems. For example, prolonged unnatural positioning compromising the patient's breathing can lead to hypoxia and hypercarbia.

Obstructing the flow of blood, for example in the legs can also increase the incidence of damage to blood vessels resulting in such conditions as thrombophlebitis and deep venous thrombosis.

Neurological complications include damage to the brachial plexus, for example when extending the shoulder for long periods of time. Any prolonged pressure or stretching of nerves has the potential to damage the nerves, potentially leading to nerve palsies (Gruendemann & Fernsebner 1995).

During positioning, there are several other factors affecting the patient which practitioners must also consider. For example maintaining normal body alignment helps to prevent nerve damage, circulation deficits and skin damage. Padding or protective devices, such as low-pressure mattresses or intermittent pressure pneumatic devices may help protect the patient (Taylor & Campbell 1998b).

Other safety considerations include the use of restraining safety straps and upholding acceptable staffing levels. Preventing pooling of skin prep solutions around equipment helps to avoid the risk of potential skin damage or inflammation of alcohol based solutions. The patient should not be able to touch grounded metal objects, which may cause problems with electrosurgery burns (see Chapters 2 and 5). Practitioners should protect catheters and intravenous cannulae from stretching, pulling or unintentional removal. Preoperative assessment of patients may identify risks such as obesity, low body weight, potential for skin damage, incontinence, stiff joints and other physical conditions which may affect positioning.

Postoperative evaluation of the patient's response to positioning is an important part of patient care. Erythema or changes in skin integrity at bony prominences and pressure areas may be signs of lasting pressure damage and pressure sore development. There may be evidence of strained muscles or ligaments if the patient complains of stiff or aching limbs or joints. Excessive damage may result in instability or dislocation of joints or altered range of motion. Compressed or injured nerves can display themselves through numbness or tingling.

The practitioner should record, in the patient's medical notes, the position, details of equipment used and any signs or symptoms of harm suffered by positioning and the patient should be told of any potential injuries (Box 9.1).

Box 9.1   Potential complications of surgical positioning

- Peripheral nerve injuries
- Skin injuries
- Eye or ear injuries
- Finger injuries
- Ligament damage
- Cardiovascular effects
- Venous air embolism
- Respiratory effects

Common surgical positions

There are four common surgical positions for the patient – supine, lithotomy, prone and lateral. Several variations of these four positions have developed to address local requirements.

Supine position

The supine position and its variants are common positions for surgery. The patient lies on the back, with arms on arm boards at a 90° angle or less to the body (Figure 9.3). Alternatively, the arms may remain parallel to the body and held in place by arm-rests or padded straps. A small pillow or pad may stabilise the head and prevent neck strain. Legs should be parallel and uncrossed to prevent pressure on calf muscles and compression of circulation. Padding helps to avoid pressure damage to areas such as sacrum, heels, elbows and bony prominences.

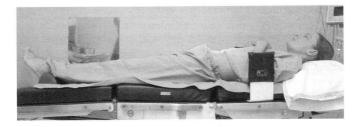

Fig. 9.3 Supine position.

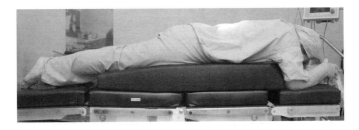

Fig. 9.4 Prone position with arms by the head.

Backache and neck ache are common problems associated with this position. Neck ache can occur following extreme or prolonged neck rotation or pressure from straps, masks or other items of anaesthetic equipment, and as a result of vigorous lifting of the jaw while establishing an airway. Backache can occur because of prolonged tension in the sacrolumbar region. This occurs because of flattening of the vertebrae as the paraspinal muscles relax under the influence of muscle relaxants and other anaesthetic drugs. Placing a small support in the space beneath the small of the back reduces this condition by helping to support the normal lumbar curve (Gruendemann & Fernsebner 1995).

Trendelenburg's position involves lowering the head and raising the feet. The downwards angle should not be excessive since only friction stops the patient from sliding off the table. Shoulder pads are inadvisable because of the danger of compressing the brachial plexus, so the practitioner must secure the patient by other means, such as straps. Reverse Trendelenburg involves a head-up and foot-down position. A footboard can prevent the patient sliding down the table and helps to prevent foot drop or plantar flexion.

Arms need special consideration in any of these positions. The anaesthetic team need access to peripheral lines and to the upper arm for blood pressure readings. The surgical team need unobstructed access to the surgical site. The common positions for arms are parallel to the body, across the chest or on arm boards at an angle to body according to the procedures taking place.

When placed on arm boards there are several considerations for the practitioner. The angle of the arm to the body must be a maximum of 90°, ideally with the palms turned upwards. Hyperabduction of the arm results in stretching of subclavian and axillary blood vessels resulting in thrombosis and vessel wall damage and stretching of the brachial plexus, ulnar nerve and other superficial nerves in the arm.

Severe hypotension can result from this position, especially if the patient is pregnant. This occurs because of pressure on the vena cava caused by the weight of the internal organs or the fetus. Tilting the patient to the side reduces pressure on the vena cavae, either by tilting the table or by placing pillows or pads in strategic positions underneath the patient (Hind & Wicker 2000).

Patients adopt a highly modified supine position if they need treatment on a traction table. The traction table places fractured legs into traction while undergoing internal fixation. An image intensifier displays the fracture in real-time using X-rays, and the large C-arm of this machine must have access close to the site of surgery. The patient is normally supine and the unaffected leg abducted to 90° at the hip and knee. A well-padded perineal post attached to the table braces against the perineum. Stretching the leg through fittings at the foot of the table applies traction to reduce the fracture to its normal alignment. Flexing and abducting the arm on the unaffected side across the chest helps C-arm access. The practitioner must watch carefully for potential complications since this position is so extreme and can place great stress on the patient's body if wrongly carried out.

Prone position

The patient adopts this position for surgery on the dorsal surface. The patient is anaesthetised in the supine position and then practitioners roll the patient over into the face down position. Several practitioners should help in this procedure because of the danger of twisting limbs or compromising the airway. The patient's arms are either rotated through their normal range of movement to rest beside the head (Figure 9.4), or left at the side of the body. The head is protected from abnormal movement and the eyes and ears padded to prevent pressure damage. Pads or pillows placed under the chest and hip regions ease breathing by allowing expansion of the diaphragm. A pad placed under the lower legs and ankles also helps to prevent foot drop.

When adopting this position for laminectomies or surgery on the spine, using a frame can stabilise the spine and open the laminar arches for easier surgical access.

There are several variations to this position including, for example, the jackknife, knee–chest and prone sitting positions, used for specialised neurosurgical or proctological procedures.

Lateral position

Patients adopt this position for lateral surgical access during procedures such as hip arthroplasty, kidney surgery and some chest surgery (Taylor & Campbell 1999b). The patient is anaesthetised supine and then turned on the side. This procedure needs several practitioners to perform safely. Supporting the head on a pillow, and the torso with supports or posts helps to keep spinal alignment. Placing a pillow between the legs relieves the pressure of the upper leg on the lower leg and flexing both legs slightly helps to improve stability.

Bringing the lower shoulder forward slightly relieves pressure on the brachial plexus, and the lower arm is either placed on an arm board or flexed to rest beside the patient's head. The upper arm often rests on a raised arm board and is placed above the head to keep it away from the surgical field. Protecting pressure points with padding reduces the risk of harm.

A special rest may be placed under the patient's hip for procedures on the kidney. This 'kidney rest' elevates the space between the 12th rib and the iliac crest, exposing the surgical area. Flexing the table at this point increases the angulation of the patient's body.

The peroneal nerve leaves the posterior aspect of the knee and travels laterally around the head of the fibula. Enough padding of the lateral knee is therefore essential because it is susceptible to pressure in this area because of the weight of the leg on the operating table.

Lithotomy position

Patients adopt the lithotomy position for gynaecological and lower bowel surgery. This is a highly unnatural position which therefore carries with it risks because of stretching and pressure on nerves, joints and tendons.

From the supine position, practitioners raise the patient's legs, flex the hips and knees, abduct and externally rotate the thighs, and place the feet in stirrups attached to poles. Surgical access to the patient's perineal area is achieved by removing the end of the table.

The arms are either placed over the abdomen or crossed over on the chest and in either case secured using straps or armrests. To help venous access one arm may be placed on an arm board at less than a 90° angle to the body.

When placing the patient in this position, practitioners must raise and lower both legs simultaneously to prevent leg and back strain. Practitioners must also take care to ensure the legs can move through the required range, especially where move-ment is compromised, for example when the patient has had a hip replacement. Pressure should be avoided on areas such as the inner leg from the posts and on the feet from the stirrups. This position also restricts breathing to a degree because of increased pressure of the viscera on the diaphragm (Beesley & Pirie 2005).

Lloyd-Davies stirrups can be used in place of lithotomy poles to offer popliteal and ankle support. Using these stirrups during prolonged procedures reduces the risk of pressure damage to the legs.

SURGICAL SKILLS

The scrub practitioner role is challenging but satisfying. The role challenges practitioners to use their knowledge of anatomy and surgical technique in the direct treatment of the patient's con-dition. Here, on the operating table, is where the focus of the patient's care resides. The whole point of the surgical patient's admission is to undergo a surgical procedure and it is here, at the operating table, that the scrub practitioner can engage directly in the patient's return to health. The experienced scrub practitioner can make the difference between a procedure that progresses slowly, with many delays, to one which is smooth and efficient.

To achieve this aim, the scrub practitioner calls on many com-petencies, such as those discussed in Chapter 6. Three areas of perioperative care which the scrub practitioner must develop competence in are:

- managing recordable items;
- haemostasis;
- wound closure, dressings and drains.

Managing recordable items

Managing items used during a surgical procedure is one of the core roles of the scrub practitioner (NATN 1998) and remains an area of high risk. All items used in a procedure are accountable and some, for example swabs and instruments, are also recordable. There are many different approaches to this procedure and many different items that need recording, therefore, practitioners need to be fully aware of local policies and procedures.

The purpose of counting and recording items is to avoid retaining any in the patient's wound. A retained swab or instrument is a potential source of infection and can interfere with the anatomy of the wound area, leading to bleeding, loss of function or pain. The potential for psychological damage to the patient is also high because of worry about the error and its future implications. The patient will also need to undergo more surgery to remove the item and face the extra risks which this poses.

Errors in managing surgical items have often resulted in litigation (NATN 1998; Woodhead 2005). The patient may claim that the surgical team have been negligent in their duties and can often claim damages for loss of earning, pain, psychological and physiological stress and inconvenience. Patients may sue the hospital directly, with members of the surgical team involved in the blame for any errors. All members of the team, not just the surgeon, are accountable for this check. The practitioner's role is to make the surgeon aware of the status of the surgical items. Any act (for example, carrying out a false check) or omission (for example, failing to tell the surgeon of an incorrect count) may leave the practitioner open to the charge of negligence (NATN 1998; Beesley & Pirie 2005).

Every item used during surgery is accountable at every stage of surgery. Most items are also recordable on the swab board or perioperative care record. Recordable items include, for example:

- swabs;
- muslin packs;
- pledglets;

- instruments;
- sutures;
- blades;
- bulldog clips;
- tapes or slings;
- electrosurgery tips.

The operating department should have a policy that specifies which items are recordable and the documentation, counting and recording procedures (NATN 1998).

Principles for managing recordable items

Practitioners must count recordable items for every surgical procedure to improve patient safety and reduce the risk of items left accidentally in the wound. This also includes minor cases when there is little possibility of loss, since a lost item may interfere with a count for a following case.

The scrub practitioner decides when the checks take place, which can include:

- before the surgical procedure;
- on receiving extra packs of swabs or other items;
- at the closure of a body cavity such as the stomach;
- at the start of wound closure;
- at the start of skin closure;
- following completion of the case.

The circulating practitioner records items on the swab board, in the intraoperative record and on the tray list. The swab board is usually a large white-board which displays the recordable items used during the surgical procedure. Since the practitioner wipes the swab board clean after every case, an intraoperative record and tray list provide permanent documentary evidence of the counts. The scrub and circulating practitioners count and record items together. One of these two practitioners should be a qualified and experienced member of the team.

The practitioners should check the instrument tray on opening and before first use of the instruments. Instruments that come in several parts should have each part independently identified. The scrub practitioner must be satisfied that every item is complete, and there are no missing parts, before use.

A combined count usually occurs regardless of the number of procedures which the patient is undergoing. This helps to reduce errors caused by mixing of items between trays or surgical sites (NATN 1998).

There are various ways of recording recordable item checks in the operating room. In most procedures, the swab board has swabs, packs, sutures and blades marked before the case starting. During a procedure practitioners count used items, weigh them to estimate blood loss and store them safely near the swab board.

Practitioners also mark the outcome of each count on the intraoperative care record and sign them. Removing all opened (used and unused) recordable items from the operating room at the end of the procedure helps to prevent errors in future counts.

The scrub and circulating practitioner sign their names in the relevant area of the operating record and on the perioperative care plan to show completion of a correct count and to accept accountability for the procedure. The scrub practitioner's responsibility is to tell the surgeon of the outcome of an incorrect count, while it is the surgeon's responsibility to decide what to do about unaccounted items. See Chapter 4 for further discussion on documentation.

Incorrect counts must be recorded and corrective action taken where possible. The surgeon will decide whether to continue the closure, to look inside the wound for the item or to wait until the item is found. Practitioners may check the patient, drapes, rubbish bags, linen bags, floor, specimens and swab bags at this stage. Swabs and other items can often be found in unexpected places, for example having fallen down inside boots, under the operating table or stuck to the soles of staff member's shoes.

The surgeon may arrange for an X-ray to find out whether the missing item may be inside the patient. The surgeon will not necessarily order an X-ray if there is no possibility of the missing item being inside the patient, and this decision should be recorded in the patient's notes. It is the surgeon's decision to carry on with closure even if the scrub practitioner reports the item still missing. The scrub practitioner should record missing items in the operating register and an incident form must be completed.

Surgical haemostasis

The scrub practitioner should understand the principles of surgical haemostasis to assist the operating surgeon effectively and to promote the smooth progress of the surgical procedure.

Surgical haemostasis is a complex subject which requires knowledge of anatomy and physiology as well as surgical procedures. For example, the techniques used for haemostasis of capillary bed bleeding are different from haemostasis of large blood vessels. Similarly, blood vessels can be temporarily or permanently occluded with slings, ties, tapes, tourniquets or sutures. When electrosurgery is used, a whole raft of instruments and techniques can be used, especially when the bleeding is deep within the body, or the procedure is been carried out with a laparoscope.

Arterial bleeding

Arterial bleeding can be identified because of the bright red colour of the oxygenated blood, the spurting action as the heart pumps it out of the damaged vessel; and the force with which it is pumped out of the vessel.

Major arterial bleeding can be serious because of the potential for high blood loss in a short time. For example, surgeons must control bleeding quickly during a ruptured aortic aneurysm or the patient may only have minutes to live. Often the only way to stop major arterial bleeds is to clamp the damaged vessel and then repair it using a suture or graft.

Direct pressure or ligation often controls minor arterial bleeds.

Venous bleeding

Venous bleeding can be identified by the dark red colour of the blood, the low-pressure release of the blood from the vessel; and the turgid way in which the bleeding occurs (compared with the high-pressure of arterial bleeds).

Major venous bleeding can be serious but is more easily controlled than major arterial bleeding. Nonetheless, major venous

bleeds can occur over large areas of tissue, arising spontaneously from damaged tissue. Venous bleeding can also be
insiduous in onset, perhaps not making its presence known for
hours after surgery has finished, lulling practitioners into a false
sense of security.

Cutting through veins, venules or capillaries often causes
minor venous bleeds. The usual course of action is to tie the
vessel or coagulate it with electrosurgery. If the bleeding is
coming from a capillary bed, such as the gall bladder bed, then
electrosurgery using fulguration or spray settings, or pharmacological coagulation using collagen or gelatin sponges may be
the methods of choice.

Haemostasis procedures

The first stage in treating perioperative bleeding problems is
evaluation of the bleeding source. The method of haemostasis
then has to be determined. The experienced practitioner
can contribute to this process by anticipating the surgeon's
needs. Some of the criteria for consideration include those in
Table 9.4.

Instruments used for haemostasis

Haemostatic instruments are either permanent or temporary.
The surgeon uses temporary haemostats when the role of the
vessel will be required following the procedure, for example
when temporarily occluding a carotid artery to allow surgery to
take place. Permanent haemostats lead to complete vessel occlusion and permanent loss of function. These are used where the
vessel itself is not required, or the part of the body which the
vessel serves is either removed or becomes non-functional, for
example during bowel resection.

Temporary haemostats include:

- Bulldog clips – these small spring-loaded clips are used
  widely in vascular surgery. They gently pinch the vessel,
  occluding it. When removed, normal blood flow resumes.
- Ringed vascular clamps – similar in shape to artery forceps
  but with specialised tips which are atraumatic to vessels.
  They are available in various sizes, shapes, angles and curves.

- Tourniquets – vary from small finger or glove tourniquets, to large major limb pneumatic tourniquets.
- Vessel loops – flexible plastic slings which manipulate and stabilise blood vessels during vascular surgery and provide haemostasis when wrapped around the vessel and pulled tight.

Permanent haemostats include:

- Artery forceps – general-purpose removable clamps used for most sizes of blood vessels. The surgeon uses them to administer a method of permanent haemostasis such as ligation or electrosurgery.
- Vascular staples – metal staples, applied using special clamps. They are left in position and body tissue surrounds them during the healing process.
- Vascular glue – methylacrylate glue which bonds tissue edges together.
- Electrosurgery – this is possibly the most common way of providing haemostasis and every operating room has an electrosurgical generator as a basic item of equipment. Chapter 2 discusses this device.
- Laser – laser can provide haemostasis. Chapter 2 also contains a discussion of this device.

All surgical specialities use ligatures (ties) free-hand, dispensed from a reel, attached to artery forceps or used with a suture to transfix blood vessels. The basic technique of vessel ligation is to clamp the end of a cut vessel with artery forceps and then place a tie around the vessel under the clamp, knot it and remove the clamp. This set routine can become quick and effective when the surgeon and practitioner learn to work together in harmony. Alternative methods include passing ties underneath the vessel using artery forceps or angled clamps and tying the vessel in continuity before dividing it.

Pharmacological agents

Various pharmacological agents provide haemostasis and are especially useful where surgeons cannot use ties or sutures. These include collagen or gelatine sponges, such as Spongistan,

Table 9.4 Some considerations for deciding the method of haemostasis.

Factor affecting mode of haemostasis	Issues for consideration	Implications for the scrub practitioner
Arterial or venous source	• Major or minor artery bleed? • Serious or minor blood loss anticipated? • In venous bleeding is it a general ooze or specific vein damage?	• Ligation of artery using suture, ligature, clips or electrosurgery. • Repair of major blood vessel may be required. • Pharmacological methods may be used to control venous oozes
Size of vessel	• Is it small enough for electrosurgery? • Are there fine ligatures available?	• Clamping of the vessel using artery forceps. • Different methods of presenting ligatures
Accessibility of vessel	• Is it superficial or deep? • Can tapes or ties be passed underneath the blood vessel? • Does the ligature need to be mounted on artery forceps to pass under the vessel?	• Long and/or short artery forceps may be required. • Tapes or loops may be used to stabilise the blood vessel. • Long electrosurgery instruments may be required
Adjoining tissues	• Are the adjoining tissues likely to be damaged during haemostasis?	• Bipolar electrosurgery may be used where pinpoint electrosurgery is required (e.g. brain tissue). • The vessel may need to be dissected away from sensitive tissues
Permanent or temporary haemostasis required	• Is it essential to preserve the role of the vessel? • Can the vessel be removed without compromising the circulation to the area?	• Vascular clamps may be required. • Tourniquets may be required (finger or limb)
Absorbable or non-absorbable suture required	• Does the vessel need long-term ligation? • Is the vessel superficial?	• Large blood vessels often require non-absorbable sutures (e.g. high saphenous ligation and suturing of bowel perforations)

and may be used, for example, in the nose, on bone ends, oozing vascular surfaces such as the gall bladder bed and in the inguinal canal following herniorraphy. Sterile bone wax pressed into bone ends prevents oozing.

Wound management

Care of the surgical wound is a responsibility of the entire surgical team. Chapter 1 discussed the homeostasis of wound healing. This chapter focuses on the clinical interventions and some of the perioperative factors that affect wound healing. Wound healing directly links to areas such as handling of tissues intraoperatively, wound closure materials and methods, and choice of dressings and drains.

Surgical technique

Traumatic tissue handling can affect its healing properties since bruised and damaged tissues take longer to heal. Careful handling and retraction of tissues is therefore essential intraoperatively. Close approximation of tissues and effective haemostasis both help to prevent blood clots collecting and encourage healing.

Complications of wound healing

Prevention of infection is essential if wound closure is to progress smoothly. Incisional infections can result in delayed healing times, unsightly scars and may progress to systemic infection, further delaying the patient's discharge. Deep wound infections are serious conditions which occasionally may result in the removal of implants or the internal breakdown of tissues and surgical repairs. In vascular anastamoses this can be fatal. The source of infection is often impossible to identify but may include contaminated instruments, poor sterile technique and environmental conditions, which stresses the need for a team approach to preventing contamination.

Wound disruption occurs in some patients because of wound closure materials failing, infection or mechanical stress on the wound. Dehiscence of wounds occurs when suture lines break down and the wound opens. Contents of body spaces, such as intestines, may erupt through the wound (evisceration). This is distressing and potentially fatal for the patient and needs urgent surgery. The dehiscence may be a sign of an underlying medical problem and so further careful wound management may be necessary.

Other common complications include:

- umbilical herniation following abdominal surgery because of weakening of abdominal wall muscles;
- hypertrophic scar formation (keloid scars);
- haemorrhage;
- sinus tract or fistula formation between areas of the body, for example the vagina and the colon;
- foreign body inclusion in the wound – for example grit or dirt in trauma procedures;
- adhesions to underlying body parts, for example adhesion of the anterior abdominal wall and colon.

Wound closure

The purpose of wound closure is to remove dead space, spread tension along suture lines, support the wound until tissue has repaired, and to bring together and evert skin edges. Types of wound closure include staples, tape, adhesive and sutures. Each method has specific indications, advantages and disadvantages, and special considerations. This section mostly concerns sutures.

Suturing of tissue promotes primary wound healing by holding tissues together until enough healing occurs to withstand stress without mechanical support (Ethicon 2005).

Suture material is a foreign body which elicits a tissue reaction. During wound closure, a sterile field and meticulous aseptic technique are critical to reduce the risk of wound infection. Other complications of wound healing, such as hypertrophic scars, wide scars and wound dehiscence, may result from patient factors (for example nutritional status), incorrect suture selection, or techniques that result in excessive tension across the wound.

Providing expert support during wound closure requires knowledge of surgical techniques and the physical characteristics and properties of the suture material and needle.

Synthetic sutures (Tables 9.5–9.7)

Natural collagen-based suture materials, made from collagen of mammal's intestines are now banned in the EU. Synthetic non-absorbable sutures produce little tissue reaction – these include synthetic substances such as polyamide and polypropelene polymers.

Coating sutures with agents to improve handling characteristics allows them to pass more easily through tissues and reduces tissue injury from their passage. Dyeing sutures also increases visibility.

Table 9.5   Synthetic absorbable sutures (Ethicon 2005).

Type	Source	Uses and absorption
Coated Vicryl (polyglactin 910) suture	Braided multifilament suture coated with a copolymer of lactide and glycolide (polyglactin 370)	Tensile strength around 65% at 14 days post-implantation. Absorption completes in 56–70 days. These sutures cause only slight tissue reaction and may be used in the presence of infection. Used in general soft tissue approximation and vessel ligation
Monocryl (poliglecaprone 25) suture	Monofilament suture that is a copolymer of glycolide and E-caprolactone	Tensile strength is 50–60% at 7 days and nil at 21 days. Absorption is complete at 91–119 days. Used for subcuticular closure and soft tissue approximations and ligations
PDS II (polydioxanone) suture	Polyester monofilament suture made of poly (p-dioxanone).	Tensile strength is 70% at 14 days and 25% at 42 days. Used for soft tissue approximation, especially in paediatric, cardiovascular, gynaecological, ophthalmic, plastic, and gastrointestinal surgery

Table 9.6 Natural non-absorbable sutures (Ethicon 2005).

Type	Source	Uses and absorption
Surgical silk	Raw silk spun by silkworms, often coated with beeswax or silicone	Tensile strength decreases and is lost over a period of 3–6 months.
Surgical steel	Stainless steel (iron–chromium–nickel–molybdenum alloy) as a monofilament and twisted multifilament	High-tensile strength with little loss over time and low tissue reactivity. Used mainly in orthopaedic, neurosurgical and thoracic applications. This suture is also used in abdominal wall and sternum closure

Monofilament and multifilament sutures

Monofilament (single stranded) sutures resist harbouring of micro-organisms, tie easily and provide less resistance to passage through tissue. Monofilament sutures become weakened if crushed or crimped by poor handling.

Multifilament sutures are several monofilaments twisted or braided together, which increases tensile strength, pliability and flexibility, but unfortunately also increases friction through tissues. Absorbing fluid by capillary action may introduce pathogens into the wound. Both these features are reduced by coating the sutures with various substances, for example, Teflon.

Absorbable and non-absorbable sutures

Absorbable sutures provide temporary wound support, until the wound heals well enough to withstand stress. Absorption occurs by hydrolysis in synthetic materials.

The surgeon often uses non-absorbable sutures, such as nylon, for percutaneous skin closure, removing them after the wound has healed. Wound healing typically occurs in 6–8 days in healthy patients. When used internally, non-absorbable sutures become permanently encapsulated in tissue.

Suture selection often depends on surgeon training and preference since various suture materials are available for each

Table 9.7 Synthetic non-absorbable sutures (Ethicon 2005).

Type	Source	Uses and absorption
Nylon	Polyamide polymer suture material available in monofilament (Ethilon/Dermalon suture) and braided (Nurolon/Surgilon suture) forms	Nylon has 81% tensile strength at 1 year, 72% at 2 years, and 66% at 11 years. Elasticity makes it useful in skin closure
Polyester fibre (Mersilene/Dacron suture (uncoated) and Ethibond/Ti-cron suture (coated))	Polyester, a polymer of polyethylene terephthalate. Sometimes coated with polybutilate (Ethibond suture) or silicone (Ti-cron)	Often used for vessel anastomosis and securing prosthetic materials, for example, heart valves
Polypropylene (Prolene suture)	Monofilament suture, an isomer of a propylene polymer	Prolene suture is not subject to degradation or weakening and preserves tensile strength for up to 2 years. The material does not adhere to tissues and is useful as a pull-out suture (for example, subcuticular closure). Useful for contaminated and infected wounds, reduces sinus formation and suture extrusion. Often used in cardiovascular surgery

surgical location and need. Normally, the surgeon uses the smallest diameter suture that adequately holds the healing wound edges.

Certain general principles apply to suture selection. For example, sutures are often no longer needed when a wound has reached maximum strength therefore non-absorbable sutures are often used to close slowly healing tissues such as skin, fascia, and tendons. Absorbable sutures can close mucosal wounds, which are rapidly healing (Ethicon 2005).

Suture selection in contaminated tissues is important because of the risk of infection. For example monofilament sutures are less likely to spread infection as they harbour fewer micro-organisms than multifilament sutures. Surgeons often select the smallest diameter monofilament suture materials such as nylon or polypropylene for repairing contaminated tissues.

Wound drains

The scrub practitioner should have a clear understanding of the features of surgical wound drainage to support the surgical team. This includes competence in the use of drains, methods of insertion, prevention of complications and safe securing of drains.

The purpose of a wound drain is to remove dead spaces, foreign objects or harmful materials that may lead to wound healing complications (Baxter 2003). Drains can also provide irrigation of wounds, relieve pressure within wounds (for example in the gastrointestinal tract) and hold open or stent hollow tubes, for example bile ducts. There are two basic categories of drains in use – open and closed.

Open drains

An open drain is open to the environment and can allow passage of air and fluid between the inside and outside environment. A Penrose drain is a soft tube of rubber which the surgeon places into the wound with the end sticking out and secured with a safety pin. Wound drainage occurs through this tube by the effects of body movements and gravity.

A sump drain is a double lumen tube which allows fluids to drain out of the wound through one channel, and filtered air to enter the wound through the other channel. This exchange of fluid with air encourages the flow of the fluid. A triple lumen tube allows the injecting of irrigations or medications into the wound site. Gentle suction is sometimes applied to sump drains to enable them to drain more effectively. A T-tube drain is a hollow tube in the shape of a T which is often used for drainage of bile fluid from the common bile duct.

Closed drains

Vacuum drains are 'active' because they gently suck the exudates out of the wound. Vacuum drains only work in closed wounds as the negative pressure gradient must be maintained for them to work properly.

Although underwater seal drains are not active, they are closed because keeping the tubes under the water stops external air from entering the wound. The drainage bottle must remain below the level of the wound to ensure that water cannot syphon out of the jar and into the wound. These drains are often used in thoracic surgery as chest drains to drain air and fluid from the pleural cavity. As the patient breathes, the fluid in the submerged tube swings as the pressure in the pleural cavity changes. On removal of the air and fluid from the pleural cavity the lung expands, the pleural cavity closes and the pressure stabilises. When this happens the water in the tube stops swinging and the drain can be removed.

Surgical dressings

The perioperative practitioner should understand the principles of surgical dressings and be able to apply them properly to provide the best environment for wound healing.

Purpose of wound dressing

Wound dressings have two main roles – to protect the wound from an unfavourable environment and to immobilise it. The ideal dressing is one which promotes the best environment for healing, provides a barrier to contamination, supports the wound and allows removal without further damage to the wound (Baxter 2003).

Wounds heal best under moist conditions, therefore a primary role of the dressing is to prevent excess drying out of the wound. The dressing also protects the wound from external contamination to prevent wound infection. Wounds can produce large amounts of exudates which can damage surrounding skin if allowed to collect. Therefore several dressings absorb and hold exudate, keeping it from damaging surrounding tissues.

Other features of dressings include helping with haemostasis, drainage and debridement of dead tissue, and acting as a carrier for therapeutic agents, such as antibiotics or antiseptics.

Types of dressing

Consideration of wound treatment must include a holistic assessment of the patient, since nutrition, illness and the patient's physical and psychological state can have an effect on wound healing. Wound healing has improved over the last 100 years not only for medical reasons but also for social reasons such as better nutrition and housing and the arrival of the welfare state.

The choice of dressing, however, is still important to ensure ideal conditions for wound healing. The wound should remain moist but not macerated, free from infection, toxins and particles from the dressing itself, undisturbed from frequent dressing changes, and kept at an optimum pH value (Baxter 2003).

Soft dressings are used for uncomplicated wounds which are closed by primary intention. Most surgical wounds fall into this category. These dressings normally consist of three layers. The first layer is a non-stick gauze which rests on the surface of the wound. It is important that this layer does not stick to the wound or new growth will be destroyed on its removal. The second layer is absorbent and can consist of relatively thicker padding which can absorb and remove the exudates from the immediate wound area. The third layer immobilises the wound area and so may be adhesive in many simple surgical dressings, or bulky and kept in position with bandages.

Single-layer dressings include semi-permeable membranes such as Opsite and Tegaderm. These dressings are used for uncomplicated wounds and promote a moist, warm environment for best wound healing. Practitioners often use these for dressing cannulation sites. Spray dressings are also examples of single-layer dressings.

Wound packing is also a dressing which is used for deep wounds healing by secondary intention. The packing prevents the surface from closing up before healing of the deeper layers has completed. Packs can be made of various substances including plain gauze, impregnated gauze and hydrocolloids.

There is also a wide range of speciality dressings which are used for complex wounds and are therefore more common during longer episodes of patient care.

REFERENCES
Baxter, H. (2003) Management of surgical wounds. *Nursing Times* **99** (13), 66.

Beesley, J. & Pirie, S. (2005) *Standards and Recommendations for Safe Perioperative Practice*. National Association of Theatre Nurses, Harrogate.

Doebbeling, B.N., Stanley, G.L., Sheetz, C.T., Pfaller, M.A., Houston, A.K., Annis, L., Li, N. & Wenzel, R.P. (1992) Comparative efficacy of alternative hand-washing agents in reducing nosocomial infections in intensive care units. *New England Journal of Medicine* **327** (2), 88–93.

Clarke, P. & Jones, J. (1998) *Brigden's Operating Department Practice*. Churchill Livingstone, Edinburgh.

Ethicon (2005) *Wound Closure Manual*. Ethicon, Edinburgh.

Fell, C. (2000) Health and safety – Hand washing. *British Journal of Perioperative Nursing* **10** (9), 461–5.

Gruendemann, J.G. & Fernsebner, B. (1995) *Comprehensive Perioperative Nursing, Vol 1*. Jones and Bartlett, Boston.

Gruendemann, B.J. & Mangum, S.S. (2001) *Infection Prevention in Surgical Settings*. Saunders, New York.

Hind, M. & Wicker, P. (2000) *Principles of Perioperative Practice*. Churchill Livingstone, Edinburgh.

Line, S. (2003) Decontamination and control of infection in theatre. *British Journal of Perioperative Nursing* **13** (2), 70–5.

Lipp, A. & Edwards, P. (2002) Disposable surgical face masks for preventing surgical wound infection in clean surgery. In: *The Cochrane Library*, Issue 1, Update Software, Oxford.

NATN (1998) *Safeguards for Invasive Procedures: The Management of Risks*. National Association of Theatre Nurses, Harrogate.

NATN (2004) *Risk and Quality Management System*. National Association of Theatre Nurses, Harrogate.

NHS Estates (2000) *Decontamination Review: Report on A Survey of Current Decontamination Practices in Healthcare Premises in England*. NHS Estates, London. www.decontamination.nhsestates.gov.uk/downloads/decontamination_review.pdf

Pearson, T. (2000) The Wearing of Facial Protection in High Risk Environments. *British Journal of Perioperative Nursing* **10** (3), 163–6.

Pinney, E. (2000) Back to basics – Hand washing. *British Journal of Perioperative Nursing*. **10** (6), 328–31.

Surgical Tutor (2005a) *Sources of Surgical Infection*. Accessed: 1st February 2005. www.surgical-tutor.org.uk/default-home.htm?principles/microbiology/surgical_infection.htm~right.

Surgical Tutor (2005b) *Asepsis and Antisepsis.* Accessed 1st February 2005. www.surgical-tutor.org.uk/default-home.htm?core/preop1/asepsis.htm~right

Taylor, M. & Campbell, C. (1999a) Back to basics: The multi-disciplinary team in the operating department. *British Journal of Theatre Nursing* **9** (4), 178–83.

Taylor, M. & Campbell, C. (1999b) Back to basics: Patient care in the operating department (1) *British Journal of Theatre Nursing* **9** (6), 272–5.

Wicker, P. (1991) Universal precautions: Infection control in a high risk environment. *British Journal of Theatre Nursing* **1** (9) 16–18.

Woodhead, K. (2005) Managing risk of swab and instrument retention. *Clinical Services Journal* **4** (1), 49–51.

Patient Care during Recovery

10

LEARNING OUTCOMES
❑ Discuss the *role of the practitioner during postoperative recovery*.
❑ Identify the main *postoperative problems*.
❑ Discuss the *key clinical skills* and *underpinning knowledge* required of recovery practitioners.

ROLE OF THE RECOVERY PRACTITIONER
Chapter 6 'A route to enhanced competence in perioperative care' outlines the competencies displayed by recovery practitioners, and shows the need for skills such as patient assessment, airway maintenance, wound care and the skills to respond to developing postoperative problems. The working party discovered that all perioperative practitioners share many of the skills and much of the knowledge displayed by experienced recovery practitioners. Therefore, the reader should refer to other parts of this book to explore some of the areas discussed in this chapter.

However, while practitioners in anaesthetic, scrub and circulating roles also display many of the skills found in recovery, the unique environment of the recovery room lends a new aspect to the role. The lack of immediate medical support in the recovery room means that practitioners work in a more autonomous role than any other area of the operating department. Under these circumstances, practitioners have to be able to support the postoperative patient at a stage of their treatment when they are vulnerable. Recovery practitioners must be able to recognise changes in the patient's condition, start suitable supportive therapies and oversee their effects, often with no immediate medical support.

The recovery practitioner efficiently and continually assesses, plans, carries out and evaluates individual care and treatment for the postoperative patient to meet the patient's individual needs. A main aim of the role is to aid in creating a calm therapeutic environment, using available resources in a safe and effective manner to reduce anxiety in postoperative patients.

The practitioner must effectively communicate within a multidisciplinary team. This includes providing information to all healthcare workers interacting with the patient to aid continuity of care and cooperation between recovery and other departments.

Recovery room environment

The practitioner's main role in the recovery room is to detect and prevent postoperative complications and to provide supportive interventions. Local policies often define the qualified staffing needed in recovery. The Association of Anaesthetists of Great Britain and Ireland (AAGBI 1998; AAGBI 2002) recommends this to be of the ratio of one qualified carer to one unconscious patient, with a minimum of two staff present when a patient is in the recovery area.

Arranging beds into individual bays promotes easy viewing of the patient and can provide easy access to the necessary equipment for patient care. Efficiency and effectiveness of movement are essential when time becomes critical for the safety of the patient. Therefore the basic equipment for patient monitoring, airway maintenance, assisted ventilation and resuscitation must be available at the patient's head in each recovery bay (Box 10.1).

The design of the bed is important for ensuring safe postoperative care. For example the bed should be able to tilt head-down to help increase cerebral blood flow during episodes of hypotension. It will also need cot sides or other methods for preventing patients from falling out of bed, and fittings for suction and IV stands. The practitioner should assess each patient's needs and suitable means for patient support and transport should be provided.

Protection and support of the patient's airway is of primary importance during the immediate postoperative period. A developing airway obstruction may require the use of equipment such as face masks, airways and suction. The

---

Box 10.1   Minimum equipment required for the recovery room

Fully equipped bed or trolley, for example:

- Oxygen supply
- Apparatus tilt mechanism
- Cot-sides
- Brakes
- Suction
- Attachments for IV stands

Equipment to help maintain the patient's airway and normal respiration, for example:

- Oxygen supply (wall-mounted with tubing), face masks, Venturi masks and pocket masks (Figures 10.1 and 10.2)
- A T-piece system and a full range of oropharyngeal and nasopharyngeal airways
- Suction with tubing
- Yankauer oropharyngeal suckers and tracheobronchial suction catheters
- Intubation equipment
- Ambubag (self-inflating) and range of face masks
- Monitoring equipment, such as oxygen saturation monitors, CO_2 monitor and other invasive monitors

Monitors to assess the patient's haemodynamic state, for example:

- Sphygmomanometer and stethoscope or automatic blood pressure monitor
- Central venous pressure
- ECG

Cardiac arrest trolley with all the necessary equipment, for example:

- Defibrillator and ECG monitor
- Intubation equipment
- Emergency drugs
- Sundry items (such as scissors, tape, pen and paper)

Patient heating device, for example:

- Electric heating blanket
- Forced air warmer (Bair Hugger)
- Ripple mattress

---

practitioner may also monitor the patient's haemodynamic state to identify conditions such as low blood pressure, low pulse and postoperative bleeding, requiring the use of equipment such as central venous pressure monitors, pulse oximeter and ECG monitor.

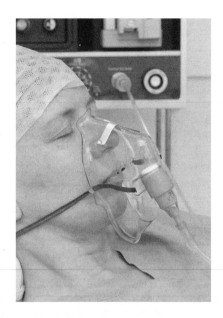

Fig. 10.1 Patient with a Venturi mask.

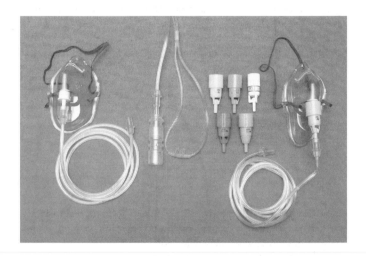

Fig. 10.2 Selection of Venturi masks.

Various items of emergency equipment need to be readily available to help in the rapid and effective treatment of emergency conditions. For example, a fully stocked cardiac arrest trolley may have items such as a defibrillator, IV equipment and emergency drugs such as adrenaline and atropine.

Recovery rooms will also need to stock equipment to warm the patient and help prevent postoperative shivering or accidental hypothermia, such as Bair Huggers, electric blankets and fluid warmers.

Transfer of patient from the operating room to recovery

An anaesthetist and a qualified practitioner usually transfer the patient from the operating room to the recovery room. Patients may be on their beds with the usual equipment for airway protection.

Early assessment of the patient's condition is an important skill for the recovery practitioner to master. This includes receiving a full handover of the patient's care and treatment in the operating room, and a physical assessment of the patient's condition on admission to the recovery room. A full handover of information ensures the early identification of potential problems, effective treatment and prevention of complications. It is also essential for the practitioner to know anything relevant in the preoperative history that may be significant, for example, the patient may be hard of hearing, epileptic or allergic to certain medications.

A handover may include information such as:

- airway condition during surgery;
- vital signs;
- surgery performed and medical diagnosis;
- patient's general condition;
- anaesthetic and other medications used: narcotics, muscle relaxant, antibiotics;
- any untoward problems that occurred in the operating room that might influence postoperative care (for example, extensive haemorrhage, cardiac arrest);
- abnormal pathology;
- any tubing, drains, catheters or other supportive aids;

- specific information to report to the surgeon or anaesthetist (for example falling blood pressure or increasing loss from drains).

The practitioner carries out the preliminary assessment of patients on admission to the recovery room to ensure that their condition is stable and to provide a baseline for future observations (AAGBI 2005). This may include an evaluation of:

- airway patency;
- depth and nature of respirations;
- skin colour;
- pulse volume and regularity;
- oxygen saturation;
- level of consciousness and the ability of the patient to respond to commands;
- evidence of haemorrhage or drainage from the operative site;
- temperature.

Care of the patient in recovery

The immediate care of the patient in recovery is a complex mix of many skills and a diverse range of knowledge. After early assessment a 'settling in' period follows where the practitioner starts observations, starts treatment and stabilises the patient's condition. Postoperative instructions from the anaesthetist and surgeon should be checked as soon as is practical. The practitioner may consider the following areas during this time.

The practitioner assesses the patency of the airway, gives oxygen as prescribed and positions the patient to maintain the airway. It is important to identify baseline recordings of respiration rate, depth and rhythm to assess the patient's condition before the anaesthetist hands over care (Starritt 1999).

There is a high potential for rapid changes to the patient's haemodynamic state during the immediate postoperative period. Therefore the practitioner should measure the pulse, recording the rate, rhythm and depth. Normally the patient has blood pressure recorded regularly (5–10 minutes). Normally, blood pressure should show a slow return to preoperative levels; however, the practitioner should not assess the reading by itself, but should assess it alongside other observations which form part of the overall assessment of the patient. For example, an anxious patient may have a raised blood pressure, despite excessive blood loss from a wound.

The practitioner should check wound sites, dressings and drains for signs of drainage, since excessive bleeding may need further investigation by the surgeon and possible return to surgery.

Fluid balance is important in the immediate postoperative period because of blood loss during surgery and the hypotensive effects of several anaesthetic drugs. The practitioner should ensure that intravenous infusions are running at the prescribed rate and should record input or output from, for example, drains, catheters or IVs. Various fluids may be given during the patient's recovery including, for example, crystalloids, blood products and plasma expanders.

The postoperative patient may need various drugs during recovery, including anti-emetics, opiates, antihypertensives and antibiotics. The anaesthetic chart usually lists any medications that the anaesthetist has prescribed for the immediate postoperative period. The practitioner should also check the patient's prescription sheet for postoperative drug regimes which the anaesthetist may have prescribed before surgery. Checking the intraoperative record before giving any drugs ensures that doses of the drug have not already been given. Recording the effect of drugs given is essential to ensure that they produce the desired effect.

Postoperative pain can lead to further complications such as hypoxia, anxiety and restlessness. Good postoperative analgesia will encourage a rapid recovery (O'Neill 1998; Starritt 2000). The practitioner must carry out a formal pain assessment and give prescribed analgesia as required, noting the effect. Giving anti-emetics helps reduce the emetic side effect of opiates.

A practitioner should remain with the conscious or semiconscious patient since confused and disorientated patients may cause harm to themselves while awakening. The practitioner should assess the level of consciousness, observing for returning reflexes, for example swallowing, tear secretion, eyelash and eyelid reflexes and response to stimuli both physical (not painful) and verbal. The patient should be oriented to time and place as often as is necessary. Patients are often disorientated and confused on waking. To reduce anxiety and increase cooperation, it is important to keep patients informed of all procedures, regardless of seeming unresponsiveness, as hearing returns before the ability to respond physically.

The patient should be positioned safely and comfortably. This is likely to be in the recovery position, which is lateral with the head on a pillow, and the upper leg resting on a pillow bent over the top of the lower leg. Keeping the patient comfortable may help relieve pain and help to prevent complications caused by abnormal positioning of limbs.

Postoperative hypothermia is a recognised complication of surgery and should be avoided as it leads to other complications such as delayed wound healing, infection and eventually organ failure. The patient must be kept warm and a space blanket or Bair Hugger applied if needed. The recovery room environment should be kept at a warm temperature, above 21°C.

Assessment for discharge

The time that patients stay in the recovery room is dependent on the rate at which their condition returns to the physical, mental and emotional state where they can be left unattended between routine observations, and the absence of any postoperative problems which can be resolved during the immediate postoperative recovery (Starritt 1999). The practitioner should inform the anaesthetist of the patient's health status before the patient leaves the recovery area and follow the unit's discharge protocols to ensure efficient and safe patient care.

Common postoperative problems

Table 10.1 and Box 10.2 indicate some of the common postoperative problems and the patient's expected state on discharge. Under certain circumstances, for example during extended periods of ventilation, the patient's condition will vary from that described.

The main areas of concern for the recovery practitioner are neurological status, airway management, respiratory and cardiovascular function, pain relief and wound care (Kehlet & Dahl 2003). Often, only the combined actions of the recovery

Table 10.1 Common postoperative problems.

Problem	Possible causes	Possible actions required (practitioner, surgeon or anaesthetist)
Airway obstruction	• Tongue occluding the airway because of poor positioning. • Foreign material, for example blood, secretions, vomit, or swollen airway tissues. • Laryngeal spasm. • Bronchospasm.	• Maintain recovery position supporting the jaw if unconscious or sit up if awake. Insert oral airway. Use suction to remove obstruction. Consider reintubation if required.
Hypoventilation	• Respiratory depression from anaesthetic agents such as opiates, volatile anaesthetics or barbiturates. • Decreased respiratory drive caused by abnormal pCO_2. • Loss of hypoxic drive in patients with chronic pulmonary disease. • Neuromuscular blockade from continued action of non-depolarising muscle relaxants caused by electrolyte imbalance, impaired excretion with renal or liver disease or hypothermia.	• Ensure oxygen therapy is in place. Ventilate by hand if required using an Ambu bag and mask. Ensure complete reversal of anaesthetic agents. Monitor pO_2 and other blood gases.
Hypotension	• Hypovolaemia caused by anaesthetic drugs (depression of the cardiovascular system or vasodilation), or blood loss during surgery	• Lay the patient flat and raise legs to increase return blood flow to the heart and increase cerebral circulation. • Wake patient up to stimulate the cardiovascular system. • Check for blood loss from the wound site or drains in case of continuing bleeding. • Increase rate of intravenous infusion to help replace fluids. • Consider the need for blood transfusion.

Cont.

Table 10.1 *Continued.*

Problem	Possible causes	Possible actions required (practitioner, surgeon or anaesthetist)
Hypertension	• Pain. • Carbon dioxide retention caused by poor ventilation. • Distended bladder leading to pain or discomfort, caused by blocked or kinked catheters or obstruction caused by damage to tissues during surgery. • Action of some anaesthetic drugs.	• Assess the patient for pain and give prescribed analgesia. Check for bladder distension. Monitor respirations.
Bradycardia	• May be the normal preoperative pulse rate in fit patients. • Depression of the cardiovascular system caused by action of opiates. • Anticholinesterases such as atropine. • Pain stimuli.	• Be aware of potential cardiac arrest and assess action required.
Tachycardia	• Hypovolaemia causing the heart to compensate by beating faster. • Pain stimuli. • Fluid overload, for example caused by IV infusions. • Fear or anxiety. • Septicaemia. • Actions of some anaesthetic drugs.	• Be aware of possible cardiac arrest. Assess cause and act suitably according to local protocols. Check ECG and assess rhythm. Check blood pressure and central venous pressure.

Nausea and vomiting	• Side effects of opiates. • Hypotension. • Abdominal surgery. • Pain.	• Prepare a vomit bowl and oral suction to protect the patient's airway. Place patient in suitable position for preserving or protecting the airway. Assess nausea score and give anti-emetic as prescribed. Ensure the patient is not hypoxic.
Pain	• Anxiety and restlessness causing increased pain from the operation site. • Surgical trauma, for example at the wound site. • Inadequate intraoperative or postoperative analgesia. • Intraoperative harm to the patient not caused by surgery – for example inadequate positioning.	• Speak to patient and assess cause of anxiety. Assess pain score, the nature and cause of pain and adjust pain relief. Give prescribed analgesia as required.
Hypothermia	• Vasodilatation or vasoconstriction. • A recognised complication following surgery. • Large infusions of blood and fluids.	• Warm patient according to local protocols and with the equipment available. Be aware of the potential problems associated with heating patients too quickly.
Wound haemorrhage	• Surgical issues such as inadequate wound closure, leaking vascular anastamosis, inadequate haemostasis. • Blood disorders, for example sickle-cell anaemia or low platelet count. • Transfusion reaction leading to abnormal clotting mechanisms.	• Apply pressure to operative site and watch drains for signs of excessive leakage. • Be aware of possible surgical complications and keep surgeon informed of developments. • Ensure blood is available. Ensure availability of clip removers if wounds are closed by clips. Give fluids as needed. • Prepare patient in case of return to the operating room.

Box 10.2   The patient's expected state on discharge from the recovery area

- Conscious and oriented to a suitable level
- All normal protective airway reflexes present
- Acceptable respiratory function and normal oxygen saturation readings
- Normal pulse and blood pressure readings for at least 30 minutes before discharge
- No persistent or excessive bleeding from wound or drainage sites
- Pain reduced to an individually acceptable level as assessed by formal pain score
- Postoperative nausea and vomiting absent
- Body temperature within normal levels

---

practitioner, anaesthetist and surgeon provide the necessary care for the patient and resolve postoperative complications.

The patient must be awake, comfortable and physiologically stable before leaving the support of the recovery area (Box 10.2). The normal airway reflexes must be present to prevent problems with respiration, such as aspiration of stomach contents into the lungs, while returning to the ward or while under reduced postoperative supervision on the ward. Respiratory function must be satisfactory and oxygen saturation readings need to be within suitable levels to prevent hypoxia during the return to the ward. The patient should have also displayed normal pulse and blood pressure readings before discharge as this suggests a return to normal preoperative state, reversal of anaesthetic and absence of bleeding or other postoperative complications.

Wound and drainage sites must be free from persistent or excessive bleeding since this may be a sign of postoperative complications which may need surgical intervention. This is especially important for surgery on or near the airway, for example thyroid surgery, since excessive bleeding may compromise breathing by causing obstruction.

The patient must have satisfactory pain relief before leaving the recovery area as this may be difficult to achieve on the ward or when pain has become established. Pain may also alter the patient's opinion and understanding of surgery and may influence future decisions about hospital treatment. Inadequate pain relief can also delay longer-term postoperative recovery by compromising respiration, reducing movement and exhausting the patient physically and emotionally.

It is important to reduce the risk of vomiting or airway problems during the patient's return to the ward since the conditions for airway control are likely to be less than ideal in the corridor or lift. The bed should contain all the necessary equipment including for example, oxygen, suction, suitable monitoring and equipment for intubation or airway control.

To ensure continuity of care, the recovery practitioner must offer an accurate handover to the ward nurse collecting the patient (AAGBI 2005). Clear, written documentation must support the handover by including, for example:

- operative procedure;
- anaesthetic;
- analgesia;
- anti-emetics;
- oxygen therapy;
- intravenous therapy and fluid losses;
- drains;
- wound dressing;
- pressure area assessment, including the Waterlow pressure area assessment score, a pressure sore severity score if a pressure sore is present and any measures taken;
- pain assessment.

A good handover of information helps to tell the ward staff about the patient's condition to:

- help plan postoperative care;
- improve communication between the patient, staff and relatives;
- help identify potential postoperative problems;
- assess the effect of analgesia;
- ensure that oxygen therapy continues in the ward;
- help identify future needs related to continuing recovery.

KEY CLINICAL SKILLS

The discussion in the previous paragraphs has highlighted the role of the recovery practitioner in helping the patient to full recovery. Many of the specific skills carried out by recovery practitioners have already been discussed in other chapters of the book. Therefore, the remainder of this chapter looks at the implication for postoperative recovery in four specific areas which are essential to good practice for the recovery practitioner:

- maintaining the airway;
- managing postoperative pain;
- maintaining fluid balance;
- monitoring haemodynamic status.

The reader should refer to previous chapters of this book for discussion of other skills practised by recovery practitioners.

Maintaining the airway

This section discusses the following areas:

- assessment of breathing and respiration;
- airway suction;
- extubation;
- insertion and removal of oral airways.

Assessment of breathing and respiration

The recovery practitioner must be skilled in assessing breathing and respiration, since there is an increased risk that the postoperative patient will have respiratory complications. Refer to Chapters 1 and 6 for discussion of respiratory assessment, physiology and respiratory conditions. Assessing the rate, depth and rhythm of breathing shows the patient's ability to manage his or her own airway and ventilation. This helps monitoring of the patient's return to a normal preoperative status, and aids diagnosis of respiratory conditions, initiation of treatment, monitoring of progress and evaluation of care.

Respiratory monitors are useful in the recovery area to assess respiratory function. For example, pulse oximetry is common for monitoring pO_2 to help avoid hypoxaemic incidents. Wright's respirometer or a peak flow meter can be used to assess respirations.

Airway suction

Effective airway suction is an essential skill, since there are many possible causes of obstruction in the early postoperative period. Suction removes secretions or vomit from the pharynx in a safe and controlled manner for patients who are unable to cough effectively. Excessive mucus in the airways often produces a 'rattling' sound in the throat. Other sounds of obstruction include 'crowing' and 'whooping' and 'stridor' caused by laryngeal spasm or obstruction of the vocal cords. Secretions are sometimes cause by irritation of the vocal cords and these secretions can be sucked out using suction catheters. Airway obstruction which progresses to complete obstruction becomes quiet or silent since the patient is not passing air through the vocal cords. In complete obstruction the patient may also show signs of excessive effort as the body tries to breathe reflexively. Therefore, since 'no sound' suggests either perfect breathing or no breathing at all, other methods of assessing breathing should always be used in conjunction to hearing. Other methods of assessing breathing include, for example, the practitioner feeling for breaths on the reverse of his or her hand, watching for condensation coming and going on the inside wall of oxygen masks, observing for chest movements and intercostal indrawing and observing signs of excessive effort.

Oral or nasopharyngeal suction is the most common method of airway suction during recovery. Key points about suction include:

- Oral suction is often carried out using rigid Yankauer suckers. Soft, Y-suction catheters passed through the nose are useful if the patient clenches the teeth.
- Avoiding using contaminated suction catheters is important to reduce the risk of respiratory infections.
- High flow, high capacity suction is required to cope with potentially large amounts of secretions or vomit.
- Avoid traumatising the oral and respiratory mucosa, for example, by forcing catheters past clenched teeth.

The patient may need tracheobronchial suction, using a soft Y-suction catheter, if there are secretions deep inside the lungs, for example, if still intubated or following tracheostomy. The practitioner must be aware that this procedure can be distressing for an awake patient and may cause coughing or excessive movement in semi-conscious patients. A strict aseptic technique must be followed during this procedure because of the risk of deep respiratory infection. Only apply suction on withdrawal of the catheter, to avoid damaging the respiratory mucosa. Hypoxia is a risk because the suction draws out the patient's air supply, and the catheter itself causes a partial obstruction of the airway. The patient may therefore need preoxygenation and monitoring of pO_2 is essential during the procedure.

Extubation

Patients often enter the recovery room still intubated. Semi-conscious patients may tolerate an endotracheal tube for some time while awakening, and may remove it themselves as they wake up. This is a useful choice when managed properly and if there are no respiratory complications. Successful self-extubation suggests the patient is awake enough to maintain their own airway. During self-extubation, the practitioner should remain with the patient until extubated, cutting the ties and deflating the cuff at the right time, and performing oral suction if needed.

It may also be necessary to extubate the semi-conscious patient if the endotracheal tube is irritating the airway and making the patient restless. The patient must be able to maintain their own airway and be able to breathe adequately before extubation. The key steps in extubation include:

- Preoxygenate the patient if possible to help prevent hypoxia during extubation.
- Remove any oral packs if present.
- Apply suction to the mouth and pharynx.
- Place the patient in the recovery position.
- Remove the ties and deflate the cuff using a 20 ml syringe.
- Gently remove the tube, applying suction if necessary using a soft suction catheter.

The practitioner must watch the patient after the procedure for signs of hypoxia or respiratory distress and apply oxygen according to an assessment of the patient's condition (Hatfield & Tronson 1998).

Insertion and removal of oral airways

Guedel airways are common in recovery because they are effective at keeping the upper airway clear of obstructions. These are curved, flattened tubes which are available in sizes including 4 for large patients, 2 or 3 for adults, 1 for young children and 0 or 00 for babies or neonates. They are usually clear plastic and disposable, although reusable tubes are still available.

Insert the Guedel airway upside-down to help passage over the tongue, and let it come to rest in the back of the mouth. If the patient gags then either the airway is too big, or the patient is able to protect their own airway and so doesn't need an artificial airway.

The principles for removing oral airways are similar to those of extubation – patients should be breathing normally and protecting their own airway before removal. Similarly, the patient may need suction and should be watched for signs of hypoxia after the procedure.

Managing postoperative pain

This section discusses pain assessment, analgesic administration and treatment of complications. Most NHS Trusts produce guidelines and protocols for managing postoperative pain and practitioners should be aware of how to apply these procedures to their own specific clinical setting.

Up to 70% of patients suffer acute pain in the recovery room (Hatfield & Tronson 1998). It is important to control postoperative pain because it can interfere with ideal recovery by:

- increasing restlessness leading to increased risk of cardiovascular problems and hypoxia;
- increasing the risk of postoperative nausea and vomiting;
- interfering with normal respiration and increasing the risk of respiratory complications such as obstruction from secretions, hypoxia and pneumonia;
- increasing the metabolic response (see Chapter 1) leading to increased risk of infection and delayed wound healing;
- causing the patient distress and anxiety.

Pain is a subjective experience which is in part sensory distress (hurt caused by damage to the body) and in part emotional upset, such as distress or anxiety, caused by the patient's interpretation of the cause of the pain. Drug therapy reduces one or both of these components. For example, opiates reduce pain impulse transmission, and make the patient 'not care' about the pain itself. Local analgesics on the other hand, only reduce the sensory element of pain, doing nothing specifically for the patient's emotional state.

The analgesic regime should already have been discussed with the patient preoperatively (see Chapter 6). This is important so the patient is able to cooperate with drug therapies and understands the choices available. Five steps in effective analgesia in the recovery area are:

- identifying the cause of pain;
- asssessing the pain;
- reassuring the patient;
- giving analgesia;
- identifying and treating complications.

Identifying the cause of pain

There are many causes of pain in the recovery area, coming from several sources, for example:

- preoperative medical conditions;
- poor positioning during surgery;
- cramps or muscle pain from depolarising muscle relaxants;
- headache or other 'hangover' effects from anaesthetic drugs;
- the surgical procedure including for example, incisions, donor sites, infusion sites and catheters.

Most analgesic drugs have a systemic effect, and therefore act on pain from multiple sources. However, imagine a scenario where a patient, after a hernia repair, has a headache. The practitioner gives an opiate assuming that the patient is in pain from the wound (which may after all have been injected with a local anaesthetic and therefore be pain free) which is not the most effective treatment for the patient's main problem. The practitioner must therefore develop skill at interviewing a potentially confused and disorientated postoperative patient to identify the source of pain. This includes having good communication skills especially for identifying verbal and non-verbal clues about the source of the pain from the patient.

Assessing the pain

Regular pain assessment helps the practitioner to detect changes and assess pain when the patient does not report it verbally. The practitioner must assess the patient's pain level competently and carry out any suitable actions.

The subjective assessment of pain is simply a matter of asking the patient and believing what they say (Hatfield & Tronson 1998). This often points the way towards the analgesic therapy required and opens the way for the practitioner to offer emotional support.

The objective assessment of pain is much more difficult because there is only a general correlation between the actual damage caused to the body and the pain suffered by the patient. For example, there may be no obvious cause for a headache. Similarly, a patient with a leg wound may only complain of pain on respiration, while ignoring or not feeling pain from the leg wound. Severe pain also has systemic effects such as tachycardia, bradycardia, hypertension or hypotension, nausea, vomiting, agitation and restlessness. These signs and symptoms can mask the actual cause or presence of pain.

In semi-conscious patients, objective assessment of pain may be impossible – the patient cannot respond effectively to questions about the source or intensity of pain. Developing pain protocols, or defined courses of action according to specific criteria such as surgical procedure or patient condition, help to anticipate the patient's pain based on experiences of similar patients and researched evidence. Pain protocols can be useful because they ensure that all patients receive basic analgesic cover, therefore preventing pain developing. When the patient is awake and oriented, the protocol can be adjusted according to the objective assessment of their needs.

Therefore, several pain scoring methods have been produced which aid practitioners in the objective assessment of pain. Although there are several variations, the two main methods are the visual analogue scale and the numerical scale.

The visual analogue system is a 10 cm long line with 'no pain' at one end of the line and 'worst possible pain' at the other end. The patient simply marks the point on the line which reflects the pain he feels. The practitioner compares this to the patient's preoperative assessment to help evaluate postoperative pain intensity.

Numerical scales use more precise measurements on a scale of 1–5 or 1–10. For example, 1 = no pain or 2 = mild pain up to 5 = unbearable pain. The accurate assessment of pain using a numerical scale depends on the patient's skills at self-awareness and self-assessment, as well as numerical understanding and ability.

Observation of the signs and symptoms of pain should supplement the objective assessment of a patient's pain, especially where the patient is unable to use the tools described above, for example when disorientated, confused, where the patient is unable to understand how to use the tool, or in babies or young children.

Reassuring the patient

Anxiety can make pain worse, therefore, it makes sense to try to reduce anxiety to moderate the patient's response to pain. Reducing anxiety about the cause of the pain may help the patient to relax tense muscles, adopt a positive attitude to the pain, relieve worry and cooperate with analgesic regimes. The practitioner needs to be skilled at assessing the patient's anxiety and be able to offer information, explanations or solutions to satisfy the patient.

Giving analgesia

Analgesia can be given by various routes to provide the best pain relief. Analgesic administration in the recovery room is normally either parenteral or by local or regional analgesics, however, the recovery practitioner should be familiar with several methods of administration including IV, IM, oral, rectal, subcutaneous, epidural and patient-controlled analgesia.

Opiates are widely used in the postoperative treatment of pain, and so the practitioner must be well aware of their use, potential side effects and complications. Opiates are often given intravenously in the recovery room. This is an ideal route because onset of action is rapid, which is an advantage for patients in acute pain. Intravenous analgesia also produces its effects almost instantaneously, whereas absorption of an intramuscular dose may be erratic because of poor blood supply in a recovering postoperative patient. Patient-controlled analgesia is popular in recovery since it allows the patient to titrate small doses of analgesia themselves, according to the pain that they feel, giving an accurate level of analgesia.

Identifying and treating complications

The potential for side effects from opiate administration is high in recovery because the patient's surgery and anaesthesia already puts them at risk of the common side effects of opiates, namely cardiovascular and respiratory depression, and postoperative nausea and vomiting.

A satisfactory dose of analgesia will make the patient's pain manageable, make the patient drowsy and result in a respiratory rate of around 8 to 10 breaths per minute. However such patients may be at risk from hypoxia if the action of opiates continues to increase, for example, if an intramuscular dose is still being absorbed. The postoperative patient on opiates should therefore receive oxygen to help prevent the onset of hypoxia. Monitoring of blood pressure, pulse and pO_2 is also essential to enable early identification of side effects.

Postoperative nausea and vomiting (PONV) can arise from several causes in the recovery room, for example, hypotension, anxiety, swallowed blood, abdominal procedures and opiate side effects. Practitioners often underestimate patient distress caused by this condition, even though research suggests that patients would rather suffer pain than PONV, and would be willing to pay a substantial amount of money for an effective anti-emetic (Tramer 2003).

Conscious patients often give early signs of the onset of vomiting, for example dry retching, nausea, pallor and increased salivation immediately before vomiting. Sitting patients up if awake can help them to vomit into a container. Unconscious patients must be placed on the side, and suction used to remove the vomit. Tipping the bed so the patient is head down helps drainage out of the mouth and may prevent aspiration into the lungs. Anti-emetics may be prescribed and their effectiveness should be monitored. The practitioner should also be aware of other possible complications of PONV, such as wound dehiscence, aspiration pneumonitis, oesophageal rupture, and alveolar rupture leading to airway compromise. The lack of a universally effective anti-emetic has led one author to believe that patient assessment is one the key skills to preventing and treating PONV (Arnold 2002). See Chapter 3 for further discussion of pharmacology and administration of analgesics and anti-emetics.

Maintaining fluid balance

This section discusses postoperative fluid therapy, monitoring of fluid balance and inserting urinary catheters. See Chapter 1 for a discussion of fluid and electrolyte balance.

Postoperative fluid therapy

Normal homeostatic responses during surgery can mask postoperative hypovolaemia caused by blood loss in the operating room, but hypovolaemia can become obvious during the recovery period. This may be indicated by signs and symptoms of tachycardia, low urine output and pallor. Many postoperative patients therefore have intravenous infusions in progression on return to recovery. Infusion solutions can include dextrose 5%, sodium chloride 0.9% (normal saline) or plasma expanders such as dextran. Choice of intravenous solution is based on blood results such as levels of serum sodium, urine osmolarity and interpretation of blood loss and normal fluid requirements by the body.

Fluid balance problems that the postoperative patient may face following surgery are:

- fluid depletion or overload;
- sodium depletion or overload;
- blood volume depletion or overload.

Fluid depletion or overload

An adult, under normal circumstances, needs a minimum of 2.5 litres of fluid per day. When the trauma of surgery and anaesthesia are added this requirement normally increases. Therefore the maintenance dose of fluids given intravenously are roughly 1 litre of saline and 2 litres of dextrose daily. Signs and symptoms that suggest water depletion include high serum sodium, concentrated urine and evidence of water loss through vomiting, diarrhoea and sweating (Hatfield & Tronson 1998).

Fluid overload is normally iatrogenic and a result of over-infusion of solutions such as dextrose. Acute overload of fluids can also be caused by bladder or prostate surgery because of absorption of irrigating solutions (Rao 1987). Signs and symptoms of fluid overload are wide and varied and may include, for example, feelings of dizziness, headache and nausea, restlessness and confusion progressing to hypertension, haematuria and bradycardia. Definitive diagnosis can be made by measuring serum sodium with results of less than 130 mmoles/litre. Medical management of serious fluid overload may include oxygen therapy, a diuretic such as furosemide and dopamine to support a failing cardiovascular system.

Saline depletion and overload
Saline depletion may be treated with saline infusions. Signs of saline depletion may include low urine output, tachycardia and low central venous pressure. Vomiting, gastric fluid loss or diarrhoea may cause saline depletion.

Saline overload can result in cardiac failure and the patient will present with such signs and symptoms as raised central venous pressure, pulmonary oedema and abnormal heart sounds. A diuretic such as furosemide can be used to treat this condition.

Blood volume depletion and overload
Blood volume depletion can present as surgical shock (see Chapter 1) if severe enough. Treatment of blood depletion in recovery is usually with crystalloid solutions, blood products or colloids. Blood or colloid overload in the operating room will present in recovery as left ventricular failure. Blood or colloid stays in the circulation and therefore puts undue strain on the heart. Treatment of overload is by diuretics or phlebotomy if required.

Fluid therapy
Fluid therapy should be recorded to avoid problems such as those mentioned above. All the usual vital signs, for example

anomalies in blood pressure, pulse, respiration or pO_2, may point to problems with fluid therapy. In particular the following methods may be specifically useful in suspected conditions:

- auscultation of the chest – can show pulmonary oedema, abnormal heart sounds;
- central venous pressure – can show increased jugular venous pressure;
- chest X-ray – can show venous engorgement, lung oedema;
- blood results – identify serum sodium, potassium and other electrolyte disturbances;
- urinalysis – helps with diagnosis of saline overload or depletion.

Fluids therapy must be recorded accurately to help prevent errors in administration. This is especially important when drugs are added to infusions.

Urinary catheterisation

Many postoperative patients are catheterised to help in accurate fluid balance monitoring, and to help avoid postoperative complications. Indications for catheterisation include:

- postoperative conditions such as acute retention;
- chronic retention with renal damage;
- to help in accurate fluid balance recording in at-risk patients;
- urinary incontinence caused by nerve damage, for example, because of diabetes, spinal or neurological disease;
- to help with tissue viability during the intraoperative or postoperative periods.

Most catheters inserted for surgical reasons are intended for short-term use (1–6 weeks) and made of plastic (if removed immediately on emptying the bladder), or latex with various coatings to reduce urethral trauma and infection. Catheters are usually of the Foley design, which have an eye at the distal end to promote drainage and a balloon which prevents the catheter from falling out and reduces the chance of bypassing of urine. Speciality catheters include three-way catheters (for irrigating the bladder), double balloon (for controlling haemorrhage), and speciality tipped for example Coude (olive) tip and whistle tip.

The catheters come in lengths of 43 cm (male), 30 cm (female) and 26 cm (paediatric).

Catheter diameter is measured in Charrière (Ch) or French gauge (Fg), which are identical scales. Sizes range from 12 Ch/Fg to 24 Ch/Fg, where 12 Ch = 4 mm diameter. Paediatric catheters are available from 6 Ch/Fg to 12 Ch/Fg. Balloon size varies from 3 ml to 30 ml. The practitioner should always identify the correct balloon size and use the correct amount of sterile water to fill the balloon. All the relevant information should be recorded in the patient's notes.

It is important to use an aseptic technique and maintain good hygiene when managing catheters because of the risk of urinary tract infection (UTI). Between 1 and 4% of catheterised patients who develop a UTI go on to develop bacteraemia and septicaemia, of whom 13–30% die.

Urinary tract infection associated with catheterisation can occur because of contamination during the catheterisation procedure, by contamination from peri-urethral space, and from contamination of the internal lumen of the catheter, from the drainage bag or a connection port. The recovery practitioner can help prevent UTIs by ensuring a satisfactory fluid intake, inserting the catheter aseptically and by teaching the patient catheter care (if appropriate, for example in day surgery). The catheter should be removed as soon as possible and prophylactic antibiotics should be considered in at-risk patients.

The practitioner should always use lubrication such as Instillagel, a water-based gel that contains 2% lidocaine for anaesthetic action and chlorhexidine for antiseptic cover. Instillagel leaves the patient pain free within 3–5 minutes, reduces urethral trauma to a minimum and reduces contamination by bacteria. Box 10.3 details correct catherisation procedure.

There are many problems associated with catheterisation. Trauma caused by rough insertion of the catheter can cause bleeding. This can lead to pain and discomfort, anxiety and blockage of the catheter. The practitioner should always insert catheters gently to help prevent damage to the urethra. Catheters can become blocked by encrustations (biofilm) or by bleeding, especially following surgery on the renal and urinary systems. Pain can be caused by spasm of the urethra, trauma, irritation, allergy and so on. The cause of the pain must always be assessed and suitable measures taken. The catheter may be pulled out by semi-conscious or confused patients, or when transferring the patient from bed to table. This is especially painful and dangerous when the balloon is still inflated. A non-deflating balloon is also dangerous and may need surgery to remove the catheter. The balloon may also burst leading to the risk of retained latex fragments and painful removal of the catheter.

Box 10.3   Catheterisation procedure

The procedure should be carried out aseptically and the patient should be socially clean before starting.

(1) Initiating male catheterisation
- Place patient supine with legs straight.
- Retract foreskin and clean with saline 0.9%, clean from tip of penis towards glans.
- Change sterile gloves if necessary.
- Insert 11 ml of Instillagel, hold glans firmly between thumb and forefinger to prevent reflux and wait 2–3 minutes.

(2) Initiating female catheterisation
- Place patient supine, legs abducted and bent at the knees, heels together.
- Spread the labia and find the urethral opening.
- Clean area from front to back.
- Be aware of possibility of false placing of the catheter into the vagina. Folds of skin may also be mistaken for the urethra.

(3) Catheterisation procedure
- Select correct size and catheter.
- Gently insert a size 12–14 Fg catheter into the urethra.
- Gently feed the catheter along the urethra only touching the outside plastic covering and not the catheter itself, until urine drains.
- Attach bag or spigot.
- Gently advance the catheter and ensure all the balloon is in the bladder.
- If resistance is felt do not force catheter, remove it and send for help.
- Take a urine sample for microbiology at this point if needed.
- Inflate the balloon with the correct amount of sterile water watching the patient for verbal and non-verbal signs of pain.
- Aseptically connect to drainage bag and secure to patient's leg.
- In males, retract the foreskin and ensure area is clean and dry, then replace foreskin in normal position. Be aware of risk of paraphimosis.

Monitoring haemodynamic status

This section discusses the use of monitoring in recovery, in particular, blood gases, blood pressure, central venous pressure and pulse oximetry.

Much of the recovery practitioner's time involves recording patients' physiological measurements. Monitors can supplement the visual and verbal signs and symptoms of developing complications by providing objective evidence of particular measurements. Chapter 2 discusses the use of equipment, and Chapter 1 considers several of the physiological parameters, including ECG. This section focuses on the practical use of monitors in the recovery environment.

Monitoring blood gases

Recovery practitioners are increasingly becoming involved in this procedure. Arterial blood gases can be taken from an arterial cannula, or from the radial, femoral, brachial or dorsalis pedis arteries, in order of preference. Care should be taken to assess the suitability of the artery chosen and the practitioner must consider systemic factors such as diabetes or vascular disease. The practitioner must be able to undertake an Allen's test before cannulation of the radial artery. This test involves occluding the radial and ulnar arteries in turn and observing for flushing of the hand when one is released. If either is occluded then neither can be used for blood gases because of the danger of damage to the blood supply to the hand.

Arterial monitoring kits are available to help obtain the sample. The blood must be stored in a cool container and sent to the labs as soon as possible. The form accompanying the sample must be fully and carefully completed, because of the importance of the readings. Applying a pressure pad should help to stop bleeding over the puncture site and the practitioner should watch the site carefully for bleeding over the next few minutes.

Blood gases can make various physiological measurements, for example, pH, pO_2, pCO_2 and bicarbonate among others. The practitioner must be familiar with normal levels and be able to respond quickly to abnormal results.

Monitoring blood pressure

Most recovery areas now have automatic blood pressure monitors; however, it is a useful skill to be able to monitor blood pressure using a manual sphygmanometer. In brief, the following procedure may be used to take manual blood pressure:

- Explain to the patient what you are doing as you attach the cuff to the upper arm.
- Place your fingers on the radial pulse.
- Inflate the cuff to about 30 mmHg above the point at which the pulse disappears.
- Take your finger off the radial pulse and listen with a stethoscope to the blood flow returning to the brachial artery in the cubital fossa.

The point where the first sound is heard is the systolic pressure, the diastolic pressure is when the sound disappears completely.

Manual blood pressure measurements are prone to errors because of factors such as the patient moving, agitation and excessive movement, wrong size of cuff used, inaccurate readings being taken and so on. An alternative is to use an oscillometric blood pressure monitor which automatically inflates and deflates the cuff at intervals. This device is now widely used in the recovery areas and has largely superseded manual methods of blood pressure monitoring (Ramsey 1991). It helpfully alerts the user to kinks in the tube or errors in cuff placement. Again, errors are possible in these readings although the automatic function makes it a useful monitor for busy practitioners (Burton 2000).

A potentially more accurate way of measuring blood pressure is to use an arterial catheter connected to a transducer. Errors can occur using this method because of false calibration or faulty setup, however, it is generally accepted to be the most accurate way of assessing blood pressure. The practitioner should remember that it is not individual readings that are important during patient recovery, it is the trend, which can show an improving or worsening condition. Readings from blood pressure monitors should also be supplemented by a holistic assessment of the patient. For example, a patient sitting up in bed, conversing with a practitioner, is unlikely to have a blood pressure of 60/40 mmHg, regardless of what the equipment records.

Central venous pressure

Central venous pressure (CVP) monitors are used to measure filling of the right side of the heart and can point out signs of fluid imbalance. These monitors also help to guide fluid replacement, to infuse drugs and to give venous access when peripheral cannulation is difficult. The normal reading for CVP is between 0 and 5 cm H_2O. The measurement is taken by measuring the distance a column of water is pushed up a measuring tube by the central venous pressure. The practitioner should refer to manufacturer's manuals or Trust procedures to ensure the correct setting up of the equipment, since various errors in setting up the equipment can lead to false readings. In brief:

- Medical staff insert the central venous catheter.
- Identify a zero reference point – the zero of the measuring tube should be level with the right side of the heart, which is roughly midway between the anterior and posterior of the chest (mid-axillary line). Mark the point for future reference with a permanent pen.
- Ensure there is a continuously flowing infusion to prevent occlusion of the catheter.
- Open the tap in both directions – this shuts off the infusion and opens a direct pathway between the measuring tube and the patient.
- Measure and record the distance up the tube the water is pushed.
- Close the tap to the tube, opening it to the infusion.

The CVP is especially useful in a bleeding patient since venous pressure alters before arterial pressure. As blood volume falls, the CVP also falls, sometimes rapidly, before arterial pressure is affected. Comparison of CVP readings to arterial blood pressure can help with the diagnosis of conditions such as hypovolaemia, shock, cardiac failure and abnormalities in fluid balance. Complications of CVP include infection, pneumothorax, arterial puncture and air embolism caused by disconnection in the system.

Pulse oximeters

Pulse oximeters are useful in the postoperative patient since they are non-invasive, quick and easy to apply, give an accurate indication of pO_2 and are a good guide to whether the patient is hypoxic (Pedersen *et al.*, 2002; Wright 2003). Readings should be approaching 100% when on oxygen, or greater than 90% when breathing room air, in an otherwise healthy patient, before discharge from the recovery room. In most circumstances haemoglobin saturation greater than 90% means the patient is not hypoxic. However, pO_2 also depends on the pH of the blood and if the patient is acidotic, saturation can remain high, but pO_2 may be low. Therefore, again the practitioner should not rely on this monitor by itself, but must use it as part of the holistic patient assessment. In all situations, a falling reading of less than 90% should be investigated because of the increasing danger of hypoxia as saturation decreases.

REFERENCES

Arnold, A. (2002) Postoperative nausea and vomiting in the perioperative setting. *British Journal of Perioperative Nursing* **12** (1), 24–30.

Association of Anaesthetists of Great Britain and Ireland (1998) *The Anaesthesia Team*. AAGBI, London.

Association of Anaesthetists of Great Britain and Ireland (2002) *Immediate Postanaesthetic Recovery*. AAGBI London.

Association of Anaesthetists of Great Britain and Ireland (2005) *Day Surgery*, (revised edn). AAGBI, London.

Burton, J. (2000) Oscillometric blood pressure monitors. *British Journal of Perioperative Nursing* **10** (12), 624–6.

Hatfield, A. & Tronson, M. (1998) *The Complete Recovery Book*. Oxford University Press, New York.

Kehlet, H. & Dahl, J. (2003) Anaesthesia, surgery, and challenges in postoperative recovery. *The Lancet* **362**, 1921–8.

O'Neill, O. (1998) The efficacy of oral analgesia for postoperative pain. *British Journal of Perioperative Nursing* **8** (9), 5–8.

Pedersen, T., Dyrlund Pedersen, B. & Møller, A.M. (2002) Pulse oximetry for perioperative monitoring (Cochrane Review). In: *The Cochrane Library*, Issue 1. Update Software, Oxford.

Ramsey, M. (1991) Blood pressure monitoring: automated oscillometric devices. *Journal of Clinical Monitoring* **7**, 56–67.

Rao, P.N. (1987) Fluid absorption during urological endoscopy. *British Journal of Urology* **60**, 93–9.

Starritt, T. (1999) Patient assessment in recovery. *British Journal of Perioperative Nursing* **9** (12), 593–5.

Starritt, T. (2000) Pain management in recovery. *British Journal of Perioperative Nursing* **10** (2), 115–19.

Tramer, M.R. (2003) The treatment of postoperative nausea and vomiting. *British Medical Journal (International edition)* **327** (7418), 762.

Wright, J. (2003) Introduction to pulse oximetry. *British Journal of Perioperative Nursing* **13** (11), 456–60.

Index